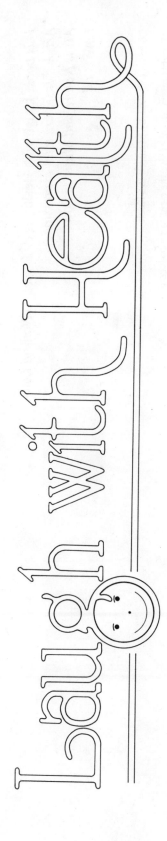

Laugh With Health

NUTRITION + LIFE

FACT + REALITY

Manfred urs Koch

An Owl Book
HOLT, RINEHART AND WINSTON
New York

This book, Laugh with Health, is dedicated to Natural Law.

Art + Music are total expression.

Art is Nature and Music is Love.

Love is all.

First published in the United States in 1984 by Holt, Rinehart and Winston, 383 Madison Avenue, New York, New York 10017.

ISBN: 0-03-071308-0

Published simultaneously in Canada by Holt, Rinehart and Winston of Canada, Limited.

Originally published in Australia, designed and produced by Renaissance & New Age Creations.

Library of Congress Cataloging in Publication Data

Koch, Manfred Urs.
 Laugh with health.
 Bibliography: p.
 1. Nutrition. 2. Food, Natural. I. Title.
 TX353.K7 1984   613.26   84-3750
 ISBN: 0-03-071308-0

First American Edition

Designer: Manfred urs Koch

Printed in the United States of America

10 9 8 7 6 5 4 3 2 1

Cover Watercolor by Mr. Lance Sullivan of Victoria, Australia.

ISBN 0-03-071308-0

FOREWORD

Every aspect of Life is a development of Energy. Even realizing you are Alive requires Energy. The Human Body has the capacity to Live for a few hundred years; however, nobody ever lives that long due to a multitude of interfering factors, and possibly the main one is sickness. Without the right Energy, sickness will develop. Every illness is a lack of certain Energy at a specific time. By considering the average duration of human life and the relationship with all the moments that make up that life, we can appreciate the abundance of human Energy. Everyone has a mind of thoughts and decisions that directs their own aspirations throughout life. Is sickness part of that decision? Our knowledge today has the ability to help all people to live in good Health. All you need is the knowledge to help you appreciate Nature's goodness. Humans have the ability of directing their Energy into more than a million directions. Without sufficient knowledge of Nutrition, you may struggle with sickness that will distract you from enjoying a satisfying Life. Within the boundaries of this book, *Laugh with Health*, the information contained is designed to broaden your appreciation and perspective of Natural foods. Without Nature's assistance, we would all die. Nature is Energy. Nature gives Energy. "If you don't turn on the switch, you may never see the picture." As simple as a fuse to fix, it can be easy, it can be hard, all depending on what you know and what you do with that knowledge. Nature gives, so we can Live.

—Manfred urs Koch

INTRODUCTION TO TABLE OF CONTENTS

TABLE OF CONTENTS

CHAPTER ONE

INTRODUCTION

COMPOSITION OF THE HUMAN BODY

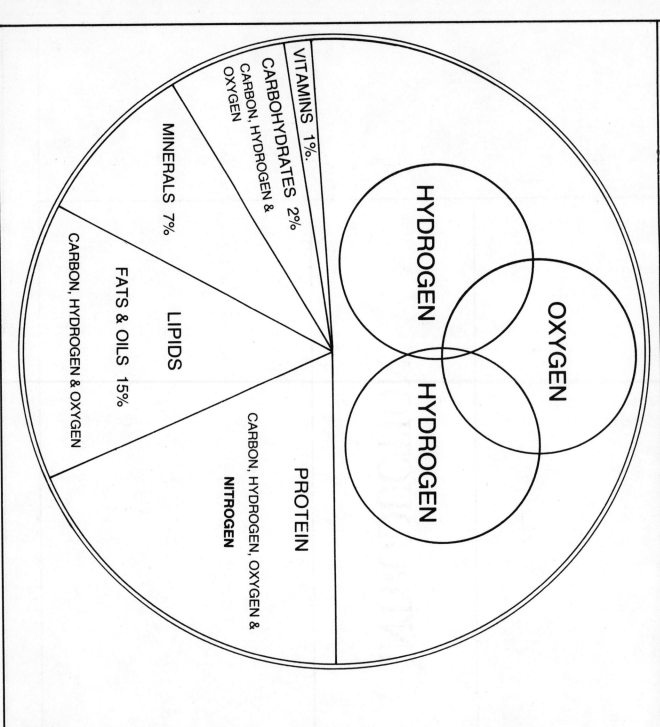

VITAMINS 1%.

CARBOHYDRATES 2%
CARBON, HYDROGEN &
OXYGEN

MINERALS 7%

LIPIDS

FATS & OILS 15%

CARBON, HYDROGEN & OXYGEN

PROTEIN

CARBON, HYDROGEN, OXYGEN &
NITROGEN

HYDROGEN

OXYGEN

HYDROGEN

The illustration on the left, shows the relationship of the various Elements that make up the structure of the Human body. The other two gaseous Elements, that is Nitrogen and Carbon are interrelated with the three main food groups; Carbohydrates, Proteins & Lipids. Proteins differ from Carbohydrates and Lipids as they contain Nitrogen, as well as Carbon, Hydrogen & Oxygen. The Minerals & Vitamins have special qualities. See pages 138–198 for details.

A comparison of the Human body in relation to the Function & Average Daily Nutrient requirements, shows a marked difference in the group of Carbohydrates.

The reason is that Carbohydrates are used as the main Energy–Fuel food for everyday and every minute use. Carbohydrates are used by the body as soon as the digestive processes have taken place, which is about 2–3 hours. Carbohydrate foods include all Fruits, Vegetables, Whole Grains and Legumes. These 4 Carbohydrate food groups are the main Energy providing foods that the body converts into Glucose–Primary fuel. The balance between the three food groups–Carbohydrates, Proteins & Lipids that are part of the daily food intake, will determine the efficiency of the body. The type of Carbohydrates that are supplied with the diet, will also influence the amount of Energy produced. Proteins & Lipids are also capable of being used as Energy, however the Carbohydrates are the main Energy Food Group.

FUNCTION & AVERAGE DAILY REQUIREMENT OF ESSENTIAL NUTRIENTS

BUILDING

20%

PROTEINS

Protein foods provide the main building material for growth and repair of all body cells. Nuts, Seeds, Grains and Legumes provide all the essential Amino acids that your body requires for growth and development.

ENERGY

60%

CARBOHYDRATES

Fresh Fruits, Vegetables, Whole Grains and Legumes are the four main Carbohydrate food groups. They also supply valuable amounts of Glucose, Minerals and Vitamins that ensure effective digestion, protection and body building qualities.

REGULATING

WATER

The average daily intake of Water for a person in a temperate climate needs to be about 3 litres per day. Water is the most precious liquid. Fresh fruits and vegetables provide 60-90% water content. A few glasses of fresh water everyday is vital for Health.

REGULATION & PROTECTION

1%

VITAMINS

The daily requirement of Vitamins is minute, but essential for protection against disease and illness. Vitamins are always combined with Natural whole foods to ensure maximum effectiveness.

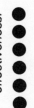

'The Vitamin Tablet is only as good as the diet that goes with it'.

PROTECTION BUILDING & REGULATING

4%

MINERALS

Minerals are required for building and regulating a multitude of body functions. All Natural foods contain a well balanced supply of Minerals in combination with other essential nutrients that ensure effective digestion, absorption and utilization for body building, regulation and protection.

HEAT

15%

FATS & OILS

Fats & Oils provide the main heat producing requirements for the body. Nuts, Seeds, Grains, Legumes, Vegetable oils, Olives and Avocadoes are the major natural source that will supply all the essential ingredients for body heat production.

HUMAN NUTRIENT REQUIREMENTS

MAIN NUTRIENTS:		INDIVIDUAL COMPONENTS OF MAIN NUTRIENTS:	TOTAL
GASEOUS ELEMENTS	60%	**HYDROGEN OXYGEN NITROGEN**	3
CARBOHYDRATES CARBON / SUGARS & STARCH		**Mono-Saccharides Di-Saccharides Poly-Saccharides** Glucose Sucrose Glycogen Fructose Maltose Cellulose Galactose Lactose Starch Pectin CARBOHYDRATES ALSO CONTAIN: CARBON, HYDROGEN & OXYGEN.	10
PROTEINS ESSENTIAL AMINO ACIDS	20%	**Arginine Histidine Isoleucine Leucine Lysine** **Methionine Phenylalanine Threonine Trypotophan Valine** PROTEINS ALSO CONTAIN: CARBON, HYDROGEN, NITROGEN,	10
OTHER AMINO ACIDS		Cystine Glutamic acid Glycine Serine Iodogorgoic acid Proline Hydroxyproline Tyrosine Alanine Aspartic	10

LIPIDS (FATS & OILS)	15%	**Mono-Unsaturated Poly-Unsaturated Saturated**
		Oleic Acid Linoleic Acid Stearic Acid
		                   Linolenic Acid
		                   Arachiodonic Acid
			5

		FATS & OILS ALSO CONTAIN: CARBON, HYDROGEN, OXYGEN	10
MINERAL ELEMENTS	4%	**Calcium Phosphorus Potassium Sulphur Chlorine Sodium** **Fluorine Magnesium Iron Manganese Silicon Copper Iodine Zinc**	14
TRACE MINERALS		Cobalt Molybdenum Selenium Vanadium	4
VITAMINS	1%	Vitamin A Vitamin B1, B2, B3, B5, B6, B12, B15. Vitamin C Vitamin D Vitamin E Vitamin K P.A.B.A. Biotin Choline Folic acid Inositol Vitamin F Vitamin T Vitamin P Vitamin U	21
		TOTAL	77

MAIN NUTRIENTS R.D.A. CHARTS

Food is required for the maintenance of Life. All forms of Life are dependant on an input of food, that varies greatly from one species to another. The Human body also has certain basic needs, some that only food can provide. The variety of Natural foods that are available does make up a very complete and enjoyable Life supporting need. Every individual type of food has specific properties and a composition of elements that is unique. If even one element was missing, the food would be different and may never have developed at all. Human Nutritional needs have only recently been analysed and stated as the RECOMMENDED DAILY ALLOWANCE. If we miss out on just one of the essential nutrients, our body may be at risk of sickness and a prolonged deficiency could lead to permanent damage and possible death. Another recent development has been the manufacture of chemically formulated foods, refined foods and other food processes and techniques, which have disturbed the Natural Balance of some peoples food intake and consequently a decline with the intake of Essential Life supporting nutrients. You may not at first understand all the statistics that are included in this book.

All you really need to know is that any food that has been chemically converted by food technologists, (processed & refined) is more than likely to be harmful for regular Human consumption. The statistics and charts that are included in this book, will give you factual information so as you may logically conclude that Natural foods are balanced, by Mother Nature for the benefit of everybody and everymind. The chart below is based on the Recommended Daily Allowance that was evaluated by the American Academy of Sciences. Complete guides to the Mineral and Vitamin R.D.A. are also supplied on pp. 157 and 198.

NUTRIENTS		CHILDREN (BOYS & GIRLS)							WOMEN				BOYS			MEN	
		0-6 months	1-3	4-6	7-10	11-14	15-18	19-22	23-50	Pregnant	Lactating	51 & Over	11-14	15-18	19-22	23-50	51 & Over
CALORIES REQUIRED FOR LIGHT ACTIVITY		770	1,100	1,600	2,200	2,300	2,300	2,000	2,000	2,000 +300	+500	1,850	2,800	3,000	3,000	2,600	2,600
CARBOHYDRATES	grams	115	165	240	330	345	345	346	300	na.	na.	277	na.	na.	na.	390	390
PROTEINS	grams	14	23	30	36	44	48	46	46	46 +30	+20	46	44	54	54	56	56
LIPIDS	grams	28	38	58	80	80	78	79	66	na.	na.	59	na.	na.	na.	87	87
MINERALS—CALCIUM	m.gramms	360	800	800	800	1,200	1,200	800	800	1,200	1,200	800	1,200	1,200	800	800	800
MINERALS—PHOSPHORUS		240	800	800	800	1,200	1,200	800	800	1,200	1,200	800	1,200	1,200	800	800	800
VITAMINS—THIAMINE, B1		0.3	0.7	0.9	1.2	1.2	1.1	1.1	1.0	+.3	.3	1.0	1.4	1.5	1.5	1.2	1.2

SUNLIGHT, AIR, WATER

GASEOUS & MINERAL COMPOSITION OF THE BODY

GASEOUS ELEMENTS	BODY WEIGHT	MINERAL ELEMENTS	BODY WEIGHT
OXYGEN	65%	CHLORINE	0.25%
CARBON	18%	SODIUM	0.25%.
HYDROGEN	10%	FLUORINE	0.20%
NITROGEN	3%	MAGNESIUM	0.05%
WATER H2O	75%	IRON	0.008%
CALCIUM	2%	MANGANESE	0.003%
PHOSPHORUS	1%	SILICON	0.002%
POTASSIUM	0.4%	COPPER	0.002%
SULPHUR	0.25%	IODINE	0.00004%

Our everyday lifestyle should be a worthwhile investment. Throughout the pages of this book, the information contained is designed to give you an intellectual and practical guide to Health and with this knowledge, your body and mind will work together to keep you living with Natural foods and hopefully a Natural lifestyle.

Nutritional deficiencies go hand in hand with unnatural foods and the unnatural lifestyle. A prolonged use of those refined unnatural foods will eventually lead to nutritional deficiencies that can only be restored by a diet of Natural whole foods.

Without Health your Life will be sick. For some people, the revival to Natural foods and Natural living may seem to be impossible. It is unfortunate that some of those people have never been brought up to experience the variety of Natural foods and some delicious recipes. This book will give you a basic idea of Natural recipes to serve you as a guide to better Health. There are numerous other books available on natural food preparation. Natural whole foods are the best value. The cost of processing, refinement, profit markup, etcetera, will soon add up to sell you a product ten times the price of the original natural whole food, that has the benefit of giving you Health and Life.

Nutritional knowledge today will verify that all Human Nutritional requirements are obtainable directly from Nature. The balance of Elements contained in a food is most important. Whole Natural foods are precisely balanced to ensure maximum nutritional benefits. Natural foods: fruits, vegetables, whole grains, legumes, nuts, and seeds. Sunshine, Air, and Water are also essential. Many factors are important in supplying our body and mind with Health and positive satisfaction with Life. The surrounding environment that you live in has a great influence on your lifestyle, type of diet, health, and happiness. A city environment can have a most distracting and detrimental influence on Natural living and Natural food intake. The temptation of eating take-out foods, processed and refined foods, and drinks can become so over-powering that a regular routine may develop. There are many ways to avoid those unnatural eating habits and retain Natural satisfaction. Save your money and give yourself Health with the variety of Natural foods that are designed for human consumption. Processed and refined foods lack enzymes—the spark of all Life.

Nature supplies all our needs, with 3 of the main elements being obtainable directly. However, with the fourth element, Earth, Nature has designed an intermediate assistant, Plant Life, to extract those essential nutrients that are part of the Earth and the basis of all Human nutritional needs. All forms of Plant Life need Sunshine, Air, and Water. The main difference is that plants are adapted to living directly from those Mineral Elements in the soil (Inorganic Elements). Humans are not adapted to use Inorganic Mineral Elements. We need plant life to survive. All forms of Human food start with plant life.

The best foods for Man are obtainable directly from plant life (Fruits, Vegetables, Grains, Legumes, Nuts, and Seeds). These foods are composed from certain Elements that are in balance only when the food is obtained directly from the Original Plant source, as Nature planned.

Before food processing factories and the business world took over, Man obtained all food directly from the Natural source.

NATURAL FOOD GROUPS

13

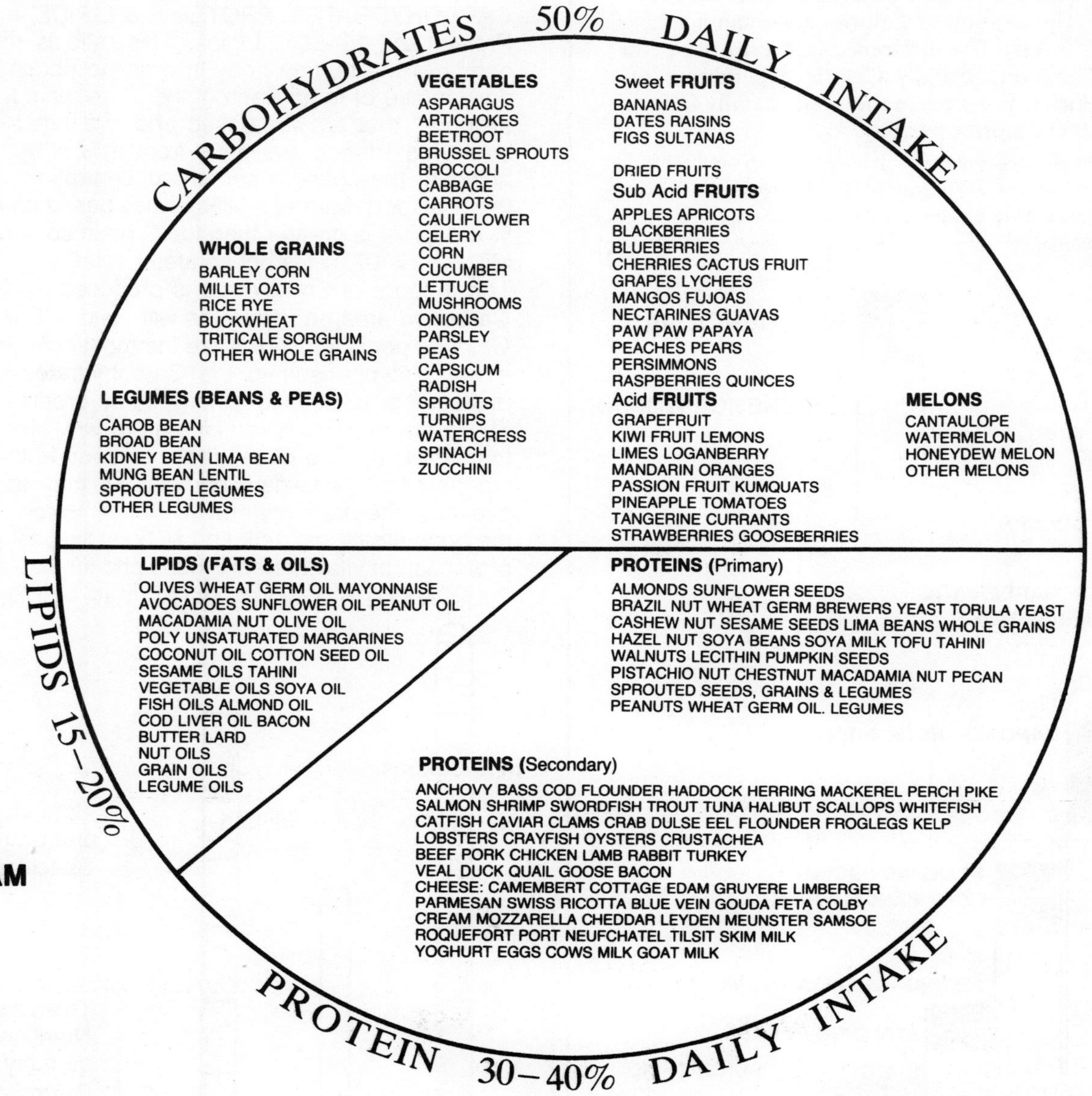

CARBOHYDRATES 50% DAILY INTAKE

VEGETABLES

ASPARAGUS
ARTICHOKES
BEETROOT
BRUSSEL SPROUTS
BROCCOLI
CABBAGE
CARROTS
CAULIFLOWER
CELERY
CORN
CUCUMBER
LETTUCE
MUSHROOMS
ONIONS
PARSLEY
PEAS
CAPSICUM
RADISH
SPROUTS
TURNIPS
WATERCRESS
SPINACH
ZUCCHINI

WHOLE GRAINS

BARLEY CORN
MILLET OATS
RICE RYE
BUCKWHEAT
TRITICALE SORGHUM
OTHER WHOLE GRAINS

LEGUMES (BEANS & PEAS)

CAROB BEAN
BROAD BEAN
KIDNEY BEAN LIMA BEAN
MUNG BEAN LENTIL
SPROUTED LEGUMES
OTHER LEGUMES

Sweet FRUITS

BANANAS
DATES RAISINS
FIGS SULTANAS

DRIED FRUITS
Sub Acid FRUITS
APPLES APRICOTS
BLACKBERRIES
BLUEBERRIES
CHERRIES CACTUS FRUIT
GRAPES LYCHEES
MANGOS FIJOAS
NECTARINES GUAVAS
PAW PAW PAPAYA
PEACHES PEARS
PERSIMMONS
RASPBERRIES QUINCES
Acid FRUITS
GRAPEFRUIT
KIWI FRUIT LEMONS
LIMES LOGANBERRY
MANDARIN ORANGES
PASSION FRUIT KUMQUATS
PINEAPPLE TOMATOES
TANGERINE CURRANTS
STRAWBERRIES GOOSEBERRIES

MELONS
CANTALOUPE
WATERMELON
HONEYDEW MELON
OTHER MELONS

LIPIDS 15-20%

LIPIDS (FATS & OILS)

OLIVES WHEAT GERM OIL MAYONNAISE
AVOCADOES SUNFLOWER OIL PEANUT OIL
MACADAMIA NUT OLIVE OIL
POLY UNSATURATED MARGARINES
COCONUT OIL COTTON SEED OIL
SESAME OILS TAHINI
VEGETABLE OILS SOYA OIL
FISH OILS ALMOND OIL
COD LIVER OIL BACON
BUTTER LARD
NUT OILS
GRAIN OILS
LEGUME OILS

PROTEIN 30-40% DAILY INTAKE

PROTEINS (Primary)

ALMONDS SUNFLOWER SEEDS
BRAZIL NUT WHEAT GERM BREWERS YEAST TORULA YEAST
CASHEW NUT SESAME SEEDS LIMA BEANS WHOLE GRAINS
HAZEL NUT SOYA BEANS SOYA MILK TOFU TAHINI
WALNUTS LECITHIN PUMPKIN SEEDS
PISTACHIO NUT CHESTNUT MACADAMIA NUT PECAN
SPROUTED SEEDS, GRAINS & LEGUMES
PEANUTS WHEAT GERM OIL. LEGUMES

PROTEINS (Secondary)

ANCHOVY BASS COD FLOUNDER HADDOCK HERRING MACKEREL PERCH PIKE
SALMON SHRIMP SWORDFISH TROUT TUNA HALIBUT SCALLOPS WHITEFISH
CATFISH CAVIAR CLAMS CRAB DULSE EEL FLOUNDER FROGLEGS KELP
LOBSTERS CRAYFISH OYSTERS CRUSTACHEA
BEEF PORK CHICKEN LAMB RABBIT TURKEY
VEAL DUCK QUAIL GOOSE BACON
CHEESE: CAMEMBERT COTTAGE EDAM GRUYERE LIMBERGER
PARMESAN SWISS RICOTTA BLUE VEIN GOUDA FETA COLBY
CREAM MOZZARELLA CHEDDAR LEYDEN MEUNSTER SAMSOE
ROQUEFORT PORT NEUFCHATEL TILSIT SKIM MILK
YOGHURT EGGS COWS MILK GOAT MILK

4 CALORIES PER GRAM

CARBOHYDRATES
FRUITS
VEGETABLES
4 CALORIES PER GRAM
WHOLE GRAINS
LEGUMES
4 CALORIES

PROTEIN
NUTS
SEEDS
YEAST
WHOLE GRAINS
LEGUMES
EGGS FISH
YOGHURT
CHEESE MEAT

LIPIDS
SEED OILS
VEG. OILS
FISH OILS
NUT OILS
9 CALORIES PER GRAM

CALORIE INTRODUCTION

Illustration below; represents the approx. amount of CALORIES expended per minute with various activities. The amount of Calories a woman needs to do the same work as a man is 20% less. The difference is due to the extra (average) weight of the male. The average daily Calorie expenditure for males ranges from 2,400-4,000 Calories. For woman the average daily Calorie expenditure ranges from 1,600-3,000 Calories per day.

The Reference man is 22 years of age, physically Healthy and weighs 70 kilograms. He also lives in a temperate climate of 18 Celcius. The Reference woman is also 22 years of age, physically Healthy and weighs 58 kilograms,

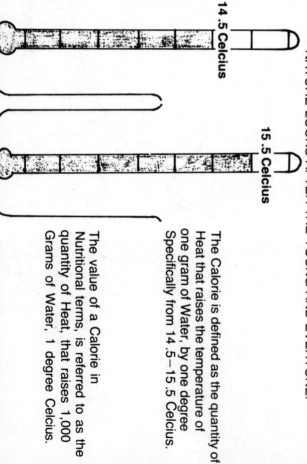

CALORIES PER MINUTE

1 2 3 4 5 6 7 8 9 10 11 12 13 14

SKIING WALKING UPSTAIRS, CARRYING A 14 lb.weight

CROSS COUNTRY RUNNING COMPETITIVE SPORT

SQUASH, SWIMMING

FOOTBALL, SOCCER

HEAVY GARDENING & MANUAL WORK

DANCING—ROCK & ROLL

STANDING, DOING LIGHT MANUAL WORK

SITTING—CLERICAL WORK

STANDING AT EASE

SUNBATHING

AT EASE

The **BASAL METABOLIC RATE**, is related to a persons Calorie requirement at a complete mental & physical rest, comfortable temperature and clothing, with at least 12 hours since the last meal.

REFERENCE MAN

REFERENCE WOMAN

The illustration on page 13 shows the ratio of the three main food groups. **CARBOHYDRATES, PROTEINS & LIPIDS**, in the ratio of 50% **C.**, 25–35% **Protein** and 15–20% **Lipids**. This ratio is related to the basic nutritional needs of the human body in order to obtain maximum efficiency from the daily intake of food. Each of the three main food groups has a wide variety of foods, that are discussed and evaluated in the following pages of this book. Most foods are made from a % of all three food groups: **C. P. & L.** however they have a certain concentration, within one of the groups. The Original food,-Mother's Milk, is also based on all 3 food groups, however the % of Lipids, is greater than the Protein content. For 100 Grams of Human Milk— 7.07 Carbohydrates, 1.06 Protein and 4.5 Lipids.

The amount of Energy that is produced by the 3 main groups is different. Carbohydrates and Proteins will yield 4 Calories per gram. Lipids yield 9 Calories per gram. Lipids are the most concentrated source of Energy, however in comparison to the Carbohydrates, Lipids require more complex digestive processes for Energy to be produced.

There are numerous reasons as to why Human Milk supplies more Lipids than Protein. One of the main reasons is that Lipids are vital in the early stages of a childs development, as they assist in supplying and making available the main mineral—Calcium, which is essential in the formation of the bone structure, teeth and all body tissues. Lipids are also required for the protection of vital internal organs and for insulation and storage of body heat.

NATURE LOOKS AFTER THE YOUNG AND EVERYONE.

14.5 Celcius

15.5 Celcius

The Calorie is defined as the quantity of Heat that raises the temperature of one gram of Water, by one degree Specifically from 14.5-15.5 Celcius.

The value of a Calorie in Nutritional terms, is referred to as the quantity of Heat that raises 1,000 Grams of Water, 1 degree Celcius.

NOTE: 1 Kilojule = 4.2 Calories approx.

'Laugh with Health' is a book designed to broaden your perspective and appreciation of Natural foods. Carbohydrates are the first main food group that are given a comprehensive description and evaluation. All forms of Life are dependant on Carbohydrate foods as a starting point for their food requirements. Humans have such a wide variety of Carbohydrate foods to choose from — over 100 individual species of plant life are available for Human consumption. Carbohydrates are classed into four main groups — **GRAINS, LEGUMES, FRUITS and VEGETABLES.** Our Health depends on Carbohydrate foods. In fact, our Lives depend in a multitude of ways on Carbohydrates. Carbohydrates are our main source of Energy foods.

Every moment of living is a development of Energy.

CARBOHYDRATE foods are formed from a combination of the four main Elements — SUN, AIR, WATER and EARTH, all part of the Energy cycle. A fair majority of people seem to be unaware of the simple and almost 'common sense' reasons for food, effects of food and especially the benefits of Natural foods in their Natural undisturbed state. Many people consider a breakfast should come from a carton or other food packaged form. A food starts off simple, with the Elements of Nature working in harmony. All forms of packaged food and drinks are the result of the effects of the business world, with profit in mind and with little, if any, consideration towards people, their Health and Life. One cannot appreciate Health unless one is in a Healthy condition. A combination of Mind and Body is a way to describe the Human. Harmony-satisfaction with Life, relies on mind and body harmony. If you continuously feed your body with processed, refined and other unnatural foods and drinks, your body will react with a corresponding decline in Health. GLUCOSE is the main food for the Nervous system and Brain. All Carbohydrates in their Natural whole state are the major source of Human Glucose requirements. A deficiency of Glucose foods — Grains, Legumes, Fruits and Vegetables, will lead to a daily lack of Energy and the long term effects of inadequate nutrition for the Nervous system and Brain are so numerous that only a list of modern diseases and illnesses would show. Would there be over 1,000 varieties of 'food' supplied in packaged form? Yes, that's right, over 1,000 ways to get your body into an unnatural state. The minority of Natural foods supplied in packaged form is a reflection of the freedom of Nature, Natural Living and Natural Foods. Every stage of processing etc. will be an added cost to the product, so if you think you are doing well when a 10 cent discount is given on a processed food, think twice about the expense and also your Health. A visit to the doctor could be ten times the cost of the processed product. Good value is what determines a product's versatility, level of sales and market appeal. Natural foods are supplied free by Nature, with some Human effort involved to assist the process of development, apart from that, there should be little or no need for the extra expense of processing, refinement, chemical preservatives, factory work, machinery and all other overheads. The value of a food is directly related to the benefits it contributes to people, for Health and for Life. Save on expensive shopping bills and Live and learn to use Natural foods.

CHAPTER TWO

CARBOHYDRATES

CARBOHYDRATE INTRODUCTION

CARBOHYDRATES are produced in plants by the action of Carbon dioxide with Sunlight and forms into Natural sugars, fibres, gums and starches.

Carbohydrates contain the elements; CARBON, HYDROGEN and OXYGEN.

Carbohydrates yield 4 Calories per gram.

Carbohydrate foods should supply 50% of our daily Energy requirements.

Carbohydrates are the main energy-providing food group. The four main Carbohydrate food groups are: fruits, vegetables, whole grains and legumes, comprising a total of over 100 individual foods, all provided by Nature, for human energy requirements and a healthy life. A well balanced diet should include foods from each Carbohydrate food group and because each main group provides different ingredients and requires different digestion to be converted into energy, it is valuable to know the basic requirements of each food for digestion so as to ensure positive value from the foods eaten and to maintain complete health.

Fruits are not fattening as the Natural sugar content is protected with Minerals and Vitamins, that regulate and protect your body against excess weight.

When *Refined* Carbohydrates are eaten, the body will crave to get the essential Natural daily nutrient requirements (that are lacking in processed and refined foods), this often leads to excess eating so as to satisfy the body's daily nutrient needs, lack of Energy due to excess eating, ill health and expensive food bills.

Carbohydrate digestion begins in the mouth, with the Saliva, which converts the Starches into Sugars and the Sugars into a simpler digestible form.

Carbohydrate foods that are poorly prepared in the mouth and stomach will lead to fermentation, flatulence, indigestion, stomach pains and lack of Energy. *Refined* Carbohydrates and *processed* foods lack the essential nutrients and combinations of minerals and vitamins, that ensure proper digestion. Carbohydrate foods are only as good as the nutrients and combinations they supply. Fresh Fruits, Vegetables, Grains and Legumes, in their Natural undisturbed state are a complete form of Life and food. Any additions (sugar) or extractions (processing and refinement) affects the totality of the nutrients that have been supplied by Nature for Health and Life.

Proper combination of Carbohydrate foods is most important for maintenance of good health and also after dinner satisfaction.

PHOTOSYNTHESIS

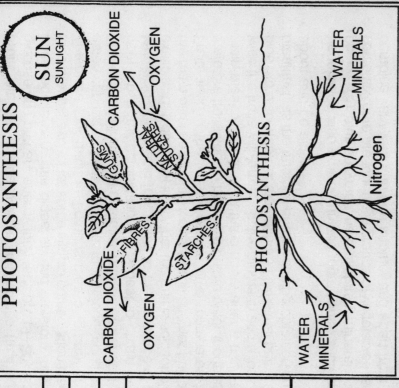

SALIVA is produced by three pairs of Salivary Glands. Saliva's function is to moisten food; a lubricant, aiding swallowing of food particles. Saliva is constantly produced in the mouth even without the addition of food, but as food enters the mouth, special nerves connected to the Salivary glands, send messages to the brain, advising of the type of food and for an increased amount of Saliva.

Saliva is an alkaline fluid consisting of; 99% Water and the Enzyme PTYALIN. Ptyalin's function is to act on Carbohydrate foods (especially Grains and Legumes) in preparation for other processes of Digestion. Adequate chewing of food is essential for Health.

PAROTID

SUBLINGUAL

SUBMANDIBULAR

CARBOHYDRATE FOOD GROUPS

Fruits are the unique provider of fructose (fruit sugar), which is very similar to glucose (the primary energy fuel) (see pp. 19–20). Because of the fructose content, fruits require very little digestion and therefore they are not compatible with other food groups, except for some simple combinations (see pp. 203 and 205 for details). There are four main fruit-groups (see diagram). The group of melons should be eaten separately from any other fruit or food group as they require unique digestion. The sub-acid fruits will combine with either the acid fruits or the sweet fruits. Apart from those fruit-combinations it is best to obtain fruits from the same group. The term acid or sub-acid fruit refers to the presence of organic acids: citric, malic and oxalic acid. It does not imply that the fruit is acid forming, in fact, fruits are classed as the main alkaline forming foods, that is another fruit benefit (see pages 44 and 163). Fruits require the least digestive time, compared to the other food groups and therefore fruits should be eaten before other foods and definitely not directly after a main meal. Allow at least three hours after a main meal before eating fruits otherwise the fruits will ferment in the stomach and a loss of valuable nutrients will occur, plus the discomfort of stomach and intestinal pains. The best time to eat fruits is at breakfast, as the fructose energy can be obtained quickly to help you wake up, walk about and be active.

Vegetables also provide unique ingredients, such as their chlorophyl content (see pp. 77–78), plus enzymes, natural starch, minerals, vitamins and also some protein content. There are four main groups of vegetables (see diagram). All vegetables will combine very well with one another and apart from the starch vegetables, they all combine well with whole grains or legumes and that enables the preparation of complete meals (see p. 207 for details). The starch vegetables should be limited in use with whole grains or legumes, otherwise an excess intake of starch may occur. Vegetables are the ideal companion for any animal produce meal, as they provide many essential nutrients to balance the meal. For more details on the benefits of vegetables see pages 62–79.

Whole grains and legumes require similar digestion. They are both composed of natural starch, protein, minerals, vitamins and a low fat content. Both whole grains and legumes provide long-lasting energy, as their starch content is slowly converted into glucose. Refined grains or legumes can only provide a portion of the original energy potential and over a prolonged period, refined foods will deplete the store of nutrients within the body and lead to numerous health problems (see pp. 22, 187–197 for details). Only natural Carbohydrate foods can give you all the energy you require, for a very happy, healthy life.

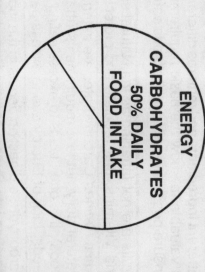

SUB ACID FRUITS		SWEET FRUITS	
Apples Apricots Blackberry Pears		Bananas Dates Figs Prunes	
Cherry Grapes Paw Paw Peaches		Raisins Dried Fruits	
Loganberry Lychees Mangoes			
ACID FRUITS		**MELONS**	
Grapefruit Limes Kiwi fruit Oranges		Cantaloupe Watermelon	
Lemons Pineapple Mandarin		Honeydew Melon Other Melons	
Tomato Passionfruit			
GRAINS		**OTHER GRAINS**	
Barley Corn		Bulgur	
Millet Oats		Sorghum	
Rice Rye		Triticale	
Wheat		Buckwheat	
		Sprouted Grains	

ENERGY

CARBOHYDRATES
50% DAILY
FOOD INTAKE

STARCH VEGETABLES		LEAFY VEGETABLES	
Beetroot Cauliflower Pumpkin		Spinach Celery Bean Sprouts	
Potato Artichoke Carrot Turnip		Watercress Lettuce	
Parsnip Radish			
OTHER VEGETABLES		**FLOWER VEGETABLES**	
Garlic Onions Egg Plant Cucumber		Broccoli Asparagus Brussel Sprouts	
Mushrooms Okra Capsicum Zucchini			
OTHER LEGUMES		**LEGUMES**	
Adzuki bean		Carob Lentil	
Asparagus bean		Chick pea Lima bean	
Black eyed pea		Kidney bean Mung bean	
Broad bean Peanut		Soya bean	
Hyacinth bean		Sprouted Legumes	
Pidgeon pea Navy bean			

CARBOHYDRATE—DIGESTION—ENERGY

Carbohydrates: fruits, vegetables, whole grains and legumes are all energy providing foods. Fruits contain fructose (fruit sugar) and that is converted directly into glucose (see p. 20). Vegetables contain varying amounts of starch and that is also converted into glucose, after some simple digestion (explained below).

For the conversion of Carbohydrates into energy, special digestive enzymes are produced and they act upon the food substance at various times within the human digestive system. The following enzymes are required for Carbohydrate digestion: ptyalin, amylase and maltose.

1. Ptyalin is produced in combination with saliva, during the action of chewing food. Ptyalin converts the starch content of cooked vegetables, grains and legumes into the form of maltose, which is termed a double sugar (see p. 20).

2a. In the stomach, ptyalin continues to convert mainly cooked starch into the form of maltose.

3. After leaving the stomach, uncooked starch is also converted into maltose by the enzyme amylase, which is produced by the pancreas.

4. Within the small intestine, millions of tiny glands produce the enzyme maltose and that converts the starch-maltose into the usable form of glucose.

5. The absorption of glucose occurs mainly within the small intestine and then it is conveyed to the liver, via the bloodstream.

6. The liver stores glucose in the form of glycogen and when the body requires glucose-energy, glycogen is reconverted into glucose.

7. In combination with glucose, a special ingredient is required to provide the spark to convert glucose into energy. The ingredient is called insulin. It is produced by cells from the pancreas, known as the islets of Langerhans. As the body requires energy, both glucose and insulin are released into the bloodstream and they travel to the various muscles, nerves and tissues, to provide a continuous supply of usable energy. The common ailment, diabetes, is related to a lack of insulin production. To ensure that you protect against diabetes it is essential to avoid refined foods and to prepare natural wholesome meals. Only natural foods can provide the correct balance of essential nutrients, to protect against such disorders. In Australia, over 100,000 people have diabetes and possibly many other people are at risk to being a diabetic if they continue to eat refined foods: white bread, white sugar, sweet biscuits, lollies, packaged breakfast foods and sugar drinks. You can be healthy tomorrow if you eat naturally today.

2b. Whole grains and legumes provide protein as well as their starch content and so extra digestive processes are required to convert the protein into usable protein - (amino acids). The most important substances secreted by the stomach glands for protein conversion are: pepsinogen and hydrochloric acid and when they combine, they form into the active enzyme: pepsin.

When whole grains or legumes enter the stomach they are first acted upon by the enzyme for starch conversion: ptyalin, after which the stomach will produce pepsin to initially convert the protein content, however the hydrochloric acid will be secreted last so as to maintain an alkaline state within the stomach, to assist proper starch conversion; as the action of ptyalin can only continue when the stomach is in the alkaline or low acid state.

After sufficient starch conversion, the stomach glands will produce more pepsinogen and acid: pepsin, which can then act upon the protein content of the grains and legumes. Once the food has left the stomach a number of other enzymes are produced within the small intestine and pancreas, to complete the protein conversion — (see page 94 for details). When concentrated protein foods: nuts, seeds or animal produce foods are combined with grains or legumes, a higher level of acid is then produced and that can interfere with initial starch conversion within the stomach, thereby causing poor digestion and incomplete preparation of the valuable starch-energy content. Also, the increased stomach acid required for concentrated protein foods will be excess for the proper digestion of the protein contained in the grains or legumes. For the best value from whole grains or legumes, fresh vegetables and some cooked vegetables are the ideal companion. By combining grains and legumes, an increased protein availability occurs and therefore no extra protein should be required. When grains and legumes receive proper digestion and preparation, they will supply valuable amounts of all essential amino acids (protein)—see pages 41, 42, 85–88 and 98.

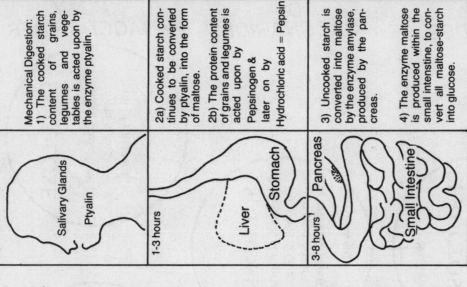

1 minute — Salivary Glands, Ptyalin

Mechanical Digestion:
1) The cooked starch content of grains, legumes and vegetables is acted upon by the enzyme ptyalin.

1-3 hours — Liver, Stomach

2a) Cooked starch continues to be converted by ptyalin, into the form of maltose.

2b) The protein content of grains and legumes is acted upon by Pepsinogen & later on by Hydrochloric acid = Pepsin.

3-8 hours — Pancreas, Small Intestine

3) Uncooked starch is converted into maltose by the enzyme amylase, produced by the pancreas.

4) The enzyme maltose is produced within the small intenstine, to convert all maltose-starch into glucose.

5) Glucose is then conveyed to the liver and stored as glycogen, until required.

6) The liver re-converts the glycogen, into glucose.

7) Both glucose and insulin combine to provide the spark of natural energy.

ILLUSTRATION OF HOW YOUR BODY CONVERTS CARBOHYDRATES INTO ENERGY

MONO--SACCHARIDES — SINGLE SUGARS

DI--SACCHARIDES — DOUBLE SUGARS

POLY--SACCHARIDES — CHAIN OF SIMPLE SUGARS

CELLULOSE
Indigestible part of the plant; most suitable form of roughage.

SUCROSE
Sucrose is converted into Fructose & Glucose by the enzymes Sucrase & Invertase.
cane sugar

FRUCTOSE
Fructose is the simplest form of fruit sugars.
fruit sugar

STARCH
Starch is initially converted by Ptyalin, (Salivary Glands) and then by the Enzyme Amylase, (Pancreas), into the form of Maltose.

DEXTRIN

MALTOSE
Maltose is converted by the enzyme Maltase directly into Glucose.
malt sugar

GLUCOSE (ENERGY)
Glucose is the simplest form of (ENERGY)

GLYCOGEN
Glycogen is stored in the Liver.
When the body requires extra energy, Glycogen is re-converted into Glucose, by the liver.

LACTOSE
Lactose is converted by the enzyme Lactase into Glucose & Galactose.
milk sugar

GALACTOSE
SIMPLE SUGAR

PECTIN
(Indigestible).
Pectin is used for the making of jam & jellies.

INTRODUCTION – NATURE – EARTH FOOD

Welcome again to the world of Nature foods! Your potential to improve both your health and range of recipes may provide you with more opportunities than for a person who has experienced nutritional knowledge and the practical application of that knowledge for many years. The first sign of health is when a person takes interest in the type of foods they are eating. It is a personal asset to recognize that all foods have different effects and benefits for your body and from that conclusion, you can vary your diet to suit your personal requirements: age group, occupation, climate, availability of food, culture and the amount of food intake. The first important point to realize and remember is that, Nature supplies all our food and nutritional requirements as well as the best environment to appreciate our life and health. Since the very beginning of time, people have lived because Nature supplied the food and the environment to exist. We are also part of Nature and our ability to adapt to the environment has developed through many time-changes. Throughout the world today, there is a vast variation with lifestyles and their general direction and for the people who have the good fortune to obtain a regular supply of food, comfortable housing, suitable clothing and a friendly environment, they have some advantages that other people may never live to experience. There is one problem that the 'fortunate people' may encounter and it is based on a direct link with the modern technological age and the production of factory-produced foods and drinks, a problem that you can easily solve, you choose the foods you eat, you can avoid all food that is factory-produced: packaged, processed, refined, canned and bottled food-substitutes. Remember that all food is provided by Nature. Even factory-produced foods have at one time developed from a natural source: fruits, vegetables, whole grains, legumes, nuts or seeds. Think about the foods you have at home and about their origin, they most certainly developed from a natural source, if not, from where did they originate? The main reason for a factory-produced food is profit, apart from that, a factory-produced food may have developed for the basic reason of convenience, just open the can, bottle or carton and you get food, no need to prepare, just swallow and have another if you like, there are plenty of supplies and they are on special this week, six for the price of two, hurry! hurry!, the bargain only lasts till the stock is cleared. That's a sample of common advertisement used to excite people into a buying-spree. Does anyone or any advertisement ever give you such enthusiasm about the world of Nature foods, maybe the supermarket has the occasional special for tomatoes or over-ripe bananas, that's their business – for their benefit. Have you any idea of how many hospitals there are and how many people are hidden away in such a caring environment, the answer is – too many! The human body is designed to live in health, sickness can be avoided and so can all those factory-produced foods, you decide for yourself and that reflects in others. Parents have a double obligation, children eat the food you provide, you give them a sweet-lollie to be good, and, at the same time you're not. Give them a Nature-food now. For those people who have a limited idea about the world of Nature foods, this book will describe all the main Nature-foods, their main benefits and various healthful recipes. On your next shopping day, discover for yourself how many Nature foods you can obtain and then let Nature give you life. Nature-foods are the best value, they maintain and promote health and they are essential for life. Always use the whole Nature food and your life and health will be complete with all living benefits.

GRAINS

INTRODUCTION

GRAINS have been used for thousands of years as a main supplier of food and nourishment. The discovery of Grains as a source of food, by primative Man, was a most influencing evolutionary factor, as it enable people to settle in one place and rely on a regular food supply from the 'food that did not wander'. Those people learned to share the task of crop cultivation until such time that the modern world took over. Nowadays some people have never seen a field of Grains, and most important of all, many people rarely even eat the Whole Grain. Processed and refined foods seem to be taking over. Grains are classed as a Carbohydrate food, an Energy source. For many people the regular diet will include only one main Grain, usually Wheat as in sandwiches. Rice is also a common addition to the diet, however the other Grains never get a chance to contribute their Nutritional benefits, unique taste and range of recipes. Your Health is based on the food you eat. Your diet is based on the recipes you know. Health is often poor due to the lack of knowledge on Natural Whole Grain recipes. In this book, Grains are the first food group for you to broaden your understanding of, with facts of history, nutrient benefits and also some simple recipes, so as you may use the information directly with your next meal and others to follow. The routine of modern day living has a most detrimental effect on a majority of people's Health. Time goes so quickly in the morning that some people compensate by relying on the quickest and most convenient packaged breakfast foods, with little if any thought of the effects of that meal with their activities throughout that day, and also the effects of a prolonged use of such foods. As explained in the previous pages, Carbohydrate foods are the main Energy foods. You need Energy to get you through a busy day, so give it to your body, and the best time is with the morning meal. Grains supply long lasting Energy. Apart from being an excellent source of Carbohydrates, Grains also supply a fair percentage of Primary Protein. Many people are unaware of the variety of foods that supply Protein. It is often the case that a person will rely heavily on Secondary Proteins for their daily requirements, often to the extent that an excess intake of Proteins occurs and follows to produce the widespread occurrence of obesity and associated ill effects. One meal a day should be based around Whole Grains. There are many forms of the Whole Grain, some of which are seldom included or even thought of as part of the daily diet. Whole rolled Millet, Oats, Barley, Rye and Wheat are just one example of an excellent substitute for the commercially prepared and refined breakfast cereals. A Rolled Grain is a Whole Grain, with all the essential nutrients that only Nature can provide in proper balance. Only recently has Nutritional knowledge been capable of analyzing individual foods for their composition of nutrients and effects of prolonged nutrient deficiencies been proven. Another recent development is the processing, refinement, conversion and commercial packaging of food. Many people find it hard to choose one packet from another as they are the same size, price and weight, sometimes the only difference is the brand name and other forms of decoration used to attract some people's attention. Common sense must be on a very low scale of intelligence, for a mass of people continually rely on a refined product that needs thousands of dollars advertisement for it to sell, giving little if any nutritional benefit and with the added expense of processing, refinement, labour, storage, advertising and profit

Live with Life, with Nature and Learn to use Natural Foods.

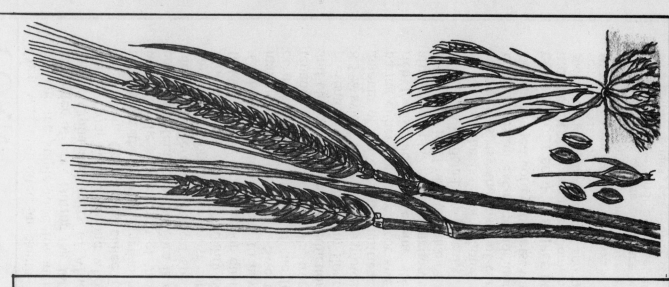

BARLEY

Barley was grown in Egypt over 8,000 years ago and for the early Greek, Roman and Hebrew civilizations, Barley was well respected and used for the making of their daily bread. The Barley grain was also used by the Chinese people thousands of years ago and even then, they recognized numerous therapeutic benefits associated with regular use of Barley. The Barley grain was later introduced throughout many European countries and it became the staple grain for those people living in the colder climates like Scotland, Switzerland and Denmark. Captain Cook on his voyage to Australia is reported to have fed his crew with sprouted Barley and that was most valuable when fresh fruits and vegetables were not available as the sprouted Barley supplied sufficient vitamin C and other essential nutrients, that protected his men against the development of scurvy and other diseases. Today, Barley is used throughout most parts of the world and it is available in various forms such as the original whole grain, that is obtained from either the two row or six row Barley plant. Apart from the original whole grain, Barley is also prepared into whole rolled Barley or Barley flakes, whole grain Barley flour and home made Barley sprouts all of which are a valuable addition to the diet and should at least occasionally, provide the range of nutrients that only Barley in the whole grain from supplies as well as the various traditional and modern recipes that are based on the Barley grain. Compared with other Grains, Barley heads the list for heat-producing qualities. For those people who feel the chill of winter, Barley meals will help you stay warm for many hours. Try some whole grain Barley meals next winter and you will discover the warming and body building benefits of Barley. Many people throughout the colder regions of the world use Barley as a staple food with such dishes as: soups, muesli, muffins, fruit cakes, vegetable pies and a delicious sweet-nutty tasting whole grain bread.

Barley is easier to digest than other Grains and it supplies valuable amounts of the minerals: phosphorus — promotes healthy nerves, potassium — muscle development, iron — protection from colds and cleansing of the blood, sodium — promotes carbohydrate digestion and protects against excess body acidity, magnesium — healthy and strong teeth, nerves and glands, manganese — blood development, chlorine — protects against obesity, sulphur — protein metabolism and cleansing of the digestive system. Whole grain Barley is also a good source of vitamins: B1 — healthy nerves, B2 — good eyesight, B3 — improves blood circulation, protects against digestive disorders, B5 — is the most dominant B group vitamin with the whole Barley grain that promotes digestion and metabolism of fats and may account for the heat producing qualities associated with Barley as Vitamin B5 will stimulate the body to use fats effectively. Vitamin B5 is heat sensitive and so are most other B group vitamins. Regular use of whole grain and rolled Barley or Barley sprouts as a breakfast cereal or with any meal of the day will promote repair and development of nerves, skin, blood, muscles and protect you against the chills of winter. See chapter seven for Barley recipes, also page 32 and some other natural food recipe books. Barley was once used as a barter-currency, today it could be your best investment.

CORN

Corn was cultivated in South America over 10,000 years ago and it has developed to become the staple food for millions of people. The American Indians termed Corn as the 'daughter of life'. During the 16th century, Corn was introduced to such countries as India, Japan, China and parts of Africa. The daily bread of Mexicans is called Tortillo, this is made from coarse ground whole Corn meal. The North American people make a similar bread from Corn, it is called Hominy. The word 'corn' has developed various meanings throughout the world. English people use the word corn to mean wheat as 'corne' is the word for the staple grain of their country, that is nowadays wheat. When a Scotsman says corn, he refers to oats. Corn is often called Maize, both are identical crops. Corn is available in 5 different botanical species: dent corn, flour corn, flint corn, pop corn and sweet corn. Dent corn is the most common type, it is mainly used as a flour for bread making. Flour corn is the best quality corn for bread making. Flint corn is mainly used as animal fodder. Pop corn is a poor quality food. Sweet corn is the most delicious of all varieties. 'Corn on the cob' seems to have developed in America and it is now popular throughout many parts of the world. Sweet corn is abundant in vitamin A and the whole grain flour corn is a good source of the following nutrients: phosphorus — promotes growth, maintenance and repair of cells, iron — blood development, potassium — muscle development and chlorine — weight reduction. Small amounts of the essential B group vitamins are alos present in the whole grain flour corn and sweet corn. The protein content of flour corn is 8.5%, sweet corn is 3.3% protein. Compared to other Grains, Corn supplies only a minimal amount of the essential nutrients and it is very low in the main mineral calcium. When preparing either corn bread or sweet corn it would be advisable to always add some calcium rich foods such as sesame seeds, tahini, sunflower seeds, almonds, parsley, broccoli or alfalfa sprouts. A combination of whole grain Corn flour with wheat, soya, rye or triticale flour is an ideal way to enhance the nutritional value of home made Corn bread. Corn Oil is discussed in detail on page 133. Whole grain flour corn is available at some natural food stores, try the taste of a home made corn bread with an avocado dip and for those cold winter days, try the taste of corn sprout soup, a simple meal to prepare and digest. Sweet corn makes an excellent addition for a home made quiche, a complete protein meal. Avoid buying canned corn products, wait until you can obtain fresh corn, try today.

CORN SPROUT SOUP — SIMPLE RECIPE — IDEAL WINTER MEAL.

INGREDIENTS: 2 ears fresh Corn, 1 cup of buckwheat, lentil, mung or soya sprouts, 1 medium carrot, 2 sticks celery, ½ cup chopped spring onions, 2 cups of prepared soya milk, vegetable salt and spices to suit the occasion.

METHOD: Slice Corn off the cob with a sharp knife and place in a cooking pot with grated or chopped carrot, celery and spring onions. Prepare soya milk and add to the corn and vegetables. Then add sprouts of your choice and place on the stove. Cooking time should be no more than 10 minutes and the mixture should not boil. Keep the stove switched on low position. Other vegetables such as broccoli, pumpkin, leek, cauliflower or cabbage can also be included. Serve with whole grain bread.

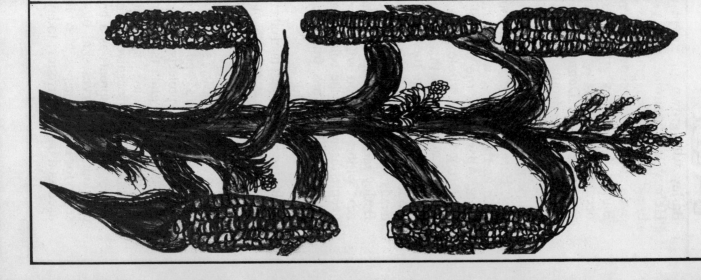

MILLET

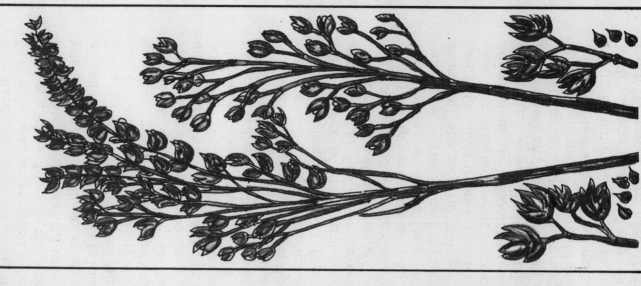

Millet has been used as a staple grain in China for about 12,000 years and may possibly be the oldest cultivated grain. Millet belongs to the Sorghum family of Grains and there are three main types of Millet: foxtail millet, pearl millet and prosso millet. Whole grain Millet has a very hard outer casing and that is usually removed and then sold as hulled millet. Today, Millet is used throughout many areas of the world especially India — with 40 million acres under cultivation, China, Russia, Argentina, America and some European and Asian countries. Apart from the whole grain Millet, you can obtain rolled millet, millet grits, millet flour and millet meal. The benefits associated with regular use of the millet grain are as follows: Millet is the best grain-source of the mineral Iron with 7 mg. per 100 gram portion. Everyday your body needs a supply of iron for the development of new blood cells and for protection from colds, influenza, hepatitis and other types of infection. Regular consumption of coffee, tea, refined bread and processed foods will lead to a deficiency of the mineral iron and also other nutrients such as vitamin E — healthy heart muscles, protection from pollution and cigarette smoke, repair of damaged skin tissue and internal organs. Millet is an excellent grain-source of vitamin E and it is one of the few alkaline forming grains and thereby supplies an abundance of alkaline body building and healing minerals such as: potassium, sodium, magnesium iron and manganese. Millet is the best grain-source of potassium — the muscle building mineral. Millet is also the best grain-source of magnesium — the mineral of the nerves. Regular consumption of alcohol and refined foods will deplete your store of magnesium and a prolonged deficiency of magnesium can lead to any of the following ailments: arteriosclerosis, diabetes, heart disease, nervousness, diarrhea and tooth decay. A Millet meal will help your nerves get the right nutrition. Millet is the best grain-source of the mineral silicon — promotes growth of hair, protects against the development of arthritis, promotes the functions of the main mineral calcium and is vital for insulation of delicate nerve fibres. Millet is also a good source of primary protein and when combined with legumes, a Millet meal will supply complete protein with an excellent balance of amino acids — the building blocks of body cells. Millet has a low fat content and is highly recommended for those people who are obese, have excess body acidity and require a gluten free diet. Millet is the ideal substitute for bran as it provides a very gentle and soothing action whereas bran is fairly rough on the linings of the intestines. Millet is also a good source of lecithin and this can protect you against the development of arterial damage. If you have never tried Millet before, your health will surely improve when you do. Millet may not replace the supermarket range of processed cereals today, but, do you care more for the wealth of the supermarket owner or for the health of your own body. Try some rolled Millet with fresh fruits for breakfast and various other millet recipes regularly for health. Try the taste of a millet vegetable pie, millet cookies, millet muesli, home made millet bread, millet soup and a millet casserole. See page 32, chapter seven or refer to other natural food recipe books. Millet is as versatile as your imagination.

OATS

Oats have been used since the days of the Roman empire and compared to other Grains, Oats have a short recorded history. It was not until the mid 17th century that Oats were used as a staple food by the people of Scotland. Apart from the whole grain Oats, you can obtain rolled oats, steel-cut oats, hulled or gritted oats and quick cook oats.

Whole Oats are available at some natural food stores and they provide the best range of essential nutrients such as calcium — Oats are the best grain-source of the main mineral calcium and in combination with the excellent supply of the minerals phosphorus and silicon, Oats can be considered the best grain for development and maintenance of strong bones, teeth and heart muscles as well as promoting a healthy nervous system. An old time nerve tonic was based on raw Oats. Dr Bircher Benner, a leading Swiss nutritionist was the first to develop the recipe for Muesli and this was based on raw Oats, fresh fruits, nuts and milk. Dr Benner designed the recipe to restore the health of elderly patients in the best way possible — with good nutrition and a pleasant mountain air environment. Most modern day Muesli imitations are very acid forming due to poor combinations of refined and heat affected mixed grains. Home made Bircher-Muesli is an excellent food for anytime of the day and it supplies all the essential daily nutrients in correct balance. Dr Benner would hesitate to claim fame over the recent Muesli boom and it's effects as he sought after maximum nutrition and not a half-hearted mixture of natural-processed and refined grains. Whole Oats are an excellent source of B group vitamins especially B1 and Inositol. Whole and rolled Oats are one of the richest source of Inositol and this can be most beneficial for proper metabolism of fats (Oats have the highest fat content of all grains), reduction of blood cholesterol levels, prevents hardening of the arteries and it is essential for brain cell nutrition and treatment of constipation, baldness and heart disease. Oats are the second best grain-source of primary protein, they supply near 14%complete protein. Regular use of whole grain and rolled Oats for breakfast will ensure that you start the day with a good balance of protein, carbohydrates, lipids, minerals and vitamins. Oats are a very good source of the mineral iron — healthy blood development, essential for proper protein metabolism and improves respiratory functions, potassium — muscle development, healthy skin, regulates the heartbeat, sodium — promotes carbohydrate digestion and improves the condition of the blood. One of the best food-medicines for prevention and relief from arthritis is whole grain or rolled Oats. The abundant supply of the minerals: calcium, phosphorus, silicon and sodium all contribute to promote healthy bone formation and they protect against a buildup of inorganic and toxic elements within the bloodstream and bone structure of the body. Daily use of raw Oats can be highly recommended for protection from arthritis and also baldness. Do not boil Oats, they need very little cooking and for maximum nutrition the Oats should be soaked overnight and served in the natural state with fresh seasonal fruits and nuts. Oats should have a dominant role with your nutrition and range of recipes. See page 32 and chapter seven for some delicious whole Oat recipes.

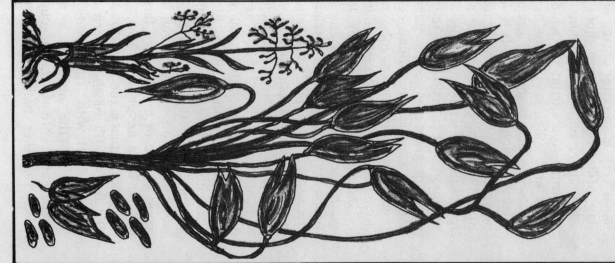

RYE

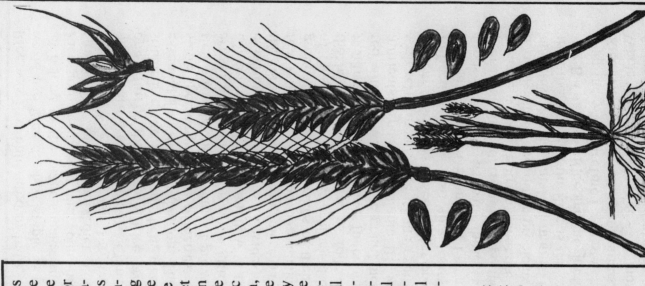

Rye was the staple grain throughout Europe during the Middle Ages and it has remained as the dominant grain for people in Germany, Scandinavian countries, Russia and some Eastern European countries. Today, over 90% of the Rye cultivation areas of the world are situated in the European countries. The Rye plant is most suited to a cold climate and for this reason it has and will continue to be used throughout Europe. Russia and the Scandinavian countries as the basic Grain for breadmaking. Rye is available in various forms such as the whole grain Rye, rolled Rye, whole grain Rye flour and Rye groats all of which contribute a valuable supply of essential nutrients. Rye is often termed as 'the muscle building grain' and that is due to the abundance of the mineral potassium and also vitamin E. The mineral potassium is termed as the 'muscle mineral' and vitamin E is often termed 'the heart muscle vitamin'. Rye is the second best grain-source of the mineral potassium, Millet is number one. After the digestion of food, the mineral potassium assists in the conversion of glucose to glycogen and that is stored in the liver until such time as the muscles require more fuel. Potassium is an alkaline mineral and it stimulates the kidneys to eliminate toxic waste and also helps to normalize the heartbeat in combination with the mineral sodium, that is also supplied with whole grain Rye. Vitamin E foods such as Rye increase the stamina and endurance of muscles by allowing nerves and muscles to function efficiently with a minimal supply of oxygen. Whole grain Rye is also a very good source of the minerals: phosphorus — stimulates muscle contractions such as the heartbeat, promotes repair of cells and is essential for mental development, iron — transports oxygen to every cell in the body, magnesium — helps to regulate glandular functions, vital for muscular contraction, prevention of cramps and nervous tension, silicon — strong bone formation and promotes good blood circulation. Whole Rye is also a good source of: sulphur — the mineral that promotes a good complexion as it expels waste toxins from the body, calcium — promotes the absorption of vitamins and digestion of food. Vitamins B1, B2 and B3 are all well supplied with whole grain Rye. Apart from the minerals and vitamins, whole grain Rye supplies 12% primary protein and a low 1.7% fat content.

Various types of Rye bread are available such as the very dark pumpernickel, wholemeal Rye and the light continental Rye. The low gluten content of Rye is the main reason for the Rye bread to be more compact than the wheat bread. Some commercially produced Rye bread also contains extra gluten flour so as to produce a lighter loaf. Homemade Rye bread is enjoyable to make and delicious to taste. Rolled Rye can also be included with the morning muesli and various other whole Rye meals are worth discovering. During the 1930's an important 'new-Grain' was developed from a combination of Rye and Wheat plants: it was called Triticale, the name is derived from the following botanical names: Rye — secale, Wheat — triticum. The Triticale grain combines the benefits of both Rye and Wheat and it has an improved protein, mineral and vitamin content. Triticale flour is an ideal choice for any home made bread. Experience the numerous benefits and taste of Triticale today.

RICE

Rice was first cultivated in India, over 5,000 years ago. Today, nearly half the people in the world use Rice as their staple — main food. There are over 10,000 varieties of Rice, almost all belong to the plant species known as Sativa. One of the most beneficial aspects of the Rice grain is due to the abundance of alkaline minerals. Rice is one of the few alkaline Grains. 75% of the daily diet should be based on alkaline forming foods. Rice helps over half the people in the world to live with health. Throughout the world, over 200 million tons of Rice are grown annually. China produces nearly one third and India is second with over one fifth of the world's Rice production. The main Rice growing areas of the world are situated in the monsoon belt, where the heavy rains provide large flooded areas which are essential for Rice cultivation. The average Rice plant will grow to a height of 2 metres, some species grow to 6 metres. Rice seeds are usually developed away from the 'paddy fields' for the first month of growth and are then transplanted into the fields, just before the arrival of the monsoon rains. Often a Rice crop has been destroyed by unpredicted weather conditions and poor timing with the planting of the Rice seeds. Both India and China have experienced conditions of widespread famine, due to the failure of their Rice crop. During the 18th century, the Japanese navy began to feed their crew with refined Rice, one of the few foods they had on board, and as a result of a prolonged deficiency of especially the B group vitamins, thousands of their sailors developed a disease known as beriberi and many of those died due to a prolonged deficiency of especially vitamin B1-thiamine. Symptoms of the beriberi disease are as follows: nausea, fatigue, constipation, diarrhea, respiratory difficulties, disturbed nerve functioning, heart failure and weight loss. When the sailors were fed with the whole Rice grain, their health improved rapidly. Refined Rice is deficient in all nutrients especially vitamin B1, with over 80% of the original B1 content being destroyed with refinement. One of the main functions of vitamin B1 is to promote a healthy nervous system, also, it is essential for proper digestion and absorption of starch, sugar and alcohol. Refined Rice has also 40% less vitamin B2-riboflavin than the whole grain Rice and over 60% less vitamin B3-niacin. For many of us, it is fortunate that we have a wide variety of foods to supply us with these essential life supporting B group vitamins, however, when preparing Rice it is most important to use the whole grain Rice so as to ensure a correct balance with all nutrients that are supplied and thereby prevent such after dinner complaints as indigestion and other problems associated with a prolonged use of refined Rice such as: diabetes, diarrhea and dermatitis. If you rely on Rice everyday for food, as many people do, then the whole grain Rice is the only choice to help you live and laugh with health. Without the B vitamins, Rice has no life!. Whole grain Rice takes only 10 minutes longer to cook than the white (refined rice starch). Apart from the deficiency of B group vitamins, refined Rice has less calcium, phosphorus, potassium and iron content as well as protein content. Whole grain brown Rice is a most versatile food, it combines very well with nearly all fruits and vegetables and also as an ideal protein improver for a wide variety of Legumes.

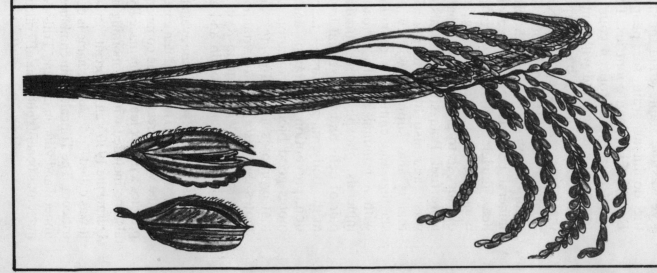

RICE

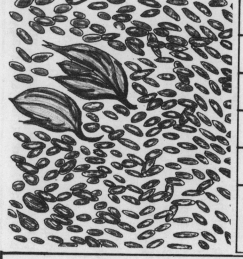

	Brown Rice.	White Rice.	Converted Rice.	Rice Polish.	Rice Flakes.
CALORIE	370	348	340	264	350
PROTEIN	7	6	6	12	6
CALCIUM	35	24	27	70	30
PHOS—PHORUS	300	130	125	1,106	135
POTAS—SIUM	150	124	153	720	185
IRON	2	.8	.8	16	1.5
VIT.B1.	.3	tr.	.15	1.8	.3
VIT.B3.	4.5	.8	3.9	28	5.2

Of all the Grains, Rice has the best percentage of available protein, 70% of the protein in Rice is usuable and when combined with Legumes, the protein availability (N.P.U.) is improved over 40%, when combined with milk, the protein (N.P.U.) of Rice is increased nearly 30%. The combination of Rice with Legumes or milk is the basis of many traditional Rice dishes from China, India and numerous other countries and this provides the main portion of their daily protein requirements. Even though Rice is classed as a Carbohydrate food, in comparison to meat, Rice has a better level of available protein. Also, the cost per usuable gram of Protein for Rice is less than one quarter the price of a porterhouse steak or lamb chop. The number of calories obtained for every gram of usable protein is more for Rice than any other Grain. On average, 69 Calories are consumed per every gram of protein, that is nearly 30 Calories more than for wheat and oats, 20 more than rye and 10 more than millet or barley. Meat on average supplies only 20 Calories per every gram of usable protein. For some people, extra Calories means that the food is fattening, that type of suggestion is far from reality when talking about whole grain Rice. There is not doubt that processed and refined foods soon add up 'empty' Calories, however, whole grain Rice is protected with the essential nutrients that prevent excess weight problems. One nutrient in particular is the B group vitamin — Biotin. Whole grain Rice is by far the best grain-source of Biotin and this vital nutrient converts unsaturated fats into the form of body fuel, promoting an active and healthy body. A prolonged deficiency of Biotin can often be the main cause of obesity, baldness, fatigue and depression.

Proper preparation of whole grain Rice is essential for obtaining all the benefits and also the unique and extremely versatile taste of the Rice grain. To obtain the maximum benefits, Rice does not need to be cooked. The sprouting of Rice will take between 3-6 days, that will soften the grains considerably and allow you to use the Rice with any cold dish such as summertime Rice pudding. The next best form of Rice is the brown natural Rice, that can also be soaked during the day to soften the grain and then allowed 30 minutes on low heat, using 2 cups of water for every cup of Rice. After 30 minutes, all the water should be absorbed into the Rice grains and then it is ready to serve you with all the benefits. Boiled Rice is not recommended. Brown Rice can also be made as soft and fluffy as refined white Rice if you allow the cooking time to be 45 minutes on low heat as well as the presoaking of the Rice during the day. The benefits of sprouted Rice and brown Rice are well worth discovering. Other forms of Rice are: converted Rice, that is prepared under steam pressure and is said to retain a majority of nutrients, (see chart for details) as the steam forces the nutrients into the centre of the grain. Homemade steamed Rice is the best alternative to that product and then you will be sure of the quality. White Rice is deficient in all essential nutrients and should not be relied upon for good nutrition. One of the best Rice products is Rice polishings, they are an excellent source of the B group vitamins, calcium, phosphorus, potassium and iron.

WHEAT

Wheat has been cultivated for nearly 10,000 years and has progressed to become the dominant Grain throughout the world. Today, over one billion people use Wheat regularly as part of their diet. The original discovery of Wheat as a food source enabled nomadic tribe people to settle in one place and rely on the Wheat crop for a major portion of their food requirements. By the year 4,000 B.C., the Egyptians were the first to discover the secrets of yeast and the preparation of Wheat and they were the first to discover the secrets of yeast and the preparation of whole Wheat bread. The Egyptians then exported Wheat to the regions of the early Roman empire and later on the Wheat Grain was introduced throughout the British empire. Many sea voyages and associated battles were partly due to the increased popularity and value of the Wheat Grain. The art of breadmaking soon became common for the people of the newly formed British empire and eventually the cultivation of the Wheat crop spread throughout America, Australia and some European and Asian countries. Over 400 million acres of Wheat are cultivated annually throughout the world and it is estimated that Wheat accounts for over one-fifth of the total calorie intake for the human race. The ability of the Wheat Grain to grow in almost any climate has led to the development of numerous 'strains of Wheat', all of which belong to the botanical species known as Triticum.

Generally speaking, whole grain Wheat is the best grain-source of primary protein and it rates third on the list for the net protein availability with a score of 60% N.P.U. Whole grain Wheat is also a good source of the essential main minerals: calcium, phosphorus, potassium, iron, sodium, magnesium, silicon, chlorine, sulphur and iodine as well as vitamins: B1, B2, B3, B5, B6 and an excellent source of vitamin E. (See nutrient composition chart for more details). The majority of Wheat products: bread, pastry, biscuits, cakes and pasta are a poor reflection of this abundant supply of nutrients and depending on the amount of 'extraction', those Wheat products may or may not be worth regular addition with your diet. The whole grain Wheat can be used in numerous ways that retain all the essential associated nutrients to ensure proper food value, digestion and maximum health benefits. Sprouted Wheat will provide maximum nutritional value and it is also one of the simplest methods of Wheat preparation. Regular use of sprouted Wheat meals is highly recommended for maintenance of health and also for regeneration of body strength, vitality and harmony, (see section on Sprouting for details). The whole Wheat grain will also retain all the essential associated nutrients when the whole grain is ground into a flour by the traditional 'stone ground' method or with the use of a home grinder. The best loaf of bread can be produced at home with the help of a hand or small mechanical grinder, that is also the least expensive way to obtain a top quality product. You could also use a home blender to prepare the whole Wheat grain for breadmaking. One of the best natural medicines is obtained from Wheat, called Wheat-grass, see section on Sprouting for details.

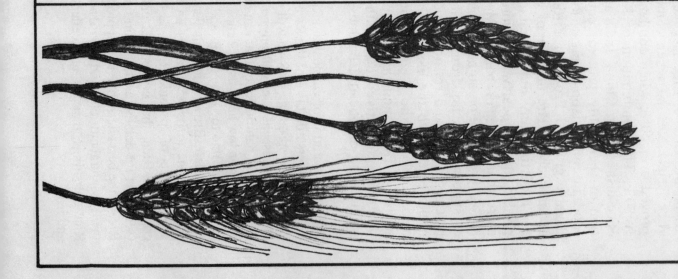

WHEAT

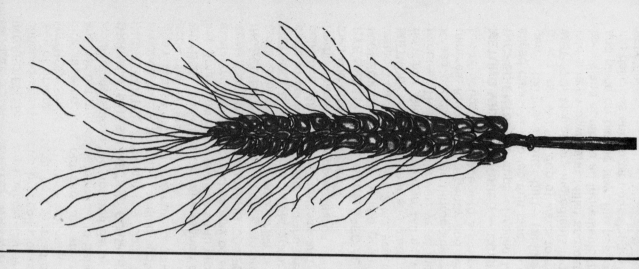

There are many varieties of commercially produced bread which are based on the whole Wheat grain and these are the best substitute for white bread, apart from the home made bread loaf. Once you have learnt to make a whole grain Wheat bread, you can avoid numerous problems that are associated with a prolonged use of especially white bread and off course, the coloured brown bread. One of the main nutrient deficiencies associated with regular use of white or brown bread and other refined foods will be vitamin E. The original Wheat grain is an excellent source of vitamin E and that promotes proper blood circulation, healthy heart muscles and protects against the effects of stress, worry, anxiety, cigarette smoking and the pollution of city air. The vitamin E content of whole Wheat is easily destroyed and often extracted during the process of refinement, as the Wheat germ oil tends to clog-up the machinery. Regular use of refined Wheat products may also lead to any of the following ailments, due to the effects of a prolonged nutrient deficiency: calcium-anemia, diabetes, diarrhoea, arteriosclerosis, arthritis and poor bone formation. Phosphorus — arteriosclerosis, arthritis and mental illness. Iron — anemia, diabetes, diarrhoea, nail problems, ulcers and leukemia. Potassium — acne, dermatitis, rheumatism, fever and headache. Magnesium — nervous disorders, hypertension and arthritis. Silicon — baldness, arthritis, poor skin condition, nervous disorders and poor eyesight. Vitamin B1 — anemia, diabetes, diarrhoea, mental illness and headaches. Vitamin B2-baldness, glaucoma and arthritis. B3 — headaches, baldness, arthritis, acne and poor blood circulation. Other common symptons of a regular — excess intake of refined Grain produce are: frequent colds, sinus problems, respiratory disorders, loss of hair, poor teeth and skin condition, obesity and poor muscular development. When a person eats large quantities of refined bread daily, their body will become saturated with 'waste starch residue' and they will also have little appetite left for the important natural whole foods: fruits, vegetables, nuts and seeds as well as whole grain and legume produce. For those people who may have difficulty at first in avoiding the daily intake of refined bread, there are numerous ways to supplement the diet, with natural whole foods, to avoid the development of any of the before mentioned ailments.

SIMPLE WHOLE GRAIN WHEAT BREAD RECIPE: 2 Loaves

INGREDIENTS: 6 cups of whole grain wheat flour, 3-4 cups of warm water (32-38d. Celsius), 2 oz fresh yeast, 1 tsp. honey, 1 tsp. brewer's yeast or 1 tblsp. rice bran.

METHOD: Place 2 oz fresh yeast into ½ cup warm water, add honey plus 1 tsp. flour, stir together, allow 2-3 minutes till ready. Place 2 cups of whole grain wheat flour into a large mixing bowl, slowly stir in 2 cups of warm water plus brewer's yeast or rice bran. Then add the cup of yeast-water to flour-mixing bowl, stir together and slowly pour in 2-3 cups of wheat flour and ½–1 cup of warm water, gently knead the flour-dough together, cut in half and then knead into shape, on a floured board to suit the shape of baking tins. Place into baking tins, allow 30 minutes to rise dough, in a warm position. Gently place into a pre-heated oven (170-180d C.) for -30 minutes, check oven temperature after 20 minutes.

BARLEY SOUP — 'WINTER WARMTH' — COMPLETE PROTEIN MEAL.
INGREDIENTS: 2 cups whole Barley grain, 1 cup chick peas, lima beans or kidney beans, 1 cup chopped celery, 1 cup broccoli pieces, 1 cup chopped capsicum, 1 cup carrot pieces, ½ cup chopped leek or onions, 1 tbl.sp. cold pressed oil. Spices to taste.
METHOD: Soak Barley and legume (chick, lima or kidney) overnight, rinse in the morning. Place Barley in a large cooking pot and turn stove on to low heat. Allow 20 minutes on low heat. Place legume in another pot and cook identical to Barley. Prepare vegetables andplace into the Barley mix, then add the legume and spices. Do not boil Barley soup. Serves 4 people. Preparation time 15-20 minutes.

ORIGINAL MUESLI RECIPE: COMPLETE PROTEIN MEAL (amount per person)
INGREDIENTS: 2 tbl.sp. raw Oats, 2 tbl.sp. natural culture yoghurt, 1 tbl.sp. raw chopped nuts: almonds, hazel, walnut. 1 grated apple, ½ cup fresh milk, 1 tsp. honey, cinnamon, extra seasonal fruits when available: pear, berries, peaches and apricots. Also raisins, sultanas and blackcurrants were added for variety.
METHOD: Soak Oats in milk-yoghurt overnight, add raw nuts, fresh fruits to the Oats-milk in the morning. Small portions were served to promote maximum health restoration. The original Muesli was served at any meal time. More Oats may be added for growing children.

SUMMERTIME RICE PUDDING COMPLETE PROTEIN MEAL.
INGREDIENTS: 2 cups whole grain brown Rice, 4 cups of prepared soya milk, ½ cup raisins, ½ cup sultanas, 2 tbl.sp. honey, 1 tsp. vanilla or almond essence. Fresh seasonal fruits.
METHOD: Either sprout whole grain Rice (see section on sprouting) or soak Rice for one day, then place in cooking pot and add the prepared 4 cups of soya milk. Allow 40 minutes onlow heat. Do not boil Rice. Add raisins, sultanas and honey 5 minutes before serving and also the essence and the freshly grated or chopped season fruits. For the sprouted Rice, cooking time is 10 minutes on low heat, then add other ingredients.

RYE BREAD: HOME MADE SPECIAL FARMER BREAD.
INGREDIENTS: 3 cups whole grain Rye flour, 1 cup whole wheat flour, ½ cup gluten flour, 3 cups water, 3 tsp. active yeast, 2 tsp. veg. salt, 2 tsp. caraway seeds, 2 tbl.sp. cold pressed vegetable oil.
METHOD: Mix Rye wheat and gluten flour together in a large mixing bowl. Form a well in the centre of flour mix. Dissolve yeast in 140 ml. warm water, add 1 tsp. molasses and place in a warm positionm. 5 minutes. Then pour water, yeast mix, oil, caraway seeds and veg. salt into the centre of flour mix. Knead dough together thoroughly — 5 minutes. Then place dough in a warm position to rise — 15 minutes. Knead again gently and place in greased baking tin. Sprinkle some more caraway seeds on top of dough and place into a pre heated oven — 200 F. for approx. 1 hour.

METUNG MILLET COOKIES — COMPLETE PROTEIN SNACK.
INGREDIENTS: 1½ cups of rolled Millet, ½ cup rolled oats, ½ cup toasted sunflower seeds, ½ cup sliced dates, ¼ cup lecithin meal, ¼ cup shredded coconut, ¼ cup raisins, ¼ cup sultanas, ¼ cup wheat germ, 100 grans better-butter (see page 147), 2 free range eggs, 2 tbl.sp. honey, ¼ tsp. cinnamon, pinch of veg. salt. Add ½ cup of water to the mix.
METHOD: Mix all dry ingredients together, toast sunflower seeds lightly, prepare dried fruits and place into a large bowl with Millet and oats. Beat two eggs and combine with better-butter. Add honey and spices and combine all ingredients throughly. Prepare large baking tray with oil. Form into little cookies and place on baking tray. Pre heat oven to 170 F and then allow 30 minutes baking time. Millet cookies are delicious and most nourishing. They should last up to two weeks in a cookie jar, depending on your appetite.

SIMPLE BREAD MAKING:

1. purchase the following: 1kg. whole wheat flour, ½kg. whole rye flour, 2ozs. fresh yeast — dry yeast. Other ingredients: cold pressed oil, veg. salt and molasses.

2. essential kitchen items: a large mixing bowl (wooden or glass), 2 bread baking-tins and one large wooden chopping board.

3. prepare kitchen sink area, the best place to start making bread.

4. place 3 cups of warm water into the mixing bowl, add 1 tsp. molasses — honey or flour into the water, sprinkle 1 tbl.sp. of fresh yeast-dry active yeast into the water. Leave for two-three minutes.

5. slowly mix into the water — yeast, 1 cup of whole wheat flour, mix in very well, then continue to add another 2 cups of whole wheat flour and 1 cup of rye flour, mix thoroughly. A soft dough will be formed.

6. sprinkle ½ cup whole wheat flour onto a wooden chopping board, take dough from the bowl and roll along the floured-board, kneading the dough, add another ½ cup of flour onto the board and continue to knead — rolling the dough for about 4 minutes, pressing firmly into the dough. Place dough back into the dry mixing bowl. Leave to rise for 20-30 minutes in a warm position, cover the top of bowl with cloth.

7. prepare baking tins with oil, spread 1 tsp. of oil per tin, after 30 minutes, take dough from the mixing bowl, cut in half, knead gently into the shape of the baking tins, place into baking tins. Light the oven, set at 350F. allow time for pre-heating the oven — 5-10 minutes, then place baking tins — dough into the oven, leave to bake for 30 minutes.

LEGUMES—

INTRODUCTION

LEGUMES is the name used to describe the family of Beans and Peas, sometimes referred to as Pulses. The following pages will provide you with information about the various types of Legumes, their nutritional value, unique recipes, historical information and methods of preparation. The main Legumes discussed are: Carob bean, Chick Pea, Kidney bean, Lentils, Lima bean and the Mung bean. On page 40, there is a section on other Legumes such as: Aduki bean, Asparagus pea, Black-eyed pea, Broad bean, Hyacinth bean, Pigeon pea, Runner bean, Peanut and Soya bean. For many people, Legumes are mainly obtainable in the dried state, only a few Legumes are available as fresh produce: French bean, Peas and Runner bean. Dried Legumes are one of nature's best store of nutrition, they are basically a seed and when water is added, new life will develop with every day of growth. Proper preparation of dried Legumes is easy, place one cupful of any of the following Legumes into a bowl: Chick peas, Kidney bean, Lentils, Lima bean, Mung bean or Soya bean, leave for approx. 8 hours, then rinse and repeat soaking, that can be done for a few days until the Legume-seed begins to sprout, otherwise the dried Legume should be soaked for at least 8 hours before preparing to cook. Pre-soaking of Legumes has many advantages, for some Legumes it is essential in order to relieve excess gas within the pea-bean-seed and also to promote better digestion. Raw-dried Legumes contain such substances as: alkaloids, glycosides and saponin and these are detrimental to the digestion and are eliminated with long soaking and proper cooking. Pre-soaking for more than a few days will greatly enhance the digestion and nutrient quality of the associated Legume. Make sure that your kitchen is always well stocked with at least these essential basic Legumes: Chick pea, Kidney bean, Lentils, Lima bean, Mung bean and Soya bean.

The variety of Legume produce is abundant and their popularity is increasing, due to the recognition of many delicious traditional recipes and their ability to supply all the essential daily protein requirements. Generally speaking, Legumes are classed as a carbohydrate food, however, when properly combined, as with many traditional recipes, Legumes in combination with whole grains, seeds or other Legumes will provide a more suitable balance of the essential Amino Acids (protein building blocks) for human absorption, metabolism and protein needs. Millions of people throughout the world rely upon Legume produce for their protein requirements and daily energy requirements. In countries where animal produce is the main source of protein, Legumes are often neglected from the diet and that combination of excess animal proteins and insufficient Legume produce is one of the main contributing factors towards the multitude of heart and arterial diseases that are so prevalent today, especially in America and Australia. If you regularly rely on animal proteins and have little knowledge about the benefits associated with Legume produce, this following chapter will assist you with valuable ideas on Legume preparation and once you have tried a few simple recipes, you will then realize how so many people throughout the world live to enjoy their Legume meals and are capable of obtaining all their daily protein requirements without having to rely on the animal kingdom. Legume meals could easily replace at least two of your animal protein meals per week. The Legume kingdom is prepared to give you protein, let nature help and continue to feed everybody.

CAROB BEAN

Carob is a member of the Locust family of plants, an evergreen tree that takes at least six years to bear fruit and may eventually grow to a height of nearly ten metres. Carob is a native plant from the Eastern Mediterranean regions such as Syria, Egypt, Spain, Palestine and Sicily and it is said to be the oldest known fruit bearing tree in those areas. Carob has supported man from the beginning of time and has been given the following descriptive titles from different generations of people: 'the staff of life', 'universal provider', 'bread that grows on trees', all of which emphasize the potential of the Carob bean in supporting human life. An extract from the Bible mentions that St. John the Baptist used Carob as a staple part of his diet during his long lifetime in the wilderness, providing him with energy, nourishment and food for thought. The name 'St. John's Bread' was also given to this remarkable life supporting food. The original method for weighing precious stones and gold was based on Carob seeds, from which the name 'carat' is derived.

Carob flour and powder supply 8% primary protein and over 70% natural carbohydrate content as well as a good source of the main minerals calcium and phosphorus. The rich natural carbohydrate content of the Carob bean is mainly in the form of fruit sugars and these have a very low fat content — 2% compared to the fat content of chocolate which is nearly 52%. Carob powder is an excellent substitute for both chocolate and coffee as it can be served either hot or cold with milk but needs no added sweetness. Carob contains no caffeine and it is an alkaline forming food which makes it valuable for reducing excess stomach acidity and could be used as an ideal replacement for the antacid tablet. Both chocolate and coffee are abundant in oxalic acid, a substance that is known to retard and sometimes completely inhibit the absorption of the main mineral calcium and with a prolonged and excessive use of both chocolate and coffee, calcium deficiencies may appear to promote such ailments as: tooth decay, nervous affliction, muscular cramps and heart palpitations. Carob is the natural substitute for any commercially prepared chocolate based drink and it can also be combined with numerous recipes that require extra sweetness. Whenever a recipe requires the use of chocolate, try using Carob instead and discover the taste similarity and economy of the Carob-chocolate powder. The pectin content of the Carob bean has proved to be most valuable in the treatment of diarrhoea and other stomach upsets. Let nature help you, laugh with health. Try a Carob milkshake or a hot cup of Carob soon.

HOT CAROB DRINK:

INGREDIENTS: ¼ cup Carob chocolate powder, ½ cup soya milk powder, 4 cups boiled water.
Optional: honey, cinnamon or nutmeg.
METHOD: Mix Carob powder and Soya milk together, Place 3 tsp. of the Carob—Soya mix per cup, slowly pour hot water and mix together.

CAROB MILKSHAKE:

INGREDIENTS: ¼ cup Carob powder, ½ cup Soya milk powder, 1 ripe banana, 4 cups of water, 1 tsp. vanilla, almond or coconut essence. Optional: honey, cinnamon, tahini or wheat germ.
METHOD: Place all ingredients in blender for 1 minute — medium speed. Serves 6 people.

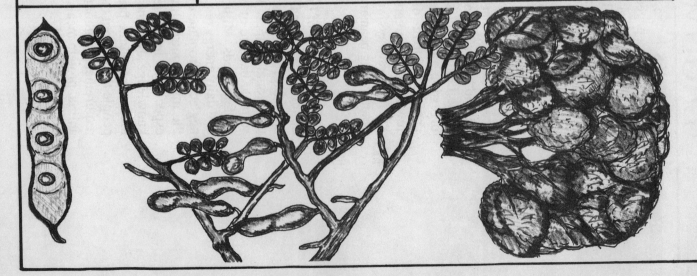

CHICK PEAS

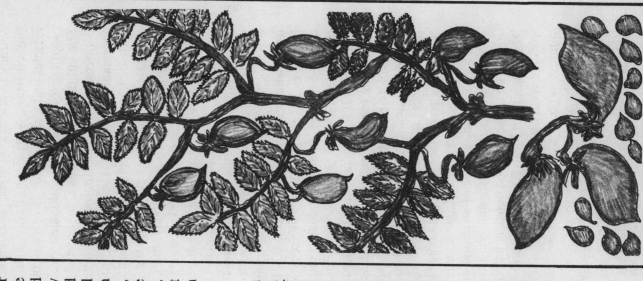

Chick Peas are also referred to as Garbanzo pea, Egyptian pea or Bengal gram and possibly a few other names, depending on their country of cultivation. Chick Peas are available in various colours such as the white, red, yellow, brown and black peas being most common, all of these having a distinctive pointed pod in which two or three peas (seeds) are found. Chick Peas were originally used by people from the early Egyptian era and were then introduced by merchant traders to people from the Mediterranian region and they have continued to use Chick Peas as an important part of their food requirements. Various traditional recipes are based on Chick Peas such as hummous, a mixture of Chick Peas, garlic, sesame, veg. oil, lemon juice and spices. In parts of Africa, Chick Peas are ground into a flour to produce the base for 'cous cous', that has now become popular throughout many parts of the world as it supplies a good amount of available protein as well as a delicious taste. Falafel, the traditional filling for Arab bread is based on Chick Peas, potato, sesame seeds, onions, parsley and various spices such as paprika, cayenne pepper and garlic, that also provide a good protein complement. Millions of people throughout the world rely upon the protein content of Chick Peas combined with whole grains for a major portion of their daily protein requirements.

When Chick Peas are combined with rice, there will be over 40% increase in protein availability, when combined with wheat: over 30% increase in protein, combined with corn: 50% increase, combined with milk: 11% increase in protein availability. Chick Peas supply 20% protein and a net protein utilization of 43% (N.P.U.). An average serve of ½ cup Chick Peas, 1 cup of rice and fresh vegetables will supply the equivalent usable protein to an 8 ounce steak, that is over half the average R.D.A. — recommended daily protein allowance. A meal of Chick Peas, rice and vegetables is one of the many ideal substitutes for the regular meat based diet. Apart from the good supply of primary protein, Chick Peas are an excellent source of mineral iron — required daily for healthy blood development, protection from infection and for promotion of protein digestion. Chick Peas supply over three times as much iron compared to a porterhouse steak. Chick Peas are an excellent source of the main mineral calcium — bone development and repair, prevents excess acidity, promotes muscle growth and aids in the utilization of the mineral iron. Chick Peas supply twenty times the amount of calcium compared to a porterhouse steak. Chick Peas are a very good source of the mineral phosphorus — required for healthy kidney functioning, healthy nerves and efficient mental activity. Chick Peas supply nearly twice as much phosphorus compared to a porterhouse steak. Chick Peas are a good source of potassium — required for nourishment of the muscular system and for regulation of the heartbeat. Chick Peas supply over three times the amount of potassium compared to a porterhouse steak. Other nutrients that are also well supplied with Chick Peas are: sodium — assists in keeping other blood minerals soluble, chlorine — helps to regulate the acid and alkali balance in the blood, vitamin A — promotes growth and repair of skin tissue, vitamin B1 — 'morale vitamin', B2 — healthy skin, hair and eyesight, B3 — healthy nerves and promotes digestion, Try Chick Peas for a healthy change and as an ideal complete protein meal.

KIDNEY BEAN

Kidney Beans belong to the botanical species – Phaseolus vulgaris, that also includes the following Beans: French Bean, Navy Bean, Pinto Bean, Haricot Bean, Snap Bean, Mexican Black Bean, Stringless Bean, Frijoles and Calico Bean. The first of the 'vulgaris' species to be used by man was the Kidney Bean, that is reported to have been cultivated over 7,000 years ago by the primitive tribes of American Indians. The vulgaris species was also reported to be growing on the island of Cuba and Honduras, around the mid 14th century when Columbus and other 'new land' explorers noted and then spread the word about the abundant growth of the vulgaris and other Legumes in those newly explored lands. During the 16th century, the Kidney Bean was introduced to European countries and shortly after, the French cultivated the bean and renamed it the 'French Bean', that prompted other people from different countries to do similar renaming and today, there are marked differences in the vulgaris bean species, due to varying climates, soil conditions and methods of cultivation. The vulgaris bean (seed) can vary in colour from white, red or black with the French bean and snap bean variety usually prepared as a fresh yellow-green vegetable. The red Kidney Bean is sold throughout the world as the most commercial canned bean: Baked Bean which line the supermarket shelves from Metung to Manhattan. Home made Baked Beans are far easy to prepare and when compared to the taste of the canned variety, home made Baked Beans are far superior, they also have a greater supply of nutrients, especially: protein, calcium, phosphorus, potassium, iron, folic acid, vitamins: A, B1, B2, B3. Apart from the better supply of essential nutrients, home made Baked Beans are free of any unnecessary preservatives and possible inferior produce and with the added expense of the canned product, you can be sure that the home made product will be a worthwhile investment, even if you only have Baked Beans twice a year. The original Baked Bean recipe was made from natural freshly prepared produce, the canned alternative can never be the same. Treat the family to a rewarding meal of freshly prepared Baked Beans and of course, home made whole grain bread, that will be a complete protein meal and for maximum benefits, serve with a freshly prepared sprout salad: alfalfa sprouts, grated carrot, beetroot and cucumber, outer green lettuce leaves, parsley and some soya mayonnaise. During the 16th century, the vulgaris Bean was considered a luxury food and even today, the freshly prepared French Green Bean is considered to be worth it's weight in taste, when served at the exclusive French restaurants. The stringless variety French Bean is a favourite and when served with a fresh fish meal and a side salad, a glass of wine and of course candlelight, you could be anywhere in France or at home, relaxing with some music and good company. When only the best will do, try natural foods. For more details on the associated benefits with the French Bean, turn to the section of Vegetables, p. 64. Both the Navy Bean and Pinto Bean are a good source of primary protein, they supply over 22 grams of protein per 100 gram (dry weight, edible portion) and have a N.P.U. – net protein utilization of near 40%. There are numerous recipes for the Navy and Pinto Bean, one such, 'quesadillas' or chilli beans will be over 40% of your daily protein requirements in one average serving. The main ingredient is whole grain rice which greatly improves the N.P.U., over 40% increase in protein availability is due to the combination of the Pinto Bean with rice. A small amount of cheese with the Pinto Bean — quesadillas recipe also promotes a 11% increase in protein availability from the Pinto Bean and when the chilli bean mix is served with tortillas (corn flatbread), there is a 50% increase in N.P.U.

discover the benefits of Natural foods.

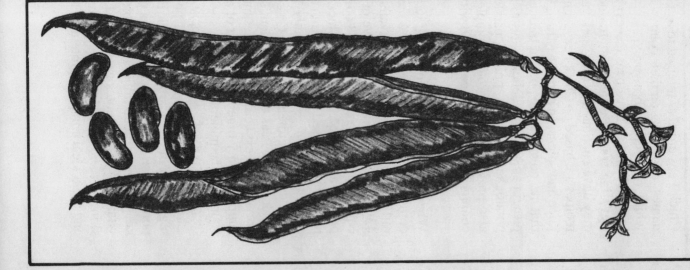

LENTILS

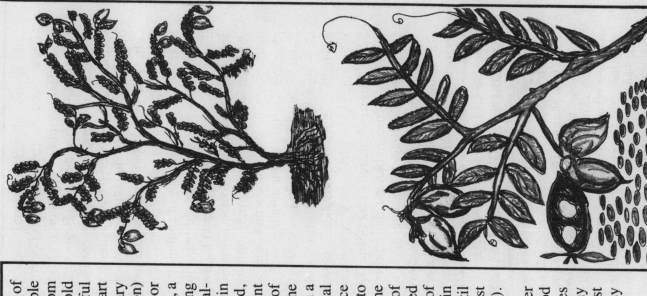

Lentils have been part of man's diet for over 4,000 years, recent evidence has discovered the remains of Lentils from ancient Egyptian tombs and some murals which date back to 1,200 BC. The Egyptian people may have developed their remarkable strength from the regular use of Lentil meals, definitely not from take-away foods. Lentils were one of the few foods that Russian soldiers had during their long and cold days on the battlefields, in the first and last world war. Sometimes for those Russian soldiers, one handful of cooked Lentils was their daily food ration. Lentils are one of the most sustaining natural foods. Apart from being an excellent carbohydrate food, Lentils are also the second best Legume source of primary protein, they supply 24% protein content and over 50% carbohydrates. The N.P.U. (net protein utilization) of Lentils is however, a very low 30%, therefore a majority of the protein content is unusable, due to a poor amino acid (protein units) structure. As will be explained in more detail in the protein section of this book, a certain composition of the individual amino acids that are contained in a food, must be supplied in varying amounts, Lentils supply insufficient amounts of the following essential amino acids: methinone, phenylal-anine and tyrosine, they are therefore termed: limiting amino acids. To obtain full benefit from the protein that is contained in Lentils, such foods as tahini, rice, wheat, corn, milk or cheese should be combined, those foods will promote a better balance of the essential amino acids. Lentils are basically an excellent energy food and one that could considerably lower your weekly shopping expense. A Lentil meal is one of the best substitutes for the 'long lasting' full stomach feeling that some people require and rely upon the animal produce, possibly without realizing the numerous benefits and delicious recipes associated with a Lentil meal and the adverse health that develops from a regular and excess intake of 'saturated' animal produce. Recent studies have shown that the people who eat less animal produce and more Legume produce — Lentils etc., have the 'cleanest coronary arteries'. Regular use of Legumes is one of the best ways to lower blood fat levels and to protect against hardening of the arteries. Apart from that, Lentils are one of the easiest Legumes to digest and they require the shortest cooking time. Apart from that, Lentils are one of the easiest Legumes to digest and they require the shortest cooking time — 1 hour medium heat. Pre-soaking of Lentils and other Legumes will reduce cooking time considerably, especially if the Legumes are developed to the sprouting stage (3–4 days), that will also reduce the excess gas that may occur after the digestion of Lentils, mainly for those people who have a slow metabolism, 'quick appetite' and have little experience in the preparation and proper food combining techniques for such unique foods as the Legumes. A Lentil salad is one of the simplest meals to prepare and digest (see recipe). Lentil soup will also be a most nourishing simple meal as well as supplying over 20% of your daily protein requirements (see recipe).

Lentils have a very low fat content and they supply an abundance of active nutrients to assist proper digestion and to protect against excess weight problems, the most dominant nutrients are: iron – blood development, resistance to infection, sodium – promotes carbohydrate digestion, magnesium – promotes protein metabolism, chlorine – promotes natural weight control and blood purifying, vitamin A – healthy skin condition, B1 – carbohydrate metabolism, B2 – absorption of the mineral iron, B3 – protects against digestive problems. Lentils are an excellent food for everyone, especially the active sportsman and busy housewife, a Lentil meal will give you all the energy you require

LIMA BEAN

Lima Beans belong to the same botanical species as the kidney bean — 'phaseolu.' a word derived from the Greek — phases, meaning aspect or appearance. The other word — 'lunatas' is de. ved from the Latin — luna, meaning moon. Together, the original names are translated to mean 'appearanc. f the moon', a very descriptive title for the Lima Bean. Other common names for the Lima Bean are: butt. bean, sieva bean, pole bean or curry bean. The Lima Bean may have developed after the kidney bean, en though both species were discovered from ancient 5,000 year old pre-Inca tombs in Peru, from where the name Lima originated. During the 17th century, the Lima Bean was one of the most popular Legumes and it was cultivated throughout America and nearly all tropical-discovered areas of the world. Since then, other Legumes were also cultivated and today, the Lima Bean is most popular in the form of 'butter beans', a favourite of many European countries and in the U.K. As well as the delicious taste of freshly prepared butter beans — Lima Beans are one of the best Legume-source of potassium — the alkaline forming mineral that is vital for regulating correct fluid level balance in body tissues, often an overweight person has a diet deficient of potassium foods. Lima Beans are also a good source of magnesium — the mineral that in combination with potassium, is most important for efficient muscular activity, without a regular supply of magnesium foods, athletes and other active people may easily develop muscular cramps, due to excess physical exertion and a deficiency of magnesium foods. Lima Beans are an excellent energy-producing food as well as supplying very good amounts of primary protein. Lima Beans provide over 60% carbohydrate content plus an abundance of active nutrients to assist in digestion and energy production: calcium, phosphorus, potassium, iron, sodium, magnesium, chlorine, vitamin A, B1, B2 and B3. Lima Beans (dry, edible portion) are 20% protein and they have a high N.P.U. (net usable protein) of 52%. A meal of cooked Lima Beans (1 cup) in combination with rice and sweet corn will provide over half the R.D.A. recommended daily protein and a well balanced supply of other essential daily nutrients. Lima Beans are easy to prepare: place 1 cup of dry Lima Beans in 2 cups of water, bring to the boil and then simmer for ¼ hour, that will yield over 2 cups of cooked Lima Beans. Make sure your kitchen is well stocked with Lima Beans, they make an excellent winter food and combine very well with any home made soup or garden salad. Lima Beans look like the moon and provide the sun's energy. Try some soon.

LIMA BEAN LOAF: PROTEIN MEAL

INGREDIENTS: 2 cups of dried Lima beans, 1 cup of whole grain wheat flour, ½ cup ground sesame seeds, ½ cup of each of the following: finely chopped celery, carrot, onion and mushrooms. 2 tbl.sp. of tahini, 1 tsp. veg. salt, 1 tsp. soya sauce and 2 cups of water. **(You could use Mung beans instead of Lima beans.)**

METHOD: Soak Lima beans overnight, then cook for 15 minutes — simmer only. Prepare all vegetables. Mash Lima beans with a fork, place into a large bowl and slowly sprinkle in whole wheat flour, also add 1 cup of water. Mix thoroughly. Then add: sesame seeds, prepared chopped vegetables, tahini, veg. salt and soya sauce to Lima beans, mix again and form into two loaves. Prepare 2 baking tins with oil, place Lima bean loaves into baking tins, then into a pre-heated over — 250F. for ½ an hour, turn oven off and leave Lima mix in for another 5 minutes. Prepare a fresh garden salad and then serve with the hot Lima loaf. Keep the other Lima loaf for another meal. It should last for nearly a week in the fridge. Preparation time is 1 hour, digestion time 3 hours and you will obtain a well balanced supply of essential daily nutrients: protein, carbohydrates, lipids, minerals and vitamins. Try a loaf today.

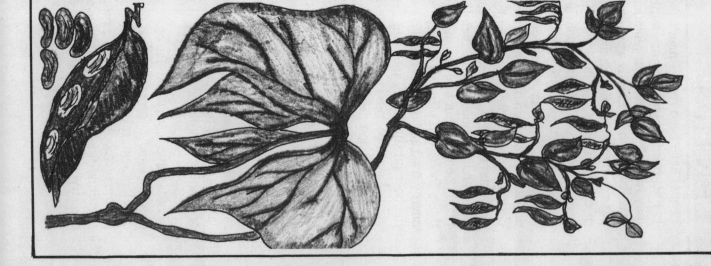

MUNG BEAN

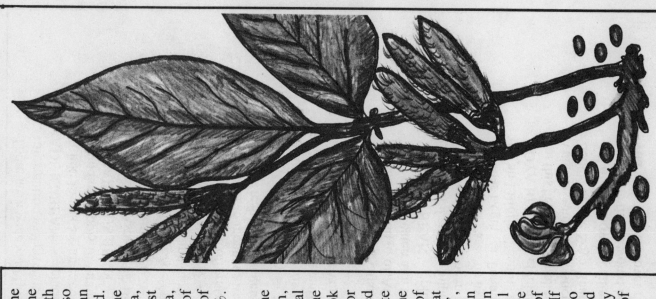

Mung Beans were first cultivated in India, possibly thousands of years before any other Legume and for the people of Asian countries, Mung Beans have provided good nutrition long before the Egyptians baked the first loaf of wheat bread. In parts of India, Mung Beans are hand ground to produce a flour, that is used with many traditional recipes and often combined with rice, fresh vegetables and nuts. The Chinese have also used the Mung Bean for thousands of years and they are well respected for a long history of Mung Bean sprouting, not until recently were the actual associated benefits of sprouting realized by the Western world. The Chinese have enjoyed Mung Beans in the best possible way, sprouting. For more information on the associated benefits of sprouting, turn to pages 103–106. Mung Beans are also referred to as: oregon pea, golden gram, black gram and green gram, depending on the colour of the Mung Bean (seed). The most common and readily available are the green Mung Beans, the other varieties are a real speciality in India, China and other Asian countries. The golden coloured Mung Beans are one of the best Legume-source of the mineral iron, the lima bean is equal number one. Mung Beans are the second best Legume source of protein, they supply 24% protein (dry, edible portion) and a very good N.P.U. net usable protein, of 57%.

Mung Beans have a very low fat content of 1% and a well balanced carbohydrate content of 60%. The Mung Bean sprouts are far richer in protein, as the carbohydrate content is converted into living protein, during the first few days of sprouting. Proper preparation of the Mung Bean should include an initial pre-soaking time of at least 8 hours, that will reduce cooking time and promote easier digestion of the Mung Bean. Most recipes for the Mung Bean are designed for the Mung sprouts, however, you can cook Mung Beans for 1 hour, after initial soaking, and combine with any recipe that requires either the sprouts or other Legumes, such as a savoury bean loaf which will provide over 35% of the R.D.A. recommended daily protein (see recipe). A Mung Bean savoury party dip is easy to make and most rewarding to taste (see recipe). Whenever you use Mung Beans, you can be sure that they are an excellent supplier of the minerals: iron, calcium – promotes digestion, regulates metabolism, potassium – promotes elimination of fluid waste via the kidneys and assists the functions of the liver, vitamin A – promotes digestion and fat metabolism, excess alcohol can severly lower vitamin A reserves. Vitamins: B1 – 'morale vitamin', sugar, alcohol and nicotene all deplete the body reserves of B1, B2 – a deficiency of both B1 and B2 can cause a considerable lack of vitality, stamina and alertness. A Mung Bean meal will ensure that you obtain these important B group vitamins in correct balance, especially with the Mung sprouts as the vitamin B1 content will double with every day of growth, until the fourth day. Mung Beans are the best Legume-source of niacin: vitamin B3 is required to process sugars and alcohol, a deficiency can occur from excess intake of refined sugar and alcohol, leading to nervous disorders, diarrhoea, dermatitis and digestive problems. If you rely on B vitamin tablets to overcome your 'socially orientated deficiencies', you may also hesitate to eat Mung Beans as your body is so adjusted to a refined diet, even the thought of eating a 'whole food' could deteriorate your nerves. The deeper you dig, the harder the way out. Mung Beans are one of the many Legumes, try them next chance you have and give you body time to adjust to the complete form of food-life.

OTHER LEGUMES

There are a wide variety of other Legumes apart from those already described in the previous pages. The following information will provide you with knowledge about the main benefits associated with other Legumes.

ADUKI BEAN — 'phaseolus angularis', a native plant from Japan where they are called the 'king of beans'. Aduki Beans are an excellent source of protein: 25%, calcium and the mineral iron are very well supplied plus an abundant supply of vitamins: B1, B2 and B3.

ASPARAGUS BEAN — 'dolichos sesquipedalis', originated in the Asian countries and it is served as a fresh green vegetable. Asparagus Beans are an excellent source of calcium and the mineral iron, they also supply good amounts of vitamin C, A, B1, B2 and B3.

ASPARAGUS PEA — 'psophocarpus tetragonolobus', also called the goa bean or winged pea, they are very low in protein content and most main nutrients. They can be eaten as a fresh green vegetable or roasted.

BLACK-EYED PEA — 'vigna unguiculata', also called the cow pea, yard-long bean or kaffir bean. They are an excellent source of protein: 23% with a N.P.U. of 45%. Black-eyed peas originated in Africa. The vitamin B1 content is abundant as well as the mineral iron and vitamin A. They can be used as a coffee substitute when ground, or as a fresh green vegetable or dried.

HYACINTH BEAN — 'lablab niger' also known as lablab bean, field bean, dolichos bean, Egyptian or Indian bean. Hyacinth Beans originated in India, they are a very good source of vitamin A and B1. They supply 22% protein. It is essential to soak and boil this bean before eating.

PEA — 'pisum sativum' also known as common pea, pois and garden pea. See section on vegetables for more details.

PIGEON PEA — 'cajanus cajan', congo pea, yellow dhal, angola pea or red gram. Grows well in hot climates, probably a native of Africa. Supplies 20% protein, and good amounts of calcium, iron, vitamin A, B1 and B3. They can be eaten as a fresh vegetable or as a cooked bean.

RUNNER BEAN — 'phaseolus coccineus' or multiflora bean and scarlet runner bean, originally cultivated for it's ornamental appeal. Supplies very good amounts of vitamin A, low in protein — 2% and good amounts of vitamin C. A very popular bean in the U.K., eaten as a fresh vegetable or cooked dried Legume.

PEANUT — 'arachis hypogae' or the ground nut. They originated in South America and are now one of the most popular Legumes. Peanuts supply 26% protein with a low N.P.U. of 43%. They are an excellent source of vitamin B3 and Biotin. Peanuts are a very acid forming food. For more details, turn to page 134.

SOYA BEANS — 'glycine max' or preta and haba soya. They have been termed 'meat of the earth', a realistic title for this bean that supplies equal protein value with top quality meat as well as supplying an abundance of minerals, vitamins and their associated benefits. Soya Beans supply 34% protein with a very high N.P.U. of 61%. For more details on the Soya Bean and Soya products, turn to pages 89–90.

All of the above mentioned Legumes have unique qualities and such a wide variety of taste, textures and available nutrients that it would be well worth trying at least one new Legume every week, with the help of some recipes, you will soon discover the life from the Legume world.

NET PROTEIN UTILIZATION:

(N.P.U.%).

- 30 – Lentils.
- 36 – Mung bean sprouts.
- 38 – Other Legumes: navy, pea bean, white bean.
- 39 – Gluten flour.
- 42 – Black bean.
- 43 – Peanut, Peanut butter, Chick pea.
- 45 – Turnip greens, Collards, Whole wheat bread, Cow peas, Mustard greens.
- 47 – Peas.
- 48 – Broad bean.
- 50 – Spinach, Chard, Brazil nut, Walnut, Pignolia nuts, Spaghetti.
- 52 – Lima bean.
- 53 – Green peas.
- 54 – Kale.
- 55 – Millet, Wheat bran.
- 56 – Soya sprouts.
- 58 – Sunflower seeds, Cashews, Rye.
- 60 – Pumpkin seeds, Bulgur, Squash seeds, Triticale, Wheat, Brussel sprouts, Barley, Potato.
- 61 – Soya beans, Soya grits, Soya flour.
- 65 – Tofu, Chicken, Lamb.
- 66 – Oatmeal.
- 67 – Wheat germ, Pork, Porterhouse.
- 69 – Sardines.
- 70 – Rice, Parmesan cheese, Swiss cheese, Camembert, Edam, Cheddar cheese.
- 72 – Corn-cob.
- 75 – Cottagecheese, Tigers milk.
- 80 – Fish.
- 82 – Milk – non fat, Milk, Yoghurt.
- 83 – Egg white.
- 94 – Egg.

PROTEIN COMBINATION RECIPES

CHICK PEA PASTE: – HUMMOUS – SUPER SALAD SANDWICH

INGREDIENTS: 2 cups of dried Chick peas, ½ cup of ground sesame seeds or ¼ cup of tahini, 1 clove garlic, 1 lemon, 1tsp. veg. salt, ¼ cup parsley. Optional: ¼ cup grated carrot, paprika and rice bran.

METHOD: Pre-soak Chick peas overnight. Place Chick peas in cooking pot and simmer for ½ hour. Finely chop garlic and parsley. Squeeze lemon and place juice into the blender, add half measures of all other ingredients to blender. Mix for 1 minute. Then prepare the other half of the mix into blender, add half measures of all other ingredients to blender plus ¼ cup water, allow Chick peas to cool, then place 1 cup of Chick peas into the blender. Chick pea paste is ideal as a party-dip, sandwich spread or use in place of mayonnaise for a fresh garden salad. Place in the fridge and have a portion every day, the mix should last two weeks.

QUESADILLAS – PROTEIN MEAL:

INGREDIENTS: 2 cups of dried Kidney beans or Pinto beans, 6 cups of water or vegetable stock, 1 onion, garlic, 2 bay leaves, 2 tbl.sp. whole wheat flour, 2 cups of brown rice, 2 tsp. chilli powder, 1 cup grated cheddar cheese. Optional: 1 dozen tortillas – corn bread or flat bread, ¼ cup parsley – chopped, ¼ cup chopped carrots, sesame meal or rice bran.

METHOD: Soak beans and rice overnight, seperately. Place beans into cooking pot and simmer for ½ hour. Also simmer rice for ½ hour. Prepare chilli + mix: add chilli powder, flour, onion, some parsley and place in pre-heated and oiled frying pan, cook for 5 minutes, stir thoroughly. Add bay leaves, onion, 2 cloves of chopped garlic to beans, simmer for another 10 minutes. Then combine beans and chilli mix together in frying pan, mix well and cook for 5 minutes. Serve the Chilli Beans with the cooked rice and serve grated cheese on top, or place cheese inside tortillas and add Chilli Beans and rice. A complete protein meal and very tasty. Serves a family of 6. Try this restaurant-meal at home, soon.

SIMPLE LENTIL MEAL: LENTIL SALAD – PROTEIN MEAL

INGREDIENTS: 2 cups of dried Lentils, ½ cup ground sesame seeds, 2 cloves of garlic or 1 large onion, sayo sauce, 1 tbl.sp. rice bran.

METHOD: Soak Lentils overnight, then rinse well. Pre-heat frying pan, add cold pressed oil, chopped onion or garlic or both, then place in cooked Lentils, cook for 10 minutes, then add soya sauce, sesame seeds and rice bran, cook for 5 more minutes. Ready to serve with a fresh garden salad and cooked brown rice. Serves 4-6 people and supplies nearly ½ of your daily protein requirements. A very inexpensive protein meal.

LENTIL SOUP: PROTEIN MEAL

INGREDIENTS: Same as above recipe, plus 1 large carrot, 1 cut chopped celery, ½ cup chopped parsley and ½ cup of soya milk powder. Optional: add chopped broccoli, cauliflower or capsicums to soup, just before serving.

METHOD: Soak Lentils overnight, rinse well. Place Lentils into large cooking pot, add 4 cups of water or vegetable stock and simmer for 15 minutes. Prepare vegetables, finely chop carrot and celery, add to Lentils. Cook for 10 minutes, then add chopped onion, ½ cup ground sesame seeds, soya milk powder and cook for 5 minutes, add parsley, soya sauce and rice bran just before serving. An ideal winter meal, serving 6 people. One serve will supply over ¼ of your daily protein requirements.

MUNG BEAN – SAVOURY PARTY DIP:

INGREDIENTS: 1 cup of dried green Mung beans, ½ cup of uncooked brown rice, ¼ cup of raw almonds, 2 tbl.sp. tahini or ¼ cup of ground sesame seeds, ¼ cup chopped parsley, onions and chives.

METHOD: Soak Mung beans and rice overnight, seperately. Place the soaked Mung beans in a cooking pot and simmer for 10 minutes, use 2 cups of water. Do the same for the rice. Prepare almonds, parsley, chives and onions. Place all ingredients into a large mixing bowl, mix thoroughly. Then place 1 cup-full of the mix into a blender, add a little water and soya sauce first, blend for ½ minute slow speed, place into party-dip bowls, serve with rye crackers, whole rye bread of corn chips. Add spices to suit the occasion. Savoury party dip will keep for over a week in the fridge. Try some as a base for a salad sandwich or mayonnaise.

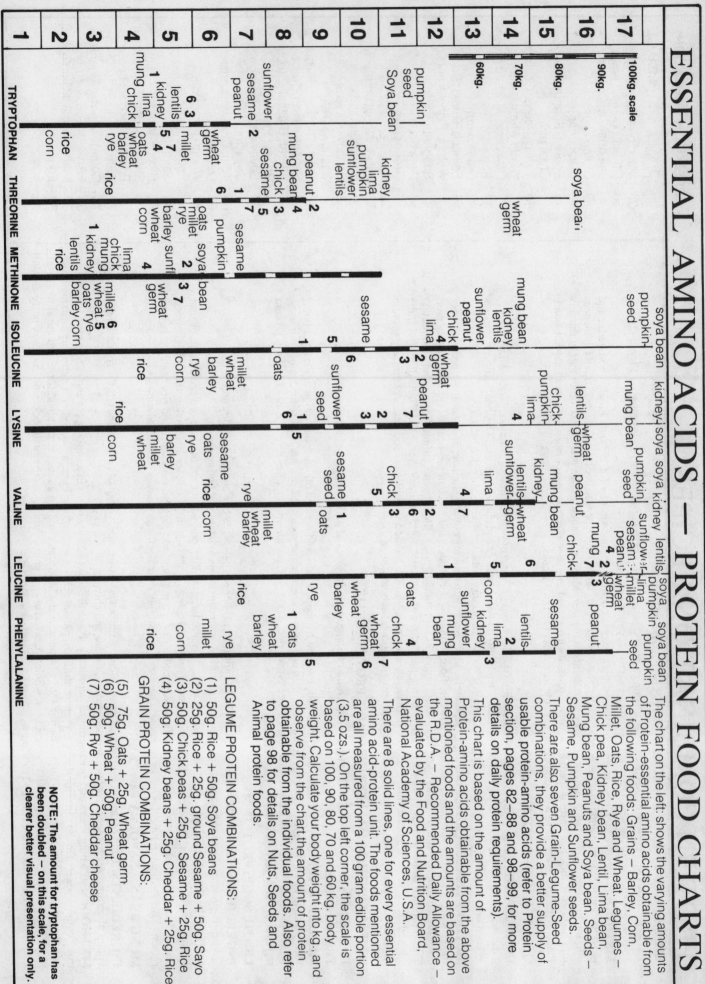

ESSENTIAL AMINO ACIDS — PROTEIN FOOD CHARTS

The chart on the left shows the varying amounts of Protein-essential amino acids obtainable from the following foods: Grains — Barley, Corn, Millet, Oats, Rice, Rye and Wheat. Legumes — Chick pea, Kidney bean, Lentil, Lima bean, Mung bean, Peanuts and Soya bean. Seeds — Sesame, Pumpkin and Sunflower seeds.

There are also seven Grain-Legume-Seed combinations, they provide a better supply of usable protein-amino acids (refer to Protein section, pages 82—88 and 98—99, for more details on daily protein requirements).

This chart is based on the amount of Protein-amino acids obtainable from the above mentioned foods and the amounts are based on the R.D.A. — Recommended Daily Allowance — evaluated by the Food and Nutrition Board, National Academy of Sciences, U.S.A.

There are 8 solid lines, one for every essential amino acid-protein unit. The foods mentioned are all measured from a 100 gram edible portion (3.5 ozs.). On the top left corner, the scale is based on 100, 90, 80, 70 and 60 kg. body weight. Calculate your body weight into kg. and observe from the chart the amount of protein obtainable from the individual foods. Also refer to page 98 for details on Nuts, Seeds and Animal protein foods.

LEGUME PROTEIN COMBINATIONS:
(1) 50g. Rice + 50g. Soya beans
(2) 25g. Rice + 25g. ground Sesame + 50g. Sayo
(3) 50g. Chick peas + 25g. Sesame + 25g. Rice
(4) 50g. Kidney beans + 25g. Cheddar + 25g. Rice

GRAIN PROTEIN COMBINATIONS:
(5) 75g. Oats + 25g. Wheat germ
(6) 50g. Wheat + 50g. Peanut
(7) 50g. Rye + 50g. Cheddar cheese

NOTE: The amount for tryptophan has been doubled — on this scale, for a clearer better visual presentation only.

GRAINS & LEGUMES - NUTRIENT CHART

	Calories	Carbohydrate	Protein	Total Fat	Calcium	Phosphorus	Potassium	Iron	Sodium	Magnesium	Chlorine	Manganese	Zinc	Silicon	Sulphur	Vit. A	Vit. E	Vit. B1	Vit. B2	Vit. B3	Vit. B5	Vit. B6	N.P.U.
Barley	348	77	9.6	1.1	34	290	296	2.7	3	35	36	1.6						.21	.07	3.7	.5	.22	60
Corn	324	84	8.5	2	5	85	296	1.8	.08							350		.2	.05	1.4			72
Millet	331	75	10	2.8	22	325	475	7		180							2	.75	.38	2.3			55
Oats	390	68	13	7.3	52	400	350	4.2	2.5	20			.8					.6	.13	1.0	.11	.01	66
Rice-white	354	78	6.5	.75	23	91	89	.9	5	6		1.5	1.2				.02	.01	.4		1		70
Rice-brown	354	76	7.4	1.8	32	216	210	1.6	8	86	2	1.6	1.8				1.5	.34	.04	4.6	1	.05	70
Rye	334	73	12	1.7	38	376	467	3.7	1	115	1			30	28			.43	.22	1.6			58
Rye Flour			16		54	540	860	4.3										.61	.22	2.7			58
Wheat germ	363	46	26	10	72	1,118	827	9.4	3	336			14				15	2	.68	4.2	2.2	.92	67
Wheat bran	240	70	16	5	130	1,400	1,200	16	10	450							0	.8	.4	20	3	.9	60
Wheat	330	69	14	2.2	36	383	370	3.1	3	160	7			46	9			.57	.12	4.3			60
Buckwheat	333	72	11	2.5	33	347	656	5	1			2					1.5	.58	.15	2.9	1.5	.57	60
Bulgur	360	77	11	1.7	29	340	233	3.7										.28	.16	6.7		.22	
Sorghum	332	73	11	3.3	28	287	350	4.4			25				12			.38	.15	3.9			
Triticale	340		19	4.6	38	540	508	5.7	7														
Carob		72	7.8	1.2	360	84																	
Chick pea	360	61	20	4.8	150	331	797	6.9	26		95					50		.31	.15	2.0			43
Kidney bean	349	63	22	1.2	135	457	984	6.4	10									.84	.21	2.2			38
Lentil	340	60	24	1.1	79	377	790	6.8		80	150					60		.37	.22	2.0			30
Lima bean	345	64	20	1.6	72	385	1529	7.8	4	180								.48	.17	1.9			52
Mung bean	340	60	24	1.3	118	340	1028	7.7	6							80		.38	.21	2.6			57
Soya bean	403	33	34	17	226	554	1677	2.8	5	265	40			27		80		1.1	.31	2.2			61
Aduki bean	325		25		252			7.6								15		.57	.18	3.2			48
Broad bean	338	58	25	1.7	27	157	471	2.2	4							220		.28	.17	1.6			
Black eyed bean	342		23		76			5.7								40		.92	.18	1.9			42
Cow pea	342	61	23	1.5	74	426	1024	5.8	35	230	60				360	30		1.05	.21	2.2			45
Peanut	564	18	26	47	69	401	674	2.1	5	206	23			5	45			1.1	.13	17.2			43
White bean	340	61	22	1.6	144	425	1196	7.8	19	170	69			25	130			.65	.22	2.4			38

NOTE: The above amounts are based on dry weight, edible portions of 100 grams — 3:5 ozs. approx.

43

FRUITS

"To each land a Fruit was given". As one man gave, another received, providing for all people. Before the days of the cities, Man was basically a Fruit eater. The forests that covered the Earth provided all Man's requirements of Food, Shelter, Fresh Air, Water and Beauty. Man's physical structure still resembles those predecessors, with various physiological facts that still relate Man as being a Fruitarian. The Digestive system is the key element in determining whether an animal (Man) be more suitable as a Fruitarian, Herbivora or Carnivorous Animal. The Digestive tract of Man is between 12-14 times the height of the body which is very similiar to all Fruit eating animals of today. The Herbivora's Digestive tract is 20 times the height of the body and the meat-eater-Carnivora has only 5 times the length. As Man's Digestive system is more suitably adapted to a Fruitarian based diet, he can also expect maximum nutritional benefits from eating Fresh Fruits. Nature planned it that way.

A total Fruitarian diet is almost unknown amongst Man, due to numerous factors of Evolutionary change that have forced Man to search for other food sources, when the supply of Fruits was limited. Fresh Fruits were not always available. Today they are. The shopping centre is usually just around the corner, with a variety of fresh Fruits, that our predecessor's would have truly cherished.

Any diet must be balanced to ensure maximum nutrition and positive Health. On average 20-30% of the daily food supply should be fresh Fruits. A variety of Fruits every week and depending on seasonal availability will supply a major portion of the essential human nutritional needs. Fruits are the best Cleansers of the body. Proper elimination of body waste is an essential factor for preservation of Health. Fruits contain a high percentage of CARBON, one of the main Gaseous elements required by Man for Life. The Carbon content of fresh Fruits acts as an incinerator of waste matter, firstly from the Digestive system, then the bloodstream, internal organs, skin tissue and finally all the body cells. All fresh Fruits are alkaline and this is vital for body development and repair. All fresh Fruits will provide you with Natural Fruit sugars — Fructose, the best source of Natural Energy. Fruits give you Energy. Fresh Fruits are the easiest food to digest especially when eaten alone and not on a full stomach. Fresh Fruits are disliked by some people, this is possibly due to poor combination of Fruits at various times. Fruits should not be combined with sugar, preservatives or secondary proteins. A fresh Fruit is a complete form of Life that has required numerous elements from the soil, sunshine, water and air to grow and fully develop. Fresh ripe Fruits eaten alone will not cause stomach upsets unless there is food in the stomach that could retard the simple preparation of the fruit and cause fermentation. Fruits are the best food for Energy requirements. The fruit-sugar known as Fructose is most easily converted into Glucose-the primary fuel. Fresh Fruits will supply you with the most delicious form of Energy. By understanding more about the individual composition of fresh Fruits you may benefit by avoiding a common distraction of Life - sickness, poor health and lack of Energy. Fresh Fruits store solar Energy.

The following pages will point out the main nutrient benefits of 22 different Fruits, this information has been compiled with the assistance of precise nutrient evaluation charts that are all based on 100 gram portions, all Fruits have a different balance of Elements and they all provide an individual set of 'dominant nutrients'. It is with this information that certain Health benefits have been determined and with regular use of those individual Fruits, you can expect to live longer and

'Laugh with Health'

INTRODUCTION

THE BENEFITS OF NATURE'S FRUITS

'A dozen Minerals'

Fructose—Natural Energy

'A handfull of Vitamins'

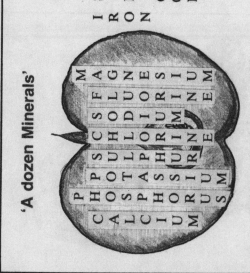

```
P C H P S C F A M
H O O U C H O L
C O T L L D U E
A L S A P O I N
L C A P O I E M
C H I S I R U I
U O R N U H N N
M R I O I M E M
    I U U S
N I P I
C E N
O R E
N
I S C I
R I O O
O L P D
```

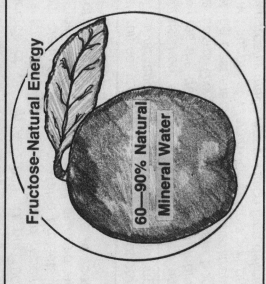

60—90% Natural
Mineral Water

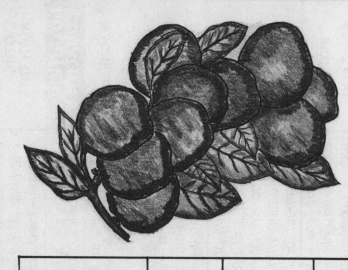

```
V V V V V   V V B
I I I I I   I I I
T T T T T   T T O
A A A A A   A A T
M M M M M   M M I
I I I I I   I I N
N N N N N   N N
A C E K B B   B B
      1 2 3   5 6
```

APPLES

pyrus malus

NUTRITIONAL QUALITIES	
	'An Apple a day keeps the doctor away' is a statement based on solid ground. A full range of essential daily nutrients are supplied with Apples - the "Queen of Fruits". As with all Fruits in the Natural whole state, the supply of nutrients - Fructose, Minerals and Vitamins is balanced, so as to ensure efficient digestion and metabolism. The quality of a Fruit is dependant on condition of soil, handling and storage. Keep Fruits in a cool place if they have been stored for over a week. A crisp Apple is the most delicious.
VITAMIN E	Apples are one of the best Fruit-source of Vitamin E. An Apple a day will help your body work efficiently, as the Vitamin E content improves the endurance and stamina of all muscles and nerves. Vitamin E will also protect your respiratory system from those harmful environmental poisons of city air.
BIOTIN **FOLIC ACID**	Apples are a very good source of Biotin and Folic acid, both B group vitamins that are required daily with the diet. Both are water soluble and cannot be stored for long periods. Biotin is a 'slimming vitamin' and Folic acid also assist by promoting a healthy appetite and clean digestive system. Eat an Apple anytime you feel hungry or have a freshly made Apple juice.
VITAMIN A **VITAMIN C**	The combination of Vitamins A and C, supplied with the Apple is most beneficial for protection from colds and infections. An Apple a day will give your body a full range of protective elements so that you can live and Laugh with Health.

The Apple gave, so that life could start.

45

APRICOTS

prunus armeniaca

NUTRITIONAL QUALITIES	
VITAMIN A	Apricots are an excellent source of Vitamin A. 2,800 I.U. per 100 grams. Vitamin A is a vital ingredient in assisting the growth and repair of body tissues and promotes smooth clean skin. Vitamin A also protects the lungs and entire respiratory tract from infections. A handfull of dried Apricots is excellent medicine in times of colds and viruses. Fresh ripe Apricots have a limited season, so get some when they are available.
PHOSPHORUS	Apricots are one of the best fruit-source of the mineral Phosphorus. This is essential for growth, healthy nerves and efficient mental functioning.
IRON COPPER MANGANESE	The combination of the minerals: Iron, Copper and Manganese are all well supplied with Apricots, promotes the development of haemoglobin, the red matter of blood cells that transports Oxygen to all parts of the body. Home made Apricot juice is one of the best medicines for the bloodstream and in combination with the abundant supply of vitamin A, Apricots will protect you from colds and infections. Try a freshly made Apricot juice for a delicious taste.
OTHER NUTRIENTS	Apricots are also a good source of the following essential nutrients: Vitamin C, Vitamins: B1, B2, B3, B5, B6 and the minerals Magnesium and Calcium. Take a few sun-dried Apricots to work or wherever you travel. The Natural sweet.

AVOCADO

persea americana

NUTRITIONAL QUALITIES	
MAGNESIUM CALCIUM PHOSPHORUS SODIUM POTASSIUM	Avocado are an excellent fruit-source of the mineral Magnesium, an alkaline mineral that is a most important activator of Enzymes that are required for proper digestion. Avocados are a complete food and should always be eaten alone, before a main meal. Digestion time is about 2 hours. The Magnesium content of the Avocado helps to promote absorption and metabolism of the minerals Calcium, Phosphorus, Sodium and Potassium all well supplied with Avocado. Have you acquired the unique taste sensation of the Avocado ?.
VITAMIN B1	Avocado supply all the essential daily B group vitamins. Thiamine is most abundant and promotes food assimilation and digestion. Thiamine is termed the 'morale vitamin' because it is most beneficial for the nerves and in combination with the excellent Magnesium content, the Avocado is Natural nourishment for the entire nervous system. Help your nerves, eat an Avocado.
BIOTIN FOLIC ACID	Avocado are a very good source of two very important B group vitamins: Biotin and Folic acid help your body to make use of the abundant supply of natural organic fat supplied with the Avocado, thereby preventing obesity. The minerals Manganese and Zinc will also protect you from adding on weight.

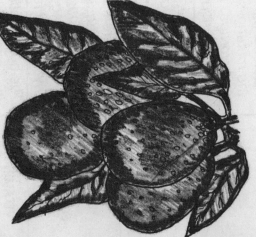

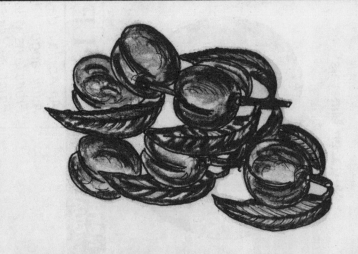

ALSO SEE SECTION ON FATS & OILS.

BANANAS
musaceae

NUTRITIONAL QUALITIES	
MANGANESE IRON COPPER	Bananas are an excellent source of the Mineral Manganese - the memory mineral and in combination with the minerals Iron and Copper, also well supplied, Bananas are an excellent food for healthy blood development.
POTASSIUM SODIUM	Bananas are an excellent source of the mineral Potassium. This mineral is required for elimination of poisonous body waste from the kidneys. Potassium also assists in regulating the heartbeat and in combination with the mineral Sodium, prevents against hardening of the arteries. Do not combine sugar with Bananas and avoid eating Bananas with bread (see pages 205 and 206).
MAGNESIUM CALCIUM PHOSPHORUS	Bananas are an excellent source of Magnesium, the mineral that promotes the absorption and metabolism of the minerals Calcium, Phosphorus and Potassium, all very well supplied with Bananas. See section on Minerals.
VITAMIN A VITAMIN C VITAMIN B6 BIOTIN	Bananas are a very good source of Vitamin A—(skin and eyes), Vitamin C-healing of scars, Vitamin E-heart muscles, Vitamin B1, B2, B3, B5 and an excellent source of Vitamin B6 - required for the production of antibodies and healthy red blood cells. The Biotin content is also very good. This is required for protection from obesity, baldness, dermatitis and sleeplesness.

BERRIES
r. fruticosus   rubus idaeus

NUTRITIONAL QUALITIES	
IRON	There are various types of Berries, all of which have similar Nutritional benefits, such as the valuable supply of the mineral Iron. Nature has combined this mineral with the essential B group vitamins to ensure proper absorption of Iron, thereby promoting healthy blood development.
SILICON	Berries are also an excellent source of Silicon - the beauty mineral. This promotes good blood circulation, keeps the eyes looking bright, protects the teeth and promotes the growth of hair. Make sure you have some berries.
VITAMIN C VITAMIN A VITAMIN F	Berries are also a valuable supplier of Vitamin C - the everyday vitamin, Vitamin A - protection from colds, healthy skin and maintenance of good eyesight. Berries are a food for nourishment of the eyes. Berries also supply Vitamin F - healthy glands, Vitamin B1, B2, B3, B5, B6, Biotin and Folic Acid.
CHLORINE SULPHUR	Berries are also a good supplier of the minerals Chlorine and Sulphur, both essential cleansing minerals. Chlorine stimulates the kidneys to eliminate harmful toxins from the body. Sulphur is another of Nature's 'beauty minerals'. It keeps the hair, skin and entire body looking youthful. Have some Berries for a real beauty treat next season. Home made Strawberry juice is most delicious.

CHERRIES

p. cerasus

NUTRITIONAL QUALITIES	
IRON	Cherries are a food for the blood. The minerals Iron, Copper and Manganese are all well supplied thereby promoting development of healthy blood. Every moment of life your body produces new blood cells and healthy ones if these minerals are obtained regularly from the diet. Regular consumption of coffee and tea will deplete your reserves of the mineral Iron and your body will lack vitality and energy. Try some Cherries next time they are available.
COPPER	
MANGANESE	
VITAMIN A	Cherries are most dominant in Vitamin A, with over 1,000 I.U. per 100 grams. Cherries also supply Vitamin C the everyday Vitamin. Buy a bag of Cherries next time you see some and prepare your body for a real treat. Vitamin A will protect you from harmful poisons that are prevalent in city air. Vitamin C will protect you every minute of the day against conditions of stress. Various types of glazed Cherries are available, they supply very little Vitamin C and A.
VITAMIN C	

CURRANTS

var. corinthiaca

NUTRITIONAL QUALITIES	
VITAMIN C	Currants are a most delicious and beneficial fruit. Various types are available with Blackcurrants being the richest fruit source of precious Vitamin C. Over 200 I.U. of Vitamin A is also supplied. Fresh Currants are not always easy to obtain. Sun dried Blackcurrants are available at most health food stores. They also stock Blackcurrant syrup that is an excellent way to obtain Vitamin C. A handfull of dried Currants per day is a sure way to give your body the most beneficial Vitamin for everyday protection from stress, pollution and poisons.
VITAMIN A	
CALCIUM	Currants are an excellent source of the minerals Calcium, Phosphorus, Potassium, Iron and Sodium. Blackcurrants are one of the sweetest health foods and well protected with the abundance of minerals to ensure positive Health. Currants are an excellent fruit to combine with Apples, Pears or any seasonal fruit. The Currant will add extra sweetness and benefits. The combination of Calcium and Phosphorus will promote development of strong bones and healthy teeth. The combination of Iron and Sodium will assist your body to eliminate harmful acid toxins from the bloodstream. All processed and refined foods and drinks contain toxins, so make sure you try some Currants and other seasonal fruits everyday. Soak some Currants overnight and serve with rolled Oats.
PHOSPHORUS	
POTASSIUM	
IRON	
SODIUM	
VITAMIN B2	Currants also supply essential B group Vitamins especially B2 and B5, both required daily for healthy nerves, good eyesight, healthy skin and absorption of the mineral Iron. Natures' foods are balanced to help you live and enjoy Health. Currants are a most delicious and beneficial addition for home made cookies.
VITAMIN B5	

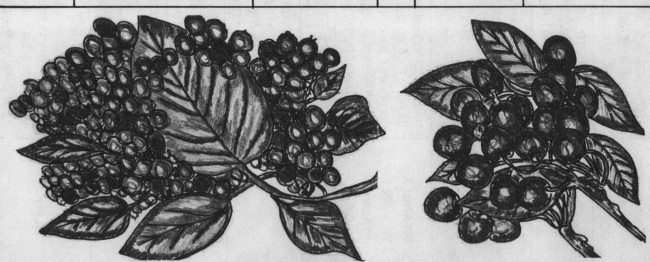

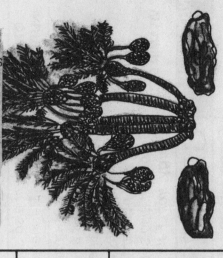

DATES *palmae*

Dates are the beneficial sweet.

Dates are one of the oldest known cultivated Fruits. Date palms flourish in desert conditions, where no other fruit tree could grow. Dates have the highest Natural sugar content of all the Dried Fruits. Dates are 72% Carbohydrate, with 240 Calories, that's real energy food.

NUTRITIONAL QUALITIES	
CALCIUM **PHOSPHORUS**	Dates are the natural food for the sweet tooth. Dates supply an abundance of the minerals Calcium and Phosphorus, both essential for strong bones, healthy teeth, prevention of tooth decay, maintenance of healthy nerves and a regular heartbeat. If you like sweets, make sure you try some Dates before your teeth fall out and your nerves deteriorate. Dates are sweet and delicious.
MAGNESIUM	Dates are also an excellent source of Magnesium the 'nerve mineral'. Regular use of coffee, tobacco, alcohol, refined foods, milk and sweets will cause a deficiency of Magnesium and may eventually lead to any of the following: arteriosclerosis, diabetes, diarrhoe, mental illness, arthritis and also bachache. Have some Dates next time for the sweetest way to Health and happiness.
VITAMIN B5 **VITAMIN B1**	Dates are the best fruit source of precious Vitamin B5. This is most beneficial when obtained regularly, for protection from stressful conditions and for promotion of hair growth. Dates are an excellent food for those people who live a busy life, like sweets and do not like baldness. Dates are also an excellent source of Vitamin B1 — healthy nerves and the minerals: Potassium — healthy heart, Copper — healthy blood. Dates are the Natural sweet.

FIGS *ficus spp.*

Fresh Figs supply 80mg Vit. A 6mg. Iron. 35mg. Calcium and 80 Calories per every 100 Gramms.

Figs are one of the Original foods, believed to have originated from the Mediterranean region around Syria.

NUTRITIONAL QUALITIES	
IRON **MANGANESE** **COPPER**	Figs are an excellent fruit source of the mineral Iron and in combination with the good supply of Manganese and Copper, Figs are a most beneficial food for maintenance of healthy blood. Fresh Figs are not always available so try some dried Figs. Soak them in water for a most delicious and sweet treat. Figs also supply valuable amounts of Vitamins B1, B2 and B6, all vital for healthy nerves.
CALCIUM **POTASSIUM** **SODIUM**	Calcium is well supplied with Figs - fresh and dried. The Combination of the minerals Calcium, Potassium and Sodium, all well supplied with Figs is most beneficial for maintenance of normal heart action, prevention of lung and chest ailments, and for efficient functioning of the nervous system.
VITAMIN B1 **VITAMIN B2** **VITAMIN B6**	Figs are also a good source of Vitamins B1, B2, B3, B5, B6 and Vitamin A. Figs are an excellent snack food, especially when eaten alone. Dried Figs can also be soaked, to enhance their digestion. The natural sugars of the Fig - Fructose, supply the body with Energy and a full range of protective elements. Fig leaves were once used as protection. They still protect you. We all need Energy and protection. Try some Figs once in a while. Slice up a few dried Figs and combine with grated apple, pear and other seasonal fruits. Serve as a complete breakfast meal or anytime of the day.

GRAPEFRUIT

poncirus trifoliata

NUTRITIONAL QUALITIES	
VITAMIN C VITAMIN E	Grapefruit are an excellent supplier of both Vitamins C and E. Vitamin C is best utilized by the body when small but regular amounts are taken. A Grapefruit for breakfast is the ideal way to start a day. Mix some Grapefruit juice with some freshly squeezed Orange juice and serve in a chilled glass.
OTHER NUTRIENTS	Grapefruit also supply these essential minerals: Phosphorus, Potassium, Iron, Sodium, Magnesium and a generous supply of the B group Vitamins.

NUTRITIONAL QUALITIES	
VITAMIN B5	Biotin is a B complex vitamin. Grapefruit are an excellent source of Natural Biotin. Without a regular supply of Biotin, your body will have difficulty in using those Fats obtained from the daily diet. Biotin is a water-soluble vitamin, so you must obtain it regularly,(daily preferably), so as your body will make use of the Fats and not carry them around. Biotin is one of the Natural slimming vitamins. Grapefruit also supply Vit. B5-Pantothenic acid, which assists in the release of Energy, from Fats & Carbohydrates. B5-healthy skin & hair-(Slimming vitamin).

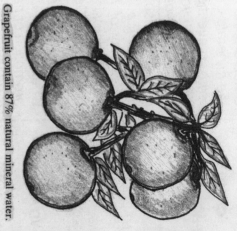

Grapefruit contain 87% natural mineral water.

GRAPES

vitaceae vitis vinifera

NUTRITIONAL QUALITIES	
MANGANESE	Grapes are one of the best fruit-source of the mineral Manganese, the 'memory chemical'. Manganese has numerous important functions of Nutrition, such as: nourishment of the nervous system and brain, maintenance of sex hormone production, production of mothers' milk, regulation of menstruation, activator of essential enzymes required for utilization of the B group Vitamins - B1,, B3, Biotin and Vitamin C, and formation of healthy red blood cells. Grape juice is excellent natural medicine and easy to make at home with a juice extractor.
SILICON	Grapes supply generous amounts of the mineral Silicon, that is essential for healthy skin, protection of teeth, promotion of hair growth, nourishment of the optic system and brain. Silicon also prevents nervous exhaustion, infectious formation, mental fatigue and is most beneficial for cases of poor blood circulation. Have some grapes regularly next time they are in season.
OTHER NUTRIENTS	Grapes are also a good source of Vitamin A - skin and eyes, Vitamins B1, B2, B3, B5, B6, Biotin and Folic Acid. The following minerals are also well supplied: Sodium, Iron, Potassium and Phosphorus. Grape juice taken regularly is most beneficial as a blood purifier and blood builder. Grape juice is also an excellent nerve tonic. Home made (blue) grape juice is one of the most delicious and beneficial drinks available. Grape juice is naturally sweet. Grape juice is also available at some health food stores. Try the taste when Grapes are not in season. Always drink any fruit juice before a meal, not after.

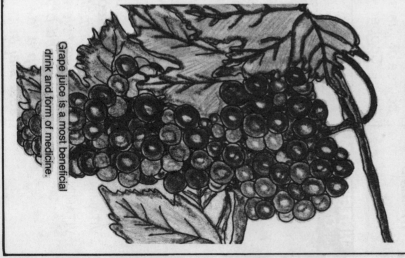

Grape juice is a most beneficial drink and form of medicine.

LEMONS

citrus limonia

NUTRITIONAL QUALITIES	
PHOSPHORUS	Lemons are an excellent fruit source of the mineral Phosphorus, required daily for repair and healthy functioning of the nervous system. Phosphorus foods rebuild and repair the brain, improve memory and promote creativity.
SODIUM	Lemons are one of the best fruit-source of the mineral Sodium, that is most beneficial for proper elimination of waste, cleansing of the lymphatic system, prevention of hardened arteries and arthritis (as Sodium keeps other minerals soluble within the bloodstream). Freshly squeezed Lemon juice taken daily will protect you and promote a healthy and clean digestive system. Try it today.
VITAMIN C VITAMIN A CALCIUM	Lemons are a rich source of vitamin C-the 'everyday vitamin'. In combination Vitamin A and the mineral Calcium: Lemons are beneficial for protection from colds and viruses, development of sound teeth and healthy gums, active blood circulation and healthy eyes. A squeeze of Lemon a day is a sure way to keep active and clean inside. A ripe Lemon needs no added sweetness. The Vitamin A and C content of Lemons is most beneficial for healthy skin.

MELONS

NUTRITIONAL QUALITIES	
SODIUM	Melons are the best fruit source of the mineral Sodium, an alkaline mineral and most beneficial for elimination of excess body acids that are a dominant cause of such ailments as: arthritis, hardened arteries and gall and kidney stones. Try a Melon on the next sunny day and discover the benefits of an alkaline meal. 75% of the daily diet should be alkaline.
OTHER NUTRIENTS VITAMIN C VITAMIN A	Melons supply an abundance of liquid that is well balanced with a full range of important nutrients such as: Calcium, Phosphorus, Potassium, Iron, Magnesium, Copper, Manganese and Zinc, plus a well balanced supply of Vitamins A and C. Melons are an excellent food for the first meal of the day. Cantaloupe are the richest fruit source of Vitamin A. 3,400 mg. per 100 grams. Have you ever tried a cool Cantaloupe or freshly made Cantaloupe juice?
CHLORINE SULPHUR	Melons are a very good source of the minerals Chlorine and Sulphur - both are termed 'cleansing minerals'. Chlorine is an excellent blood purifier and most essential for those wanting to reduce weight. A Melon will fill you up, not weigh you down. Sulphur is one of those minerals easily lost by cooking of foods. Sulphur is a natural cleanser that also protects against infection, hepatitis and baldness. Don't lose your hair over food. Melons should never be combined with any other foods as they are so easy to digest. The addition of other foods will retard digestion of the Melon and cause fermentation, indigestion pains and a loss of valuable nutrients. Home made Melon juice is very delicious.

OLIVES

oleaceae

NUTRITIONAL QUALITIES	
CALCIUM MAGNESIUM PHOSPHORUS	Olives are the best fruit source of the main mineral Calcium, with over 100 mg per 100 grams. Calcium foods are required for smooth functioning of the heart muscles, transmission of nerve impulses, assists in the process of blood clotting and muscle growth. In combination with the minerals Magnesium and Phosphorus, both well supplied with Olives, you can be assured that the Olive is an excellent food for maintenance of healthy heart muscles.
COPPER	Olives are the best fruit-source of the trace mineral Copper, that promotes formation of healthy blood, improves the absorption of the mineral Iron also very well supplied with Olives, assists in the formation of muscle fibres-elastin, promotes strong bone development and is also one of the main natural healing minerals. Olives are excellent food for healthy blood.
ZINC VITAMIN B2 VITAMIN B3 VITAMIN B6	Olives are a very good source of the trace mineral Zinc that is involved in most digestive processes, tissue respiration and as a component of Insulin. Zinc is also part of the enzyme required to break down alcohol. Olives are also a good source of the B Vitamins: B2, B3 and B6. See section on Vitamins.
SODIUM	The Sodium content of Olives is abundant, due to the addition of salt or Sodium Chloride that is used as a preservative. Fresh ripe Olives are the best.

PAPAYA

caricaceae

NUTRITIONAL QUALITIES	
VITAMIN A	Papaya are a tropical fruit, harder to obtain than most other fruits, but worth the search. The Papaya supplies one of the richest sources of the enzyme Papain, most important for protein digestion and as a promoter of the appetite. A Papaya eaten before a protein meal is especially beneficial. Papaya are an excellent source of Vitamin A and C, both are required daily. Vitamin A is most important in fighting infections, Vitamin C is required for protection from stress. A prolonged lack of Vitamin C may lead to peptic ulcers, arthritis, poor eyesight and wrinkly skin. Try a Papaya and Laugh with Health.
VITAMIN C	
SODIUM	The Sodium content of the Papaya assists the body in stimulating the appetite and producing those essential digestive juices. Sodium keeps the digestive juices at a normal consistency and also improves the quality of the blood.
OTHER NUTRIENTS	Papaya are also a good source of the minerals: Calcium, Phosphorus, Potassium, Iron and Magnesium. Try a Papaya at least once a year. Freshly made Papaya juice is a treat worth waiting for. A regular intake of Papaya will be of great benefit for your digestive system. Papaya will revitalize your entire body. Papaya for breakfast is one of the best ways to start a sunny day.

ORANGES

citrus sinensis

NUTRITIONAL QUALITIES	
	Oranges are the most convenient form of fruit drink available today. Slice an Orange in half and you have an instant nature drink for two. The benefits of freshly squeezed Orange juice are far above that of the commercially prepared substitutes. Home made Orange juice is also far better value than any other mass produced juice. On average, 50% of the commercial Orange juice is water, so why pay extra for that and also those artificial preservatives, sugar, colourings and fancy packages. Have a freshly squeezed juice and save some money. Buy some 'in season' Oranges next time they are available and make a freshly squeezed Orange juice daily. Commercial Orange juice substitutes do not satisfy the thirst as they contain some ingredients that tend to promote excess drinking. Try a natural drink. A fresh Orange juice is full of natural Life.
CALCIUM PHOSPHORUS	Oranges are one of the best fruit source of the main mineral Calcium that in combination with the minerals Phosphorus is most beneficial for protection from infections and viruses. Only when the Calcium reserves of the body are low can a virus infection occur. Calcium foods also promote smooth functioning of the heart and muscles of the small intestine. A regular intake of freshly squeezed Orange juice is also very beneficial for maintenance of healthy skin and hair.
MAGNESIUM	Oranges are a valuable supplier of the mineral Magnesium and this gives Oranges their remarkable revitalyzing power. Magnesium is a 'nerve mineral' and in combination with Calcium will promote digestion. A glass of freshly made Orange juice is an ideal way to start the day. Do not rely on expensive processed juices for health. Make your own and be sure of what you are drinking. If you smoke, drink alcohol and tend to be nervous, Orange juice will be very good natural medicine. Make the effort to squeeze an Orange today.
VITAMIN C	Oranges are well known to be a excellent supplier of precious vitamin C, on average 30-50 mg. per 100 grams are supplied. This amount applies only to freshly squeezed Orange juice and not the commercial substitutes. Up to to 90% of the vitamin C content of the commercial Orange juice is lost during processing. Vitamin C will oxidize rapidly and when exposed to heat as with most processing methods, the Orange juice will lack vitamin C- the life vitamin'.
OTHER NUTRIENTS	Oranges are also a valuable source of the following nutrients: Vitamin A for protection from colds, Vitamin E for healthy heart muscles, protection from pollution and for repair of damaged arteries due to the effects of cigarette smoking and conditions of stress, Vitamin B5 and Folic acid promote healthy skin, hair and nerves, Minerals: Potassium, Sodium, Iron, Copper, Manganese and Zinc are also well supplied with freshly made Orange juice.

NUTRITIONAL QUALITIES	PEACHES
VITAMIN A VITAMIN C	Peaches are a most delicious fruit and a valuable source of Vitamin A. In combination with the Vitamin C supply of fresh ripe Peaches, you can be assured of maximum benefits. Vitamin A is most important for healthy skin, good eyesight, protection from stress and environmental pollutants. The Vit.C content enhances all functions of Vitamin A. Make sure you have a few Peaches next time they are in season. A ripe Peach is a natural treat.
SULPHUR	Peaches are a very good source of the mineral Sulphur, this will assist your body to get one of the most important cleansing minerals. Sulphur foods prevent infection, expel harmful acid-mucus poisons from the body and are also known to improve the complexion and personality.
ZINC IODINE OTHER NUTRIENTS	Peaches are also a good source of the minerals Zinc and Iodine, both work together to assist your body in digestion of carbohydrate foods. Iodine also regulates the body's energy supply and stimulates the use of excess body fat. Zinc is essential for growth and development of the reproductive organs. Peaches give you a taste that is worth living for. Other nutrients also well supplied are Phosphorus, Iron, Magnesium, Copper, Vitamins B2 and B3.

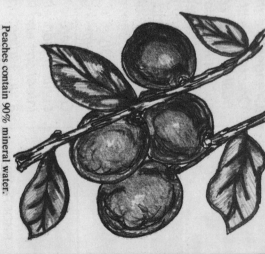

'EAT A PEACH'

Peaches contain 90% mineral water.

NUTRITIONAL QUALITIES	PEARS
SODIUM OTHER NUTRIENTS	Pears are a most valuable source of alkaline-healing and cleansing minerals: Potassium, Sodium, Calcium, Magnesium, Iron and Manganese. The Sodium content is most dominant, and this mineral is essential for the production of saliva - an alkaline liquid that promotes carbohydrate digestion. Sodium is also required regularly for proper elimination of carbon dioxide waste from the lungs. A Pear gets rid of bad air.
FOLIC ACID	Pears are a delicate fruit that have a limited shelf-life. Keep your fruit in a cool place, better still eat them direct from the tree. The benefits of freshly picked fruit is a pleasure and an experience of life. Pears are an excellent fruit source of the B group Vitamin Folic Acid, that is essential for protection and relief from unpleasant gastrointestinal disorders such as diarrhoea and constipation.
SILICON	Pears also supply the mineral Silicon, a beauty mineral that assists your body to maintain healthy teeth, hair and good eyesight. Silicon foods help you to look and feel young. Grated pear mixed with grated apple and a few raisins makes a delicious, easy to digest morning meal. Pears are a valuable aid to digestion. Whenever you have digestive problems, think about the Pear and have one, always before a main meal. Discover the benefits for yourself.

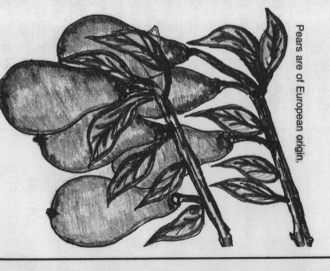

Pears are of European origin.

Pears are an excellent substitute for Bran.

PINEAPPLE

ananas comosus

NUTRITIONAL QUALITIES	
MANGANESE	Pineapples are the best fruit source of the mineral Manganese, often termed the 'memory mineral', as it helps nourish the nervous system and brain. The Manganese content is most valuable for mothers during times of lactation as it stimulates gland secretions that promote the development of mother's milk. Manganese also regulates menstruation. Freshly made Pineapple juice is one of the best drinks for women, especially those with menstruation problems.
MAGNESIUM **OTHER NUTRIENTS**	Pineapples are a good source of Magnesium the 'nerve mineral', that in combination with the excellent supply of Manganese and Vitamins B1 and B2, has most benefit for the nervous system, especially when the juice is taken regularly. (You need a juice extractor). Magnesium has an important role in all neuromuscular activity and also assists the absorption of the following nutrients: Calcium, Phosphorus, Sodium, Potassium, B Complex Vitamin and Vitamin C, all well supplied with fresh Pineapples and home made juice.
VITAMIN C **VITAMIN A**	Pineapples are a very good source of Vitamin C and A. These two work together to protect your body from all forms of stress, environmental pollutants, toxic food substances, preservatives etc. and are most valuable for maintenance of healthy skin, hair and eyesight. Look around for a fresh Pineapple.

PLUMS

prunus domestica

NUTRITIONAL QUALITIES	
	Plums are one of the few fruits that have an acidic reaction on the body. Plums are best when eaten alone. Plum jam is not a recommended food as it causes problems with the kidneys due to the addition of sugar, leading to an imbalance of all nutrients required to promote digestion and elimination of waste matter. Regular use of any jam is most detrimental for your health especially when combined with bread. Forget the jam and the pleasant memories.
IRON **POTASSIUM** **SODIUM**	Plums are a good source of the minerals: Iron, Potassium and Sodium. The combination of these minerals is most beneficial for nourishment of the muscular system and regulation of normal heartbeat. Vitamin B3 is also well supplied and this enhances the activity of minerals and is vital for good blood circulation, digestion of carbohydrates and control of cholesterol.
CALCIUM **PHOSPHORUS**	The Calcium content of Plums is well balanced with the mineral Phosphorus that is essential for effective digestion. Try the taste of Plums straight from the tree and discover the benefits of a natural fruit in the natural state. As with any acid fruits (tomatoes, oranges, lemons, pineapple, grapefruit etcetra) Plums should not be combined with grains, legumes or protein foods.

PRUNES

NUTRITIONAL QUALITIES	
	Prunes are an excellent fruit-source of the following minerals: Iron, Sodium and Magnesium. Iron works in combination with Calcium and other minerals and vitamins to improve respiratory action. Sodium combines with Potassium to regulate the acid-alkaline balance of the blood. Sodium aids elimination of body waste. The magnesium content of Prunes promotes alkalinity and a natural laxative effect. Prunes are most valuable in times of colds, viruses, digestive problems, menstruation and all forms of illness. Take a few Prunes as you would any medicine. A few Prunes a day will promote a quick recovery to Health.
IRON SODIUM MAGNESIUM	*Prunes are a concentrated food and a natural form of medicine. They are most valuable in times of colds, viruses, digestive problems, menstruation and all forms of illness. Take a few Prunes as you would any medicine. A few Prunes a day will promote a quick recovery to Health.*

TOMATO

lycopersicum esculentum

NUTRITIONAL QUALITIES	
	Tomatoes are a member of the acid fruits and they provide citric acid, malic acid and oxalic acid in moderate amounts as well as good supplies of both acid and alkaline minerals. The tomato is the best food-source of natural chlorine, an acid mineral, 1,800 mg. per 100 gram are supplied on average.
CHLORINE	*Chlorine has numerous functions such as: it stimulates the liver to filter-out waste products, it stimulates the production of gastric juices — protein digestion, and it assists weight reduction by maintaining correct fluid level retention of body cells and reduction of excess blood fat.*
VITAMIN A VITAMIN C	*Tomatoes are a good — fruit source of vitamins A and C, both these vitamins are required to protect the body against infection and to promote healthy skin condition. Freshly made Tomato juice is an excellent body cleanser and protector. Avoid using canned Tomato products, the fresh variety have all the benefits without added salt and preservatives. Tomatoes may be your favourite fruit because of their remarkable cleansing ability, even if you never knew, your body has ways to tell you!*
SULPHUR	*Tomatoes are a very good source of sulphur, also an acid mineral, it assists the liver to secrete bile and has a cleansing and antiseptic effect on the digestive system, bloodstream and skin. Sulphur is required in the formation of amino acids — protein and it is found in all body tissues and as part of blood-haemoglobin. Other minerals also well supplied by the Tomato are: potassium*
OTHER NUTRIENTS	*and sodium in combination are required to normalize the heartbeat and nourish the muscular system, phosphorus — repair of the nervous system and silicon — preserves calcium metabolism and promotes healthy hair.*

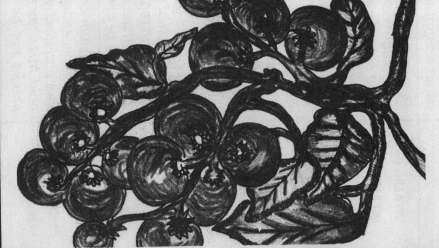
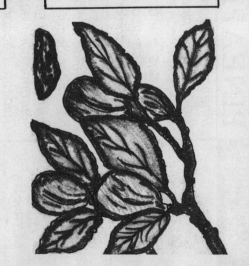

NATURAL -DAILY MEDICINE CHART

Acne	Carrot juice. Carrots. Spinach. Celery. Watercress. Grapes. Grapefruit. Apricots. Pears. Plums. Lemons. Papaya. Garlic. Tomatoes. Asparagus. Beetroot. Broccoli. Cucumber. Lettuce. Strawberries. Potatoes. Regular exercise Sunshine
Acid-Alkaline	Apples. Figs. Carrots. Chives. Celery. Garlic. Potatoes. Spinach. Radish. Dates. Watercress. Parsley. Olives. Lemons. Melons. Cucumber. Strawberries. Blackberries. Loganberries. Young Berries. Prunes. Sunshine
Arthritis	Grapefruit. Beetroot. Lemons. Cabbage. Celery. Carrots. Spinach. Cucumbers. Dates. Melons. Oranges. Tomatoes. Onion. Capsicum. Prunes. Sunshine
Bone repair	Apples. Bananas. Cherries. Olives. Peaches. Pears. Watercress. Figs. Brussel Sprouts. Cauliflower. Lettuce. Leek. Onion. Parsley. Spinach. Beetroot. Radishes. Currants Sunshine
Blood	Apricots. Avocado. Bananas. Cherries. Figs. Grapefruit. Grapes. Melons. Olives. Papaya. Beetroot. Beans. Cabbage. Celery. Cucumber. Lettuce. Leek. Onions. Peas. Potatoes. Radish. Watercress. Grapes. Lemons Prunes Berries
Brain	Bananas. Currants. Dates. Figs. Grapes. Olives. Plums. Asparagus. Radish. Tomatoes. Avocado. Garlic. Broccoli. Brussel Sprouts. Cabbage. Carrots. Cucumber. Lettuce. Parsley. Watercress. Lemons Apricots Grapes Sunshine
Complexion	Apple. Papaya. Berries. Tomatoes. Broccoli. Brussel Sprouts. Chives. Radish. Strawberries. Raisins. Grapes. Sunshine. Capsicum. Lettuce. Cucumber. Leek. Berries Regular exercise Sunshine
Carb. digestion	Apple. Pear. Pineapple. Asparagus. Green Beans. Cabbage. Celery. Leek. Parsley. Spinach. Strawberries. Cucumbers. Carrots. Lettuce. Peaches. Prunes. Garlic. Onions.
Common Cold	Figs. Lemons. Pineapple. Oranges. Peaches. Beans. Broccoli. Brussel Sprouts. Pumpkin. Blackcurrants. Cabbage. Celery Lettuce. Parsley. Onions. Garlic. Chives. Radish. Watercress. Blackberries. Strawberries. Youngberries. Apples Prunes
Constipation	Apples. Pears. Plums. Prunes. Pumpkin. Leek. Apricot. Banana. Strawberry. Grapes. Lemons. Carrots. Spinach. Cabbage. Beetroot. Raspberries. Grapes. Grapefruit. Oranges. Raisins.
Digestion	Apples. Pears. Bananas. Currants. Grapes. Melons. Olives. Papaya. Onions. Peaches. Plums. Asparagus. Beetroot. Broccoli. Cabbage.
Dandruff	Figs. Papaya. Beetroot. Broccoli. Grapes. Lemons. Oranges. Lettuce. Cucumber. Olives. Avocado. Peaches. Garlic. Onion.
Eyes	Apples. Cherries. Figs. Melons. Papaya. Peaches. Onions. Capsicum. Spinach. Asparagus. Brussel Sprouts. Carrots. Cucumber. Garlic. Lettuce. Watercress. Peaches Pears Bananas Berries Grapes
Fevers	Figs. Lemons. Olives. Oranges. Blackcurrants. Grapes. Garlic. Radish. Onions. Leek. Chives. Parsley. Berries. Spinach. Lettuce. Strawberries. Blackberries.
Blood circulation	Apricots. Avocado Bananas. Currants. Dates. Figs. Lemons. Pineapple. Plums. Carrots. Cauliflower. Chives. Spinach. Celery. Cucumber. Lettuce. Leek. Onions. Peas. Potatoes. Radish. Watercress. Grapes. Regular exercise
Hair	Apples. Bananas. Currants. Dates. Lemons. Oranges. Peaches. Peas. Lettuce. Figs. Green Beans. Brussel Sprouts. Asparagus. Cabbage. Cucumber. Spinach. Garlic.
Heart	Apples. Bananas. Oranges. Olives. Beetroot. Asparagus. Potatoes. Radish. Peas. Currants. Dates Lemons. Peaches. Pears. Parsley. Pineapple. Pumpkin. Carrots. Cauliflower. Figs Plums
Hardened arteries	Bananas. Oranges. Olives. Beetroot. Potatoes. Radish. Lemons. Avocado Celery. Carrot. Parsley. Spinach. Lettuce. Grapes.

FRUITS n' VEGIES - DAILY MEDICINE CHART

Headaches		Dates. Figs. Grapes. Papaya. Beetroot. Lettuce. Spinach. Blackcurrants. Oranges. Papaya. Berries. Peaches. Apricots.
	High blood pressure	Dates. Parsley. Lettuce. Olives. Avocados. Spinach. Grapes
Infection		Currants. Figs. Melons. Papaya. Oranges. Lemons. Pears. Broccoli. Brussel Sprouts. Cabbage. Cauliflower. Celery. Garlic. Cucumber. Lettuce. Onions. Parsley. Peas. Spinach. Pumpkin. RAdish. Watercress. Sunshine.
Kidneys		Berries. Currants. Grapes. Lemons. Melons. Asparagus. Beetroot. Celery. Lettuce. Leek. Parsley. Spinach. Pumpkin. Potatoes.
Laxative		Apples. Pears. Plums. Prunes. Garlic. Cabbage. Lettuce. Cucumber. Celery. Grapefruit. Oranges. Leek. Papaya. Melons. Beetroot. Raisins. Berries. Broccoli.
Muscles		Avocado. Grapes. Dates. Lemons. Olives. Oranges. Sunshine. Pineapple. Asparagus. Broccoli. Cauliflower. Leek. Parsley. Peas. Apples Plums Regular exercise
Memory		Currants. Dates. Olives. Figs. Lettuce. Berries. Potatoes. Apricots. Parsley. Avocado. Carrots. Asparagus. Spinach. Apples. Pineapple. Raisins. Beetroot. Bananas. Beans. Peaches. Pears.
Menstruation		Asparagus. Figs. Berries. Beetroot. Parsley. Spinach. Watercress. Potatoes. Prunes. Peaches. Lettuce. Blackberries. Raisins. Grapes. Radishes. Dates. Beans. Peas. Carrots.
Nervous System		Apples. Avocado. Cherries. Bananas. Dates. Figs. Grapes. Melons. Olives. Papaya. Oranges. Peaches. Pears. Plums. Tomatoes. Asparagus. Broccoli. Brussel Sprouts. Cabbage. Carrots. Cauliflower. Cucumber. Lettuce. Onions. Parsley. Peas. Capsicum. Spinach. Sunshine. Lemons Pineapple Apricot
	Oxygen distribution	Cherries. Currants. Grapefruit. Lemons. Currants. Cucumber. Lettuce. Parsley. Pumpkin.
Purifying		Apples. Berries. Papaya. Peaches. Pears. Lemons. Pineapple. Beetroot. Garlic. Prunes. Fasting. Broccoli. Brussel Sprouts. Cabbage Carrots. Leek. Capsicum. Spinach. Radish. Sunshine. Currants Melons Bananas Berries
	Protein digestion	Papaya. Pineapple. Prunes. Chives. Cherries. Lettuce.
Ulcers		Melons. Cabbage. Lettuce. Spinach. Apples. Pears. Grapes. Oranges.
Respiratory		Apples. Apricots. Berries. Figs. Oranges. Prunes. Exercise. Chives. Cabbage. Cauliflower. Garlic. Onions. Radish. Spinach. Potatoes. Regular exercise
Rheumatism		Currants. Grapes. Melons. Lemons. Grapefruit. Beetroot. Celery. Carrots. Figs. Olives. Cucumber. Parsley. Spinach. Apples. Lettuce. Watercress. Sunshine
Skin		Avocados. Bananas. Berries. Dates. Figs. Oranges. Asparagus. Beans. Cabbage. Carrots. Lettuce. Cucumber. Garlic. Parsley. Capsicum. Sunshine. Currants Peaches Apricots Grapes
Stress		Melons. Papaya. Lettuce. Watercress. Blackcurrants. Spinach. Sunshine. Cherries
Teeth		Apples. Berries. Grapefruit. Papaya. Pears. Figs. Carrots. Capsicum. Watercress. Cucumber. Celery. Dates
Weight Reduction		Apples. Grapefruit. Tomatoes. Chives. Lettuce. Parsley. Papaya. Pineapple. Radish. Watercress. Oranges. Lemons. Beetroot. Cucumber. Grapes. Blackcurrants. Figs. Garlic. Onions. Strawberries. Exercise. Melons Peaches Avocado
Glandular System		Bananas. Berries. Currants. Dates. Olives. Asparagus. Garlic. Lettuce. Potatoes. Grapes. Avocados. Lemons. Sunshine

SUGAR

SUGAR is one of the most abundantly consumed Carbohydrates, that not only is taken directly from the Sugar bowl but also with so many processed and refined food such as sugar coated cereals, canned and frozen fruits and vegetables, soups, mayonnaise, 'baby foods', flavoured yoghurts, ice cream, cakes, candy, biscuits, chocolate, soft drinks, beer, wine & spirits, jams, bread and cordials, to mention a few. This widespread use of sugar not only adds up the Calories per day-(for some people), but most important of all, Sugar replaces none of the essential Nutrients. Sugar is like a leach. Sugar when taken with food or drinks is quickly broken down, within the body, into the form of simple sugars—Glucose & Fructose. Our bodies are capable of handling a fair amount of Glucose-if the essential nutrients are supplied to assist absorption and utilization. Sugar supplies none of those nutrients. To put it simply, if you continually use Sugar, you will constantly deplete your body's reserves of essential nutrients.

SUGAR when taken, is absorbed directly through the Stomach wall and enters the bloodstream with little or no digestion whatsoever. This is the reason as to why some people get a quick burst of Energy, from a cup of tea or coffee. After entering the bloodstream, refined sugar will stimulate the secretion of Insulin: a hormone substance that is produced by the Pancreas-(Gland), to assist in the utilization of Glucose—(Primary fuel), which is then burnt into Carbon dioxide and Water to produce Energy. It happens every time you take sugar, in whatever form.

SUGAR consumption on average, in Australia, America and the U.K. has been estimated to be aprox.-55kg—120lb. per head. An excessively large amount, considering that Sugar supplies no Minerals or Vitamins. Sugar is the most depleted food additive on the market today. Some children are brought up as- Sugarholics. Children are often so addicted to the stimulating effects of Sugar before the age of reason, that a definite effort of will power is the only remedy to stop the well established sugar-habit. Many of these children (adults) have a very erratic Energy level that is a direct reflection of the quick and temporary stimulating effects of Sugar. You need Energy but not Sugar.

Sugar is termed as a double-sugar, as it contains both Glucose & Fructose. Fruit Sugars are simple Fructose and much easier to digest as they supply essential nutrients that promote Energy development and Health. White sugar and refined Sugar products etc. cause a sudden rise in blood sugar levels, which often only lasts 5-10 minutes and after half an hour a person will once again crave for sugar stimulation. Next time it happens try an apple or any fresh fruit and notice the Energy that Nature offers. Regular consumption of 'Sugar meals' etc. will drown out the appetite for the wide variety of Natural foods that are balanced with nutrients.

SUGAR is a pure chemical substance. The Chinese developed Sugar from the Sugar-Cane, over 2,000 years ago, however the method of extraction and processing was a Natural conversion and not a chemical formula. Sugar is a pure Carbohydrate and lacks all the nutrients that are required for Carbohydrate digestion and a Healthy Life.

CARBOHYDRATES

The Nutrient composition Chart below is based on 1tsp. Compare the Original-Sugar Cane, with the refined white & brown sugars and you will notice the effects of refinement and processing (profit making). Sugar cane is a most delicious Natural food. The refined Sugar gives you nothing except Empty Calories.

RELATIVE SUGAR SWEETNESS CONTENT

- 173 FRUCTOSE. Fruit Sugar.
- 100 SUCROSE. Table Sugar.
- 74. GLUCOSE. Simple Sugar.
- 33. MALTOSE & LACTOSE.
- 16 MILK SUGAR.

The Sugar sweetness content of the main groups of Sugar, are based on chemical analysis; Sucrose is the base used for comparison. Fructose—Fruit Sugar is by far the best source of sweetness as well as containing an adequate supply of Minerals and Vitamins to ensure efficient use of Sugar and energy for the body. Fruits, especially the sweet fruits: bananas, dates, figs, raisins, sultanas and all dried fruits are an excellent source of Natural sweetness, always have some of these fruits whenever you need energy and sweetness. Try them at breakfast or anytime of the day. If you crave for sweetnesss. remember the sweet fruits.

		CALO	CARB.	CAL.	PHOS.	POTA	IRON.	SOD.	MAG.	COP.	ZINC.	B1.	B2.	B3.	B5.	B6.	BIOT	FOLI
Cane Sugar.	tsp.	44	11	120	28	500	4.9	44	51.6	.28	.1	.01	.04	.3	.1	.05	1.8	.002
Molasses.	tsp.	44	11	137	17	585	3.2	19	51.6	.28	.1	.02	.04	.4	.1	.05	1.8	.002
Brown Sugar.	tsp.	14	12.7	7	6	trace	.6	trace.	trace	.059	trace.	003	.016	.04	trace.	trace.	trace.	trace.
White Sugar.	tsp.	46	12	0	0	trace	trace	0	0	0	0	0	0	0	0	0	0	0
Honey.	tsp.	64	17.3	1	1	11	.1	1	.6	.008	.016	.002	.014	.1	.04	.04	trace.	trace.
Maple Sugar.	tsp.	50	12.8	33	3	26	.2	3	trace.	.09	trace	trace.	trace.	trace.	trace.	trace.	trace.	trace.
Corn Sugar.	tsp.	57	14.8	.8	3	9	trace.	trace.	trace.	.07	trace.	trace.	.002	trace.	trace.	trace.	trace.	trace.
Jam, jelly.	tsp.	54	14	4	2	18	.2	2	trace.	.062	.006	trace.	.01	trace.	trace.	.005	trace.	.002

SUGAR | CARBOHYDRATES

	NUTRIENT FUNCTION;	EFFECT OF PROLONGED DEFICIENCY;
	combines with pyruvic acid, to form a co-enzyme, which is required for the conversion of Carbohydrates into Glucose-primary fuel.	Vit.B1 is known as the moral vitamin. It must be supplied regularly-(daily). A deficiency of B1, makes it hard to digest Carbohydrates and leaves you with too much pyruvic acid in the blood, which leads to a deficiency of Oxygen, that results in a loss of mental alertness, possible cardiac damage and difficulties of breathing, irritability and emotional insecurity.
B1-THIAMINE		
B2-RIBO FLAVIN	Riboflavin is required as part of a group of Enzymes, which breakdown and utilize Carbohydrates. Sugar is a pure Carbohydrate.	Required regularly for maintenance of good vision, healthy hair. A lack of B2 may lead to lack of Energy, digestive problems and loss of hair.
B3-NIACIN	Niacin is one of the most extracted Vitamins, as a result of the Sugar processing methods. Niacin acts as a co-enzyme, which assists in the breakdown of Carbohydrates-Sugar. (Proteins and Fats also).	Niacin is required for good blood circulation and for the control of blood-cholesterol levels.Niacin is also essential for the Health of the Nervous system, as are all the B complex vitamins. A prolonged deficiency of Niacin may lead to general fatigue, muscular weakness, bad breath, headaches, dermatitis, diarrhoea and numerous other nervous disorders.
BIOTIN	Sugar cane is a good source of Biotin. Refined Sugar supplies none at all. Biotin is also a co-enzyme in the oxidation of Carbohydrates. Without Biotin, you are most likely to put on excess weight. Nature protects you.	A deficiency of Biotin can lead to muscular pains, dry skin, lack of Energy, difficulties in sleeping, nervous disorders, poor appetite and obesity.
CALCIUM	CALCIUM is the main mineral of the body, which is required for activating several digestive Enzymes.(promote digestion) and utilization of the other Minerals & Vitamins. Calcium is also required to regulate the heartbeat. Calcium is extracted in the process of Sugar refinement. To prevent a Calcium deficiency your diet must supply Calcium foods for you to remain in good Health and to offset the effects of a Calcium deficiency.	The effects of a prolonged Calcium deficiency are numerous, some of which are; muscle cramps, numbness and tingling sensations in the arms and legs, bone deformation in children, osteoporosis in adults, slow pulse rate, impaired growth of children, nervous deterioration, tooth decay, slow blood clotting, arteriosclerosis, hypertension, constipation, arthritis, colds, diabetes, anemia and various types of mental illness. You need Calcium.
PHOSPHORUS	Phosphorus is required for every chemical reaction, within the body. The mineral Phosphorus is most important for the utilization of Carbohydrates,-(Sugar) Proteins and Lipids. Without Phosphorus Carbohydrates cannot be converted into Energy. Sugar supplies no Phosphorus, so your body must supply it from reserves. Niacin & Riboflavin (B group Vitamins), will not be effective, when the body lacks Phosphorus. Sugar supplies none of these. Phosphorus also helps to control fat metabolism and distribution of body fat. Phosphorus is also essential for efficient mental activity and for healthy nerves. Make sure you eat foods rich in Phosphorus to prevent a deficiency. See the section on Minerals for details, pages 144 and 158.	Sugar, supplies no Phosphorus, however Phosphorus is required in the conversion of Sugar into Energy. Your body may develop a Phosphorus deficiency, due to excess and continual use of Sugar. The effects of a deficiency can lead to Arteriosclerosis, Arthritis, Backache, Cancer, some types of mental illness, and stunted growth and poor bone formation in children. Phosphorus foods will be most beneficial.
POTASSIUM	Potassium is the main healing mineral. Potassium is a major mineral required in the conversion of Glucose to Glycogen (which is a store of Energy, in the Liver). Sugar supplies no Potassium. This mineral is also required for nourishment of the muscular system and also for the transfer of Oxygen, to all parts of the body. Potassium is also easily destroyed by Heat and cooking. Alcohol and Coffee also deplete the reserves of the mineral Potassium. See section on Potassium foods, for better Health.	Potassium is termed a 'healing mineral'. A Potassium deficiency will result when your intake of 'Sugar—foods' is regular and prolonged. A Potassium deficiency is a contributing factor to the following ailments; Hypertension, Acne, Rheumatism, Headaches, Constipation, Angina Pectoris, Polio, Poor reflexes and impaired muscular activity.

Fructose is Nature's answer for the Sweet tooth.

FRUITS NUTRIENT CHART

NOTE: The amounts for Carbohydrates, Proteins and Fat are measured in grams.

FRUITS	CALORIES	CARB	PROTEIN	FAT	CALCIUM	PHOS	POTASSIUM	IRON	SODIUM	MAGNESIUM	COPPER	MANGANESE	ZINC	A.*	C.	E.	B1	B2	B3	B5	B6	BIOTIN.*	FOLIC ACID.
Apples	32	13.5	1.4	.6	6.6	9.3	99	.27	1.1	7.9	.8	.069	.04	82	3.8	.71	.02	.018	.1	.10	.027	.97	.017
Apricots	52	13.0	1	.18	17	23	290	.4	.09	13	.10	.18	0	2800	10	na.	.028	.03	.5	.24	.70	na.	.002
Avocados	167	na.	na.	16.4	6	19	275	.5	1	24	.12	.48	.15	290	7.5	.3	.11	.2	.5	.19	.42	3	.021
Bananas	84	22	na.	na.	8	29	366	.6	1.3	32	.16	.64	.2	180	10	.4	.05	.06	.06	.26	.50	4	.028
Blackberries	55	12.4	1.0	.9	35	18	160	.8	.7	27	.15	.7	.35	193	20	na.	.026	.04	.4	.23	.04	.4	.012
Cherries	58	14.8	1.2	.34	22	19	230	.4	2	14	.12	.4	na.	1033	11	na.	.05	.06	.4	.142	.063	.4	.007
Blackcurrants	54	13.1	1.7	.1	60	40	372	1.1	3	10	.13	na.	na.	230	200	na.	.05	.05	.3	.39	.066	2.4	na.
Dates	274	72.9	.5	2.2	59	63	648	3	1	58	.22	.15	na.	50	0	na.	.09	.1	2.2	.78	.15	na.	.02
Figs	80	20	.3	1.2	35	22	194	.6	2	20	.07	.12	na.	80	2	na.	.06	.05	.4	.3	.11	na.	.01
Grapefruit	41	10.8	.5	.1	16	16	135	.4	1	12	na.	.01	na.	10	38	.26	.04	.02	.2	.28	.03	3	.01
Grapes	70	18	.6	.3	12	21	152	.4	3.2	6.4	.10	.84	na.	106	4	na.	.05	.03	.35	.8	.79	2.1	.07
Lemons	18	5.8	.78	.18	17	28	251	.54	4.5	8.7	.13	.11	na.	9	35	na.	.02	.01	.09	.17	.07	na.	.01.1
Honeydew Melon	26	6.4	.5	.2	7	10	100	.5	1	8	.04	.02	na.	590	0	na.	.03	.03	.2	.3	.06	4	.008
Melons.	32	7.6	.8	.33	14	16	255	.4	12	4.4	.06	.018	na.	40	23	na.	.04	.03	.6	.26	.056	na.	na.
Green ripe Olives.	185	3.5	1	20	105	15	25	1.5	750	17	.42	.049	.30	70	0	na.	.02	.07	.45	.014	.021	na.	na.
Papaya.	38	10	.16	.7	20	16	234	.30	3	7.6	.01	.008	na.	1750	56	na.	.04	na.	.30	.218	na.	na.	.003
Oranges.	35	9	.7	.16	30	15	145	.29	.06	10	.06	.023	.14	140	34	.21	.07	.03	.3	.25	.05	1.0	.04
Peaches	35	9.1	.5	.09	8	17	190	.4	.09	10	.08	.10	.18	1250	6	na.	.01	.04	.09	.160	.04	1.8	.003
Pears	61	15	.7	.4	8	11	130	.3	2	7	.15	.06	na.	20	4	na.	.02	.04	.1	.07	.017	.1	.014
Pineapple	54	14	.4	.2	17	8	151	na.	1.3	13	.06	1	na.	73	17	na.	.09	.03	.2	.16	.08	na.	.11
Plums	66	17	.5	tr	18	17	299	.5	2	9	.1	.1	na.	300	6	na.	.08	.03	.5	.18	.05	tr.	.006
Prunes- dried	344	91	3.3	.5	na.	na.	940	4.4	11	32	.16	.18	na.	2170	4	4	.12	.22	2.1	.35	.5	na.	.005
Strawberry	37	8.4	.7	.5	21	21	164	1	1	12	na.	na.	na.	60	59	na.	.03	.07	.6	na.	na.	na.	na.
Tomatoes	22	4.6	1.0	.2	13	28	250	.55	2.6	14	.16	.18	.13	900	22	.36	.06	.04	.065	.32	.10	1.3	.008

NOTE: All amounts are given to approximate 100 grams. All figures except for vitamin A-(I.U.) and Biotin-(mcg.) are measured in milligrams.   NOTE: When N.A. is given, figures are not yet available.

VEGETABLES

INTRODUCTION

The vegetable kingdom supplies a major portion of human nutritional requirements. This chapter on vegetables will explain in detail the main benefits that are associated with over twenty individual vegetables: asparagus, beetroot, beans, broccoli, brussel sprouts, cabbage, carrots, cauliflower, chives, capsicum, celery, cucumber, garlic, lettuce, leek, onions, parsley, peas, potatoes, pumpkin, radish, watercress and spinach. There are a few other vegetables that have not been included, however, the nutrient charts on page 79 will supply all the necessary figures for comparison of these vegetables. On pages 77 and 78 a comprehensive section of Chlorophyll is provided. All Natural foods are based on the energy of the sun, air, water and combine with the mineral elements from the soil to grow and develop. The secrets that Nature has kept for millions of years are still puzzling highly trained scientists and modern systems of chemical analysis. No one knows exactly how the 'missing link' — Chlorophyll is formed within the structure of plants. If man were to discover the essential missing ingredients that initiate the development of Chlorophyll, he may be able to assist Nature with better understanding and respect. The chemical structure of Chlorophyll — the green pigment that is highly concentrated in Vegetable produce, has a remarkable relationship with the structure of human blood. Chlorophyll and Human blood are basically one and the same. The most concentrated natural source of Chlorophyll is obtainable from the vegetable kingdom with such plants as: beetroot greens, broccoli, cabbage, chives, celery, cucumber, lettuce, parsley, peas, green pepper, spinach and watercress supplying the ultimate source of this 'sunshine liquid'. Proper preparation of these and other vegetables is most important for retention of the vital elements that are associated with the individual vegetables. Many people feel obliged to eat vegetables. Most of these people have been brought up with faulty diets and are therefore trained from an early age to exist on a limited supply of vegetables and have possibly never experienced the rewards of regular use of vegetables and home made vegetable juices. All the essential minerals and vitamins are readily available with freshly extracted juices and by including at least one glass of any fresh vegetable juice with your daily diet, you can be sure of maximum health restoring qualities as well as counteracting the detrimental effects that city living and the processed and refined foods and drinks may have had on your body over the past number of years. It takes very little time to make a fresh juice and within a month of taking daily vegetable juice, you will notice benefits that may give you a new vitality and brighter view of life. The purchase of a good quality juice extractor is a most valuable investment for your future health. Apart from the juices, Vegetables can be the most delicious foods when they are prepared with a little experience and simple food combination rules. Vegetables mix well with Grains, Legumes, Nuts, Seeds and all secondary protein foods such as, cheese, eggs, fish and meat. The benefits of combining Vegetables with secondary proteins cannot be over-emphasized. Many valuable nutrients are lacking from secondary protein foods and as a majority of people eat a great portion of such foods as cheese, eggs, fish, meat products and poultry, the advantages of a regular supply of vegetables will be to provide a better range and proper balance of essential human life supporting nutrients. Vegetables are the most simple of Natural foods to cultivate. A home garden is not complete without an area set aside for Vegetables.

Health is easy to maintain, thanks to the vegetable kingdom.

63

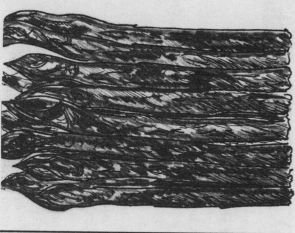
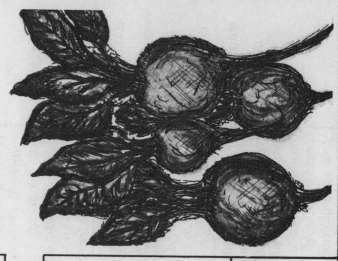

ASPARAGUS

NUTRITIONAL QUALITIES	
IODINE	Asparagus are an excellent source of the mineral Iodine and this has a most stimulating effect on the body, assisting correct thyroid activity and thereby ensuring that other glands of the body are working together in promoting efficient metabolism. The thyroid gland produces a hormone known as Thyroxine and that is composed of 65% Iodine.
CHLORINE SULPHUR	Asparagus are a good source of two dominant 'cleansing minerals', Chlorine and Sulphur impart a strong taste when obtained in the natural state and when the Asparagus is cooked, these minerals are easily destroyed and can no longer promote cleansing of the digestive system and bloodstream.
OTHER NUTRIENTS	Asparagus are also a good source of the minerals Phosphorus: healthy nerves, skin and hair, Potassium: healthy liver, active muscles and maintenance of heart muscle function. The mineral Iron in combination with the trace mineral Copper that are supplied with Asparagus, promote cleansing of the bloodstream and distribution of oxygen throughout the bloodstream. The mineral Magnesium stimulates enzyme activity, glandular functions and promotes healthy nerves.
VITAMIN E	The dominant vitamin of the Asparagus is vitamin E and that also promotes efficient use of oxygen from the bloodstream to all cells of the body. Do not boil Asparagus, use them raw or slightly steamed.

BEETROOT

NUTRITIONAL QUALITIES	
MANGANESE MAGNESIUM	Beetroot are the best vegetable source of the trace mineral Manganese and in combination with the excellent supply of Magnesium, Beetroot are a most valuable food for nourishment of the nervous system and brain. Manganese is also required for blood and bone development and vital for nursing mothers', as Manganese stimulates the production of mothers' milk. Beetroot should be obtained fresh and grated, steamed or juiced for maximum benefits. Canned Beetroot is not recommended. A small glass of Carrot, Beetroot and Parsley juice is one of the best medicines for women with menstruation problems. Manganese is termed the 'memory mineral' and Magnesium is termed the 'nerve mineral'. Remember the Beetroot and let your nerves Laugh with Health. Try the taste of freshly grated Beetroot with your next salad.
SODIUM POTASSIUM	Beetroot is a very good source of the minerals Sodium and Potassium, these two work as a team in regulating body fluid levels. Excess intake of table salt will cause cells and tissues to retain excess fluid, leading the way to overweight conditions. Table salt (sodium chloride) is said to retain 70 grams of water for every gram of salt taken. Avoid using table salt and also tinned Beetroot and other canned foods as they are often loaded with excess salt.

BEANS

NUTRITIONAL QUALITIES	
VITAMIN A	*Beans are a member of the Legume family of plants. On pages 37-48 there is a complete guide to all the main members of the Legume family; this section refers to the french bean and the yellow or green snap beans, these belong to the same botanical species as the kidney bean, however, they are cultivated for use as a fresh green vegetable-legume. In comparison to the kidney bean, fresh green beans are an excellent source of vitamin A — protects the body against infection, promotes healthy skin condition and clear eyesight,*
VITAMIN C	*green Beans are also a good source of vitamin C when obtained raw-diced, they make an excellent addition for a fresh garden salad. The following minerals are also well supplied: magnesium — regulates the functions of the glandular system, promotes healthy nerve functioning and strong tooth enamel formation, iron — assists in the transportation of oxygen and promotes healthy blood condition, calcium — promotes*
OTHER NUTRIENTS	*healthy heart action and strong bone development, manganese — in combination with the supply of iron and copper promotes blood development. Fresh green Beans also supply Vitamins E, B1, B2, B3, B5, B6 and folic acid. Avoid excess cooking of Beans, they are best when served raw with a fresh salad.*

BROCCOLI

NUTRITIONAL QUALITIES	
VITAMIN A / VITAMIN C	*Broccoli is one of the best vegetable source of both vitamin A and C. These nutrients, especially vitamin C, are heat sensitive. Prolonged cooking of Broccoli is not advised. To prepare the Broccoli properly, place the stems only, in water or preferably lightly steam the vegetable for 5 minutes. A fresh bunch of Broccoli should be used quickly and not stored for long periods. Small amounts of fresh Broccoli can be included with a fresh garden salad*
CALCIUM / PHOSPHORUS	*Broccoli is also an excellent source of the two main minerals Calcium and Phosphorus. The Calcium-Phosphorus balance of Broccoli is most valuable for building and maintenace of strong bones. Broccoli is one of the best vegetable Calcium foods as it also provides an abundance of the mineral Magnesium and vitamins: A and C, all these nutrients work together to promote efficient absorption and metabolism of the minerals Calcium and Phosphorus.*
MAGNESIUM / IRON	*Broccoli also supplies good amounts of the minerals Magnesium and Iron. Magnesium foods revitalize the body as they promote enzyme activity and nerve functioning. The Iron content of Broccoli is enhanced with the addition of vitamin C, also well supplied with Broccoli. Women, especially expectant mothers' need a daily intake of Iron foods to ensure that they overcome the regular loss of blood. A deficiency of Iron foods can lead to any of the following ailments: Nail problems, diarrhea, ulcers and gastritis.*

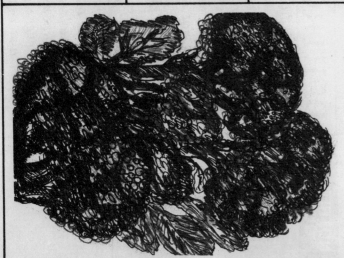

BRUSSEL SPROUTS

NUTRITIONAL QUALITIES	
SULPHUR	Brussel Sprouts are an excellent source of the mineral Sulphur and this has a cleansing and antiseptic effect on the digestive system, bloodstream and skin cells. Sulphur foods are essential for maintenance of healthy skin, nails and hair as they are a rich source of keratin, a protein substance that is also part of insulin, the hormone that promotes Carbohydrate metabolism. Brussel Sprouts should not be boiled. They can be lightly steamed or finely chopped and added to a fresh garden salad. The strong taste of raw Brussel Sprouts is due to the high Sulphur content and that can be destroyed when overcooked. Sulphur foods also promote the digestion of Protein foods.
OTHER NUTRIENTS	Brussel Sprouts are also an excellent source of the minerals: Potassium and Phosphorus and a very good source of Magnesium, Iron, B complex vitamins and a good source of vitamins (A & C when freshly obtained).

CABBAGE

NUTRITIONAL QUALITIES	
CHLORINE SULPHUR	Cabbage are an excellent source of the two 'cleansing minerals': Chlorine and Sulphur work as a team in expelling waste matter, cleansing of the blood and they also tend to reduce excess weight. A deficiency of Chlorine foods can lead to poor liver functioning and various types of conjestion such as sinusitis. Regular use of fresh Cabbage, lightly steamed or finely chopped and added to a salad will be most beneficial for protection from the common cold and virus. Also try the taste of home made Cabbage rolls and rice.
OTHER NUTRIENTS CHLOROPHYL VITAMIN U	Cabbage are also a good source of the minerals: potassium, sodium, phosphorus, silicon and zinc. The outer green leaves of Cabbage are an excellent source of Chlorophyl, the green magic medicine and a unique source of vitamin U, a recently discovered vitamin that has proved to be the best medicine for relief of peptic ulcers. (see page 205 for details). Red Cabbage is also available and that has a similar structure of nutrients, except for the Chlorophyl. Try a freshly made red Cabbage salad.
ENZYMES	Cabbage is the main ingredients of Sauerkraut, a product of German ingenuity. Sauerkraut is formed from fermented Cabbage leaves and supplies an abundance of vital enzyme elements. If not for Sauerkraut, many Germans would get very little enzyme food as they rely greatly on cooked meals for their satisfaction. All cooked, processed and refined foods are deficient in enzyme content and thereby lead the way to a sluggish digestive system and overweight conditions. Canned Sauerkraut is a poor alternative to the home made product as the canning involves heat processes, that destroys the vital enzymes and their associated benefits of renewed vitality.

CARROTS

VITAMIN A	Carrots fresh from the veggie patch are a real delight for the eyes. Apart from the excellent supply of vitamin A, fresh Carrots provide an abundance of nearly all life supporting nutrients. Carrots are the best vegetable source of vitamin A, they supply 11,000 mg. per 100 grams. Freshly extracted Carrot juice is one of the best natural medicines available for prevention from colds and viruses. Whenever you see the chance to have some cool Carrot juice, take it and you will promote your natural resistance to germs and infection. The vitamin A content of Carrots is in the form of Carotene, a substance that the body converts into the form of vitamin A. Regular intake of freshly made Carrot juice is one of the best remedies for teenage acne. The combination of vitamin A & C and the mineral silicon gives Carrots their remarkable ability to promote good eyesight, even in dim lighting. If you don't like the taste of Carrots, try a cool Carrot juice!
CHLORINE **SULPHUR**	Carrots are a very good source of the main cleansing minerals: chlorine and sulphur. Chlorine foods stimulate the functions of the liver such as elimination of toxic waste from the human system and it is also valuable in keeping the bones and joints in a youthful shape thereby providing natural protection from arthritis. Sulphur foods promote a cleansing and antiseptic effect on the digestive system and bloodstream. Sulphur is also one main component of Insulin, the hormone that is essential for the conversion of carbohydrates into energy. A cool Carrot juice will promote clear skin condition due to the abundance of cleansing minerals.
CALCIUM **PHOSPHORUS** **MAGNESIUM**	Carrots are a very good source of three major minerals: Calcium, phosphorus and magnesium work together to build strong bones and a healthy nervous system. Calcium is essential for healthy heart muscles and regulation of the heartbeat. Phosphorus is essential for healthy skin, hair and nerves. The vital Magnesium content of fresh Carrots is most beneficial for mental development, digestion of fats and the metabolism of such nutrients as: calcium, phosphorus, sodium, potassium, B complex vitamins and vitamins C & E. Magnesium is essential for the production of energy from carbohydrates. Alcohol consumption destroys Magnesium, have a Carrot juice and Laugh with Health.
VITAMIN E	Carrots are also a good vegetable source of vitamin E — the muscle vitamin. Vitamin E foods increase the efficiency of the entire muscular system by promoting efficient use of oxygen. Vitamin E also assists the transportation of blood by dilation of blood vessels thereby helping your blood to travel to all parts of the body. Carrot juice will enhance your muscular endurance.

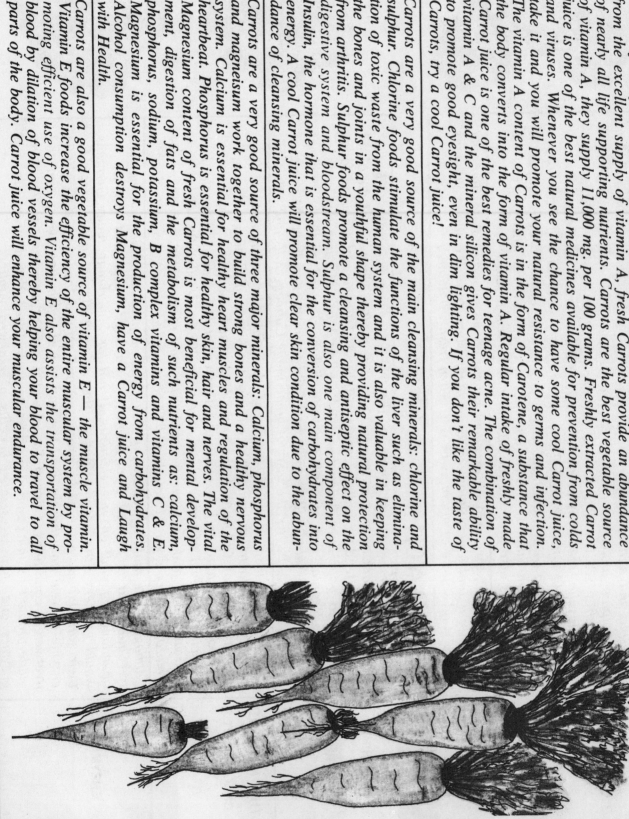

If you see a Carrot, have one and you'll see more

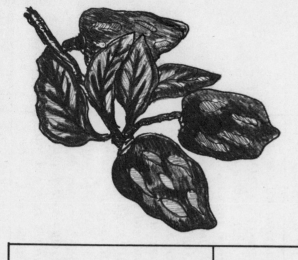

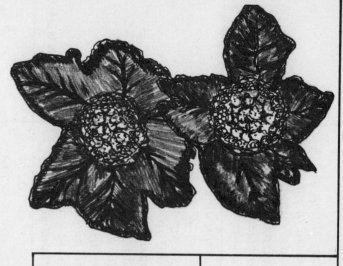

CAPSICUM

NUTRITIONAL QUALITIES	
VITAMIN C	Capsicum are one of the best vegetable source of precious vitamin C. One large Capsicum will supply a major portion of your daily vitamin C requirements. The benefits of obtaining natural vitamin C in contrast to the tablet cannot be overstressed. The action of vitamin C is dependant on a supply of bio-flavonoids, they are contained in the white part of the associated fruit or vegetable. A vitamin C tablet supplies no bio-flavonoids and therefore the action of vitamin C is greatly retarded. Various other nutrients are required for maximum vitamin C effectiveness such as the minerals calcium and magnesium. The natural form of vitamin C will also supply an abundance of enzymes that will promote the numerous functions of vitamin C. The tablet is the expensive way to get what only nature can provide in correct balance for human nutrition. Remember to buy a couple of Capsicum's this week.
BIO-FLAVONOIDS VITAMIN P IODINE VITAMIN A	Capsicum is an excellent source of bioflavonoids or vitamin P, a deficiency of vitamin P can lead to any of the following ailments: bruising, varicose veins, arteriosclerosis, arthritis and rheumatism. Vitamin P is essential for proper absorption of vitamin C. Vitamin P is vital for increasing the strength of the capillaries and thereby preventing such ailments as varicose veins. Capsicum are also a very good source of Iodine and vitamin A.

CAULIFLOWER

NUTRITIONAL QUALITIES	
POTASSIUM	Cauliflower is a member of the Cabbage family and a good source of the mineral potassium — the great muscle builder. Potassium foods assist the action of the heart muscles and promote circulation of the blood. In combination with the good iron content of fresh Cauliflower, potassium helps the body to utilize oxygen. Potassium metabolism is generated by the liver. A prolonged deficiency of potassium foods can lead to any of the following ailments: diabetes, hypertension, diarrhea, headaches, constipation, arthritis, rheumatism, acne and dermatitis. Remember to include some fresh Cauliflower with your next salad or slightly steam the Caulifloweer and serve with grated cheese for a complete protein meal.
OTHER NUTRIENTS BIOTIN	Cauliflower are also a good source of the following nutrients: magnesium — healthy nerves, phosphorus — heart muscles, healthy nerves and efficient mental functioning, Magnesium — conversion of carbohydrates into energy, Chlorine and Sulphur — cleansing minerals, Silicon — preserve calcium metabolism and protect against the development of arthritis and promote healthy hair and skin condition. Cauliflower are also a good source of vitamin C — the everyday life vitamin and an excellent source of Biotin — the slimming vitamin. Natural foods will protect you in many ways.

CELERY

NUTRITIONAL QUALITIES	
SODIUM	Celery is the richest vegetable source of the mineral Sodium with over 120 mg. per 100 grams. Sodium is a most important mineral as it keeps other mineral elements soluble within the bloodstream thereby preventing a build-up of solid deposits. Prolonged use of refined and cooked foods, especially white bread, will lead to the development of arthritic symptoms as the balance of elements with those refined foods is inadequate to support proper development of bones and connective tissues. If you have been using refined foods for a prolonged period and can feel the occasional pain in the joints, Celery juice mixed with Carrot will be the best natural medicine for repair of the damage caused and will promote elimination of those toxic substances that have deposited in various parts of the body. Regular use of Celery juice will prevent any further deposits of toxic substances and pro- vide essential alkaline mineral elements such as sodium, potassium, calcium, magnesium, iron and manganese all of which contribute valuable healing properties. Avoid the pain, have a Celery juice mixed with carrot and parsley for maximum relief and repair.
CHLORINE	Celery is also an excellent source of the mineral Chlorine and with regular use of Celery you can be assured that the beneficial action of the mineral Sodium is also enhanced to provide effective cleansing of the bloodstream and control of overweight conditions.
OTHER NUTRIENTS	Celery also supplies good amounts of the main mineral Calcium as well as phosphorus, magnesium and vitamins A & C, all of which assist in the absorption and metabolism of Calcium. Refined and processed foods are de- ficient in all the essential nutrients that enhance Calcium metabolism and a prolonged use of those foods can lead to poor bone development, weak heart muscles and arthritis. Vitamin D — the sunlight vitamin is most im- portant for correct Calcium metabolism and so if you obtain very little sun- light and eat processed and refined foods, you will be at risk of developing such bone disorders as osteoporosis and arthritis. Freshly made Celery juice will give your body a correct balance of these nutrients that enhance calcium metabolism, apart from the sunlight. Have some today.
CHLOROPHYL	
INSULIN	Celery is also an excellent source of natural insulin, an essential ingredient for the conversion of carbohydrate foods into the form of energy. Natural sugars are easily digested but for those people who regularly consume re- fined foods, especially white sugar, an increased amount of natural insulin is essential to prevent the development of diabetes. A deficiency of Insulin will retard the action of muscles and the process of carbohydrate metabolism.

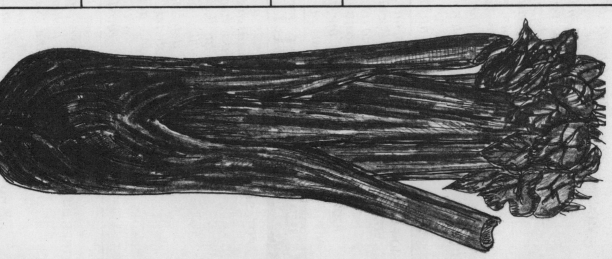

'Slim as a stick of Celery.'

CUCUMBER

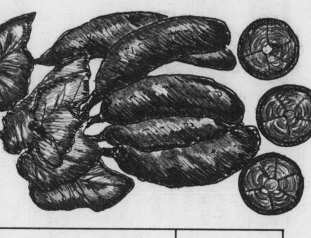

Cucumber are a beauty food.

NUTRITIONAL QUALITIES	
VITAMIN E	Cucumber are the best vegetable source of vitamin E — the muscle vitamin. A lack of vitamin E foods will retard the efficiency of muscles, especially the heart muscles. Vitamin E is termed as an antioxidant, a substance that opposes the oxidation of other nutrients within the body. Vitamin E also increases the stamina and endurance of muscles by allowing cells to function with minimum oxygen for maximum efficiency. The vitamin E content of Cucumber is also beneficial for improving circulation of the blood because it causes dilation of even the smaller blood vessels and also aids in the nourishment of cells, strengthening capillary walls and promotes the healing of damaged skin tissue. Cucumber is often used as an ingredient of facial creams and no wonder it proves to be so beneficial. Try a cool Cucumber today. Try the taste of finely sliced Cucumber and soya mayonnaise.
IODINE	Cucumber are also an excellent source of Iodine, the mineral that is essential for the functioning of the thyroid gland and that promotes the health of the hair, nails, skin and teeth. Iodine also assists the body to utilize fats and thereby protects against obesity. Cucumber are also a good source of the
OTHER NUTRIENTS	following minerals: sulphur and chlorine — cleansing minerals, silicon — growth of hair, iron — blood development and vitamin A — healthy skin.

GARLIC

It is more beneficial to smell of Garlic than to have another cold!

NUTRITIONAL QUALITIES	
SULPHUR	Garlic is a herb-vegetable, the strongest member of the onion family. The most dominant nutrient of Garlic is the mineral Sulphur. About 80% of Garlic oil is in the form of Sulphur elements, and they promote elimination of acid-mucus poisons from the lymphatic system and entire body. Sulphur foods such as Garlic are most valuable for prevention of infection and also as a form or natural penicillin. Garlic oil contains an ether like substance that is most effective in clearing up the entire respiratory and lymphatic system. Such foods as refined bread, milk, cheese and processed food and drinks as well as cigarette smoking and environmental pollutants all cause an excess buildup of mucus residue within the body. At the onset of a cold, it is a sure warning that the body needs to eliminate those excess mucus toxins and for positive results, a few cloves of fresh Garlic is the ultimate weapon. Regular use of Garlic is one of the best ways to prevent a buildup of mucus, the best way is to avoid any processed and refined foods and also to reduce the consumption of dairy produce. Once the cold symptons appear, the use of fresh Garlic will promote a rapid flow of mucus from the body, that may seem like the cold is getting worse, however, the more mucus that is eliminated today, the better off you will be tomorrow. Let Nature help you always.

NUTRITIONAL QUALITIES.	NUTRITIONAL QUALITIES.
POTASSIUM	POTASSIUM
CALCIUM	PHOSPHORUS
PHOSPHORUS	IODINE
SILICON	NICKEL
B GROUP VIT.	SILICON
SULPHUR	VITAMIN E
CHLORINE	
VITAMIN C	

LEEK

Leek are a member of the Onion family and they supply good amounts of the minerals: potassium — muscle development, healthy heart muscles, calcium — bone repair and development, aids digestion, phosphorus — mental development and repair of the nervous system, sulphur — prevention of baldness and infection, silicon — growth of hair, calcium metabolism and prevention of arthritis. Home made Leek soup is delicious, make some soon.

Leek are classed as a mild onion and can be combined with a fresh garden salad or added to any cooked meal. Leek supply good amounts of B group vitamins, especially Biotin — weight control and metabolism of fats and vitamin B6 — the vitality vitamin. Regular use of raw Leek and the occasional cooked Leek dish are valuable as a mild cleanser and for stimulating the pancreas and digestive juices. The Chlorine and Sulphur content of Leek promote cleansing of the bloodstream and lymphatic system. Leek contain more than 90% natural mineral water and supply a fair amount of vitamin C when obtained fresh. Try the unique subtle onion taste of Leek this week. Use Leek as a base for quiche, salads, soups and vegetable pies.

ONIONS

Onions supply only minimal amount of nutrients compared to other fresh vegetables, the most dominant minerals are potassium — healthy heart muscles, phosphorus — removes acids from the bloodstream and promotes repair of the nervous system, iodine — weight control and mental development. Onions are also a source of the trace mineral Nickel, that assists the utilization of sugar. Onions are a good source of the mineral Silicon and that can promote better blood circulation and prevent nervous and mental fatigue. Spring onions combine well with a fresh garden salad and cheese.

Onions are available in various shapes, sizes and potencies. All Onions contain natural antiseptic oils such as: allyl disulphate and cycloalliin and these have recently shown to be beneficial in reducing blood clots within the veins and blood vessels with encouraging results for heart patients. Onions also supply a fair amount of the heart muscle vitamin-E. There are many other natural foods that have a far greater ability to improve a weak heart condition, however, the Onion is one of the few sources of these natural antiseptic oils. Try the unique taste of home made Onion bread. Chives are also a member of the Onion family and they supply moderate amounts of the minerals; calcium, magnesium, iron, phosphorus and sulphur. Chives are an easy food to grow in the home-herb garden and they make an excellent addition for the fresh garden salad

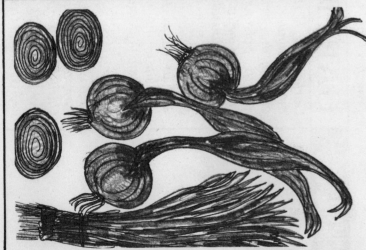
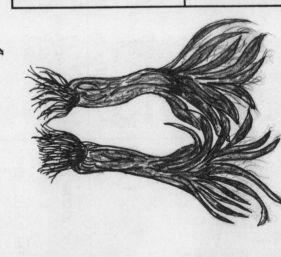

LETTUCE

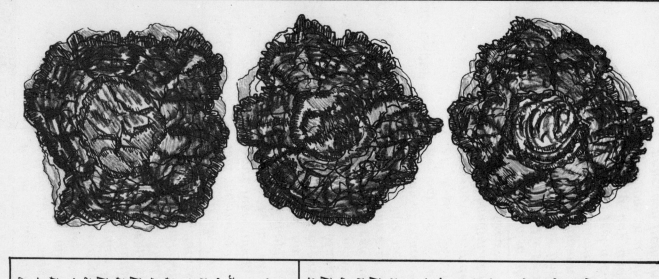

NUTRITIONAL QUALITIES	
SILICON	Lettuce are the best natural food source of the mineral Silicon, they supply over 2,000mg. per 100 grams. Apart from Oxygen, Silicon is the most abundant element in the soil. One of the main benefits of Silicon is that it enhances the functions of the main mineral of the human body, Calcium. Silicon foods preserve calcium metabolism, helping the body to distribute calcium elements and preventing the formation of calcium deposits around bone joints and thereby ensuring positive protection against the development of arthritic symptoms. Silicon elements also help to eliminate excess uric acid deposits from the bone structure and bloodstream. Regular and excess eating of meat is the major cause of uric acid accumulation and that is most detrimental as it leaches away the calcium reserves of the bone structure. Meat supplies very little calcium and great quantities of uric acid. Silicon foods will also promote the growth of hair. Daily use of fresh Lettuce, the outer green leaves are the ultimate source, will prevent the embarrasement of baldness. If you have tried everything to assist the growth of hair and have had no success, then try a glass of freshly made Lettuce, carrot and parsley juice daily and discover the natural remedy and positive results. Serve it cold.
IRON **VITAMIN E** VITAMIN C COPPER	Lettuce are one of the best vegetable source of the mineral Iron. As well as supplying an abundance of Iron, Lettuce is dominant in two essential vitamins that enhance the absorption of the mineral Iron: Vitamin E is very well supplied and good amounts of vitamin C are also available from fresh Lettuce. The mineral Iron helps the body to increase resistance to stress and disease. Lettuce also supply a correct balance of the main mineral Calcium with Phosphorus and that also enhances the absorption of the mineral Iron. Lettuce also supply good amounts of the trace mineral Copper and that is essential for Iron metabolism. A deficiency of Iron foods can lead to regular colds and any ailment that ends with the letters 'itis', such as dermatitis. Women need a regular supply of the best quality Iron foods to replace the loss during menstruation. Iron foods will protect you against poor and brittle finger nails, stomach ulcers, conjunctivitis and hepatitis.
OTHER NUTRIENTS **CHLOROPHYL** **BIOTIN**	Lettuce are a lucky vegetable as they rarely get cooked and thereby supply an abundance of heat sensitive nutrients such as the minerals potassium, sodium, sulphur and chlorine and vitamins A, C, B complex. Biotin is a B complex vitamin and Lettuce are one of the best vegetable source of this precious nutrient. Biotin is the only B group vitamin that contains the mineral sulphur and this promotes body cleansing and protection from infections. Biotin is also essential for the metabolism of fats and a deficiency of this vitamin can lead to overweight conditions, difficulty in sleeping, nervousness and dermatitis. Always remember Lettuce if you need to relax.

NUTRITIONAL QUALITIES	PARSLEY

POTASSIUM

Parsley is the richest vegetable-herb source of Potassium — the muscle mineral. Potassium foods stimulate the kidneys to eliminate poisonous waste matter, they also help to preserve proper alkalinity of the blood and body fluids and they promote a healthy skin condition. For some people, Parsley is a food to decorate a dinner plate even though they may have heart troubles, regular headaches, constipation, acne, hypertenion, rheumatism or arthritis. The nutrient content of Parsley is one of the best medicines for day to day use. One small clipping of Parsley per day will promote your health like no other food. The mineral Potassium is easily destroyed in cooking and to ensure that you are protected from a deficiency of this mineral, regular use of raw Potassium foods is essential.

MAGNESIUM
CALCIUM

Parsley is also an excellent source of the following nutrients: Magnesium — and the mineral Calcium are required in combination for proper nerve and heart functioning, daily use of Parsley is one of the best nerve medicines. Parsley is an excellent food for development of healthy blood due to the abundant supply of the three main blood building nutrients: iron, copper and manganese, they are termed as the 'blood builders'. Copper foods protect the

IRON
COPPER
MANGANESE

lungs from disease and they promote regular heart action and absorption of vitamin C. Manganese is termed as the 'memory mineral' as it helps to nourish the nervous system and brain, stimulating the transmission of impulses between nerves and their associated muscles. Parsley is also an excellent source of vitamin A — healthy skin, prevention of disease and reduc-

VITAMIN A

tion of infection, these B group vitamins are also dominant: B1 — 'the vitamin of courage', B2 — 'the youth vitamin' and B3 — 'the morale vitamin'.

B GROUP VIT.

Regular use of Parsley is one of the best ways to restore the body to a state of physical and mental strength and positive resistance to numerous degenerative disorders. Freshly made vegetable juices are always enhanced with a handful of fresh Parsley, that will be about one ounce of juice. Parsley prevents disease.

IRON
VITAMIN C

Parsley is also the best vegetable — herb source of the mineral iron and vitamin C. These two nutrients work in combination to incinerate waste matter within the body. The mineral Iron transports oxygen to every cell of the body and vitamin C enhances the activity of this function. Both the mineral iron and vitamin C are essential for protection from colds and viruses. Next time you feel a chill or cold coming on, try one large sprig of Parsley a few times a day and you will most certainly notice a reduction of the cold symptoms in a short time. Parsley is one of the best medicines available for protection from the common cold.

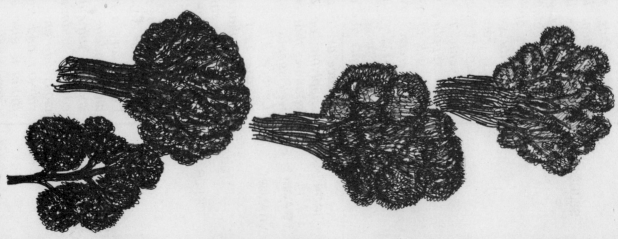

Use Parsley regularly

PEAS

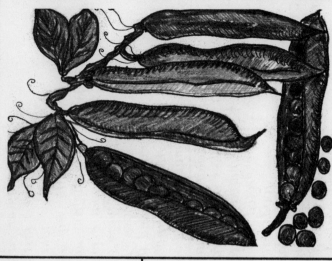

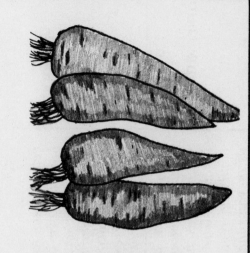

NUTRITIONAL QUALITIES	
PHOSPHORUS	Peas belong to the Legume family of plants, they are said to have originated over 4,000 years ago and were possibly one of the foods that were available in the garden of Eden. Fresh garden Peas are a most nourishing food and a good source of primary protein. Peas are an excellent source of the mineral Phosphorus and that promotes proper bone formation, kidney functioning, healthy nerves and efficient mental activity. Peas are a poor source of the main mineral Calcium and so it would be advisable to combine a top quality calcium food when serving Peas such as sesame seeds, tahini or broccoli.
VITAMIN E IRON POTASSIUM MAGNESIUM B GROUP VIT	Peas are a very good source of vitamin E and the mineral Iron. Frozen Peas are a very poor source of vitamin E as this applies to any frozen food products. A prolonged deficiency of vitamin E foods is a major cause of heart problems, arteriosclerosis and varicose veins. The good Iron content of Peas is most valuable for healthy blood development and the combination of vitamin E will greatly enhance the assimilation of the mineral Iron. Fresh Peas straight from the pod are a most valuable addition to the diet, they can be steamed or lightly cooked but should never be boiled or frozen. Peas are also a good source of the minerals: potassium — muscle mineral, sodium — keeps other minerals soluble, magnesium — nerve mineral, copper — blood development and vitamins: B1 — healthy nerves, B2 — healthy skin, hair and nails, B5 — healthy adrenal glands and vitamin C — prevention of stomach ulcers. Fresh Peas, slightly cooked are an excellent addition with rice dishes, a fresh salad, home made quiche, pasties, fresh corn or sprout salad.

PARSNIPS

NUTRITIONAL QUALITIES	
POTASSIUM PHOSPHORUS OTHER NUTRIENTS	Parsnips are classed as a tuber vegetable, they have a high carbohydrate-starch content and supply good amounts of the following nutrients: Potassium is the dominant nutrient of the Parsnip and that promotes muscle development, digestion of starches and correct fluid retention in body tissues. Parsnips supply very good amounts of the mineral phosphorus — strengthens the nervous system. Parsnips supply an abundance of the minerals chlorine and sulphur, both are vital for effective body cleansing and prevention from infections. Other nutrients also well supplied are: silicon — healthy hair, magnesium — healthy nerves, and the trace mineral bromine — healthy glands. A good range of B group vitamins and vitamins A and C are also available from fresh Parsnips.

NUTRITIONAL QUALITIES	POTATOES
POTASSIUM	*Potatoes are a Potassium food, however, the mineral potassium is one of the easiest lost in cooking. Proper preparation of the Potato is essential in order to retain this valuable 'muscle mineral'. Potatoes should be cooked with the skin on as that prevents a great loss of essential active nutrients. French fries and Potato chips are a most common food and there is no nutritional benefits associated with those adulterated Potato preparations, they are more of a health risk, as they fill the stomach with starch and have no protective elements to ensure proper digestion, the body must supply the nutrients and that leads to numerous deficiencies of especially the B group vitamins and the minerals: calcium, phosphorus, sodium, zinc and magnesium. Potatoes are one of the few real 'down to earth' foods.*
FOLIC ACID	
OTHER NUTRIENTS	*Potatoes are an excellent source of the B group vitamin Folic acid, that applies only to raw-diced Potatoes. Folic acid is one of the critical nutrients required for prevention of leukemia and pernicious anemia. The Potato can be grated and added in small quantities to any fresh garden salad. Folic acid foods are essential for proper absorption of the minerals iron and calcium and for the production of gastric juices. The Potato is also a good source of: magnesium — nerves, sulphur — heat sensitive, essential for healthy hair, silicon — protection from arthritis, beauty mineral, iodine — weight control, chlorine — purifies the blood and when obtained raw, the Potato is also a good source of vitamin C. Try the natural Potato.*

NUTRITIONAL QUALITIES	PUMPKIN
VITAMIN A **SILICON**	*Pumpkin are one of the best vegetable source of vitamin A and in combination with the excellent source of the mineral Silicon, the Pumpkin is an excellent food for prevention of infection and for promotion of healthy skin, hair and eye condition. Vitamin A foods assist in the growth and repair of skin tissue and they provide strength to cell walls, protecting the delicate mucous membranes of the mouth, nose, throat and lungs from invading infections. Silicon foods give luster to the hair and improve the condition of the brain. Freshly grated Pumpkin combines very well with a garden salad and whole Pumpkin pieces should be steamed or baked, not boiled.*
OTHER NUTRIENTS	*Pumpkin are also a good source of the following nutrients: potassium — stimulates blood circulation, iron — resistance to stress and disease, sulphur — promotes healthy skin and hair, chlorine — stimulates the functions of the liver. The Pumpkin is a most satisfying food and one that should be combined regularly with the diet. When preparing Pumpkin, save the seeds as they are the best natural source of Protein (see page 101 for details).*

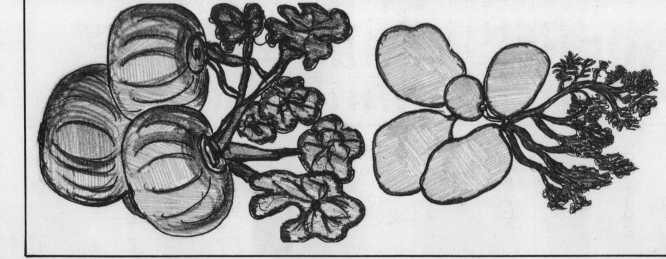

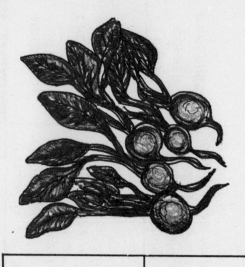

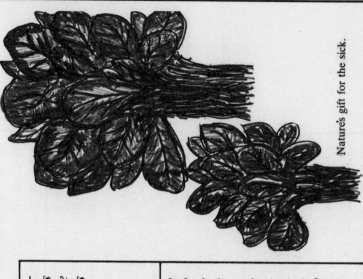

Nature's gift for the sick.

RADISH

NUTRITIONAL QUALITIES	
CHLORINE	Radish are an excellent source of the mineral Chlorine and this promotes the digestion of protein foods, as chlorine foods stimulate the production of hydrochloric acid, the vital ingredient for protein digestion. Radish are also valuable cleansers of the respiratory system as they supply good amounts of the mineral Chlorine and that assists the elimination of acid-mucus poisons from the the body. Radish also contain a volatile ether which will promote elimination of mucus from the body. A few chopped Radishes with the meal will also be beneficial for protection from infection.
SILICON	Radish are also a good source of the mineral Silicon and that is beneficial for maintenance of good teeth, healthy hair and clear vision. Silicon foods are also a good preventative of nervous exhaustion and mental fatigue. The
VITAMIN C	vitamin C content of Radish is very good and promotes such functions as good eyesight, healing of damaged skin tissue and regulation of cholesterol.
SULPHUR	The strong taste of Radish is due to the abundance of the minerals chlorine and sulphur. Add a few Radishes to your next salad.

WATERCRESS

NUTRITIONAL QUALITIES	
CALCIUM	Watercress is a member of the mustard family of plants. Apart from supplying excellent amounts of the minerals calcium and sulphur. Watercress is
SULPHUR	also an excellent vegetable source of vitamin A with over 5,000 mg. available per 100 grams. Regular use of dominant vitamin A foods such as Watercress
VITAMIN A	will promote increased resistance to virus infections and air pollutants. Watercress grows in very pure, slow moving water, around creeks and rivers. It is harder to obtain than most other vegetables but when available, Watercress should take first preference over other vegetables.
OTHER NUTRIENTS	Watercress can also be grown in the home garden, the main requirements are that the sandy-soil be kept very moist and preferable have a slow movement of water along the roots of the plants. Home grown Watercress will provide you with an abundant supply of minerals such as potassium — stimulates blood circulation and protects against the formation of cancerous tissues, sodium — protects against hardening of the arteries and promotes healthy skin condition, iron — is easily lost from the body with any excess consumption of coffee or tea, phosphorus — essential for repair and efficient functioning of the nervous system, chlorine — cleanses the blood and normalises heart muscle action, manganese — nourishment of the nervous system and brain and magnesium — bone development and strength. Watercress are also
B GROUP VIT.	a good source of vitamins; B1, B2, B3, Biotin and the mineral Iodine.

SPINACH

NUTRITIONAL QUALITIES	
MAGNESIUM	Spinach is the best vegetable source of the mineral Magnesium and as Chlorophyl is based on a magnesium atom, it stands to reason that such a dark green vegetable as Spinach would have a great concentration of this mineral. Spinach is an excellent food for nerve nutrition due to this abundance of the mineral magnesium. A prolonged deficiency of Magnesium foods can be a major cause of tooth decay, as the mineral magnesium is responsible for strengthening of the tooth enamel. Over 70% of the magnesium content of the human body is contained in the bone structure.
CHLOROPHYL	
IRON COPPER MANGANESE	Spinach supplies an abundance of the main blood building nutrients: Iron, Manganese and Copper as well as supplying excellent amounts of Calcium which is vital for maximum absorption of the mineral Iron. The bloodstream contains ten times the concentration of the mineral Iron compared to other parts of the body. Iron foods are essential for the transportation of oxygen to every cell of the body. Spinach also supplies good amounts of vitamin E and that assists the cells to make maximum use of the oxygen supplied. Fresh Spinach can be finely chopped and added to any garden salad. Freshly made Spinach juice, serve cold, is the best natural medicine for healthy blood development. One essential blood building nutrient is the trace mineral Cobalt and very few vegetables supply this nutrient. Spinach is a good source.
VITAMIN E	
OTHER NUTRIENTS	Spinach is also an excellent source of the following nutrients: chlorine — regulates the correct balance of acid and alkali in the blood, silicon — growth of hair and improved blood circulation, sodium — keeps other blood minerals soluble and regulates acid alkaline levels of the blood. Spinach are also an excellent source of vitamin A — blood formation and maintenance of good eyesight, vitamin B6 — production of antibodies and red blood cells, folic acid — required in the formation of haemoglobin and blood cells, biotin — digestion of fats, weight control and growth of children.
OXALIC ACID	Spinach, compared to other vegetables has a high oxalic acid content — .9 grams per 100 grams. The potent nutrient composition of Spinach must assist elimination of this impurity as recent reports have shown that there is no excess accumulation of oxalic acid within the kidneys after ingestion of raw Spinach juice. It has been suggested that it would take an excessive intake of cooked Spinach to cause such disorders as kidney stones. Regular use of raw vegetables in association with Spinach will surely prevent any excess build-up of oxalic acid. If you now hesitate to use Spinach, other foods such as chocolate, rhubarb, white flour, sugar, tea, coffee and other alcoholic drinks can all lead to the development of kidney stones. Chocolate and Rhubarb are very rich in oxalic acid. Raw Spinach is safe to use anytime.

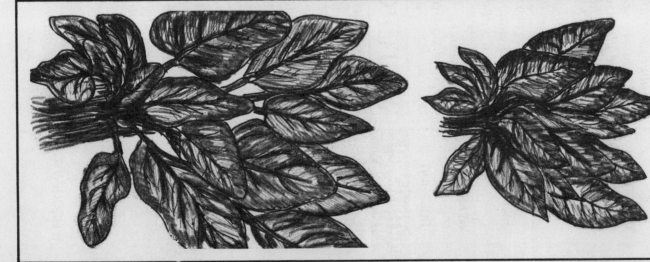

CHLOROPHYL – INTRODUCTION

CHLOROPHYL is the name used to describe the liquid substance that is found in all living plant matter. The word Chlorophyl is derived from two Greek words; Knloros – green, Phullon – leaf. Chlorophyl is produced by a process known as; PHOTO-SYNTHESIS, that is derived from three Greek words: Phos – light, Syn – sun, Thesis – developing. There are three main ingredients that are required to initiate the process of Photosynthesis, they are: SUNLIGHT, WATER and CARBON DIOXIDE.

All forms of plantlife (sea and land) are dependant on the combination of those three main elements for development and growth. Apart from the sunlight, water and carbon dioxide, some plants also utilize the elements from the soil or sea to promote their development and most important of all, they convert inorganic substances into the form of organic compounds. The Plant Kingdom provides the essential link for human nutritional requirements. The human body is unable to survive without the assistance of some plant life. When a plant obtains elements from the soil, it purifies those elements along the entire root system, stem and leaves. Without this 'purifying' and transformation of earthly elements into the form of organic compounds, by plant life, the human body could not survive. All forms of human food, natural foods, secondary produce such as: eggs, milk, cheese, meat, poultry and seafood and the majority of processed, refined and other so called 'unnatural foods', have at one time, developed with the assistance from the plant kingdom.

During this present stage of food technology, certain chemical elements may be included with some 'man made foods', those chemical elements have not developed through the process of Photosynthesis, they are classed as 'inorganic substances' and should definately be avoided in order to maintain maximum nutrition and to protect against any adverse effects that could be associated with either a minimal or prolonged intake of such inorganic chemical substances. In view of the fact that there is an increasing array of processed, refined and chemically loaded foods and drinks available throughout the majority of cities around the world and possibly one such 'processed food store' within walking distance from your home, you should take great caution before buying any packaged food item, check the label and find out exactly what chemicals may have been added to that food product. The most common additives are described as: preservatives, colouring, added salt, emulsifyers, added sugar and flavourings to mention a few. There are near 2,000 specific additives that are commonly used by the food industry today and it is estimated that the average consumption per person is between three to five pounds of chemical substance every year. There is a common guide which you could consider to be well worthwhile in practice, that is, 'the people who work at that food factory will hesitate to eat that food'. Find out from a friend, if that food is loaded with chemicals and subjected to various deteriorating processes, the answer is usually, 'I would not eat it'.

Many processed foods require a determined effort on behalf of the advertising companies, to sell. Once you have been convinced by the advertisement, about the quality of the advertising presentation, it's eye appeal and musical support, you may well be on the way to buy one such product. There is no doubt that some of those 'food advertisements' are hard to resist and even more to the point, the food itself may be so well loaded with the right chemical ingredients and associated sugar and fat content that you may within even a few hours, crave for another such food product.

Whatever amount of chemical substance you may intake per year, you can be sure that at one time or another, your body will have to eliminate those harmful toxic substances, or, be eliminated. Throughout your local town, you may often hear about those people who have 'another cold' or virus infection. The human body is designed to work at maximum efficiency and when the build-up of toxic residue (chemicals, food additives, nicotene, environmental pollutants, etcetera) within the body, is at a certain level, elimination of those substances will take place. Daily use of fresh vegetables and fruits is the best way to ensure that your body is capable of efficient cleansing and thereby protect against the occurrence of sickness. Within the city environment, it is near impossible to avoid the effects of car exhaust pollution and factory fumes, they can be a major contributing factor towards the development of sickness and to ensure that your body will eliminate those toxic substances, there is no better medicine than freshly prepared vegetable and fruit juices. Throughout the section on Fruits, pp. 44–61, and Vegetables, pp. 62–79, there is valuable information to assist you in understanding the individual and unique benefits that are associated with over 50 of the most delicious Natural foods. Both fruits and vegetables are the best natural source of the 'sunshine liquid'—Chlorophyl.

The most rewarding way to regain and maintain maximum health potential is to regularly prepare freshly extracted fruit and vegetable juices. If you are not accustomed to preparing such wonderful drinks, you may require a short starting off time to experience the full benefit and delicious combinations that are available, with the assistance of a juice extractor. Once you have obtained a good quality juice extractor, the satisfying variety of Chlorophyl based drinks: fruit and vegetable juices, will provide you with a new range of delicious, exciting and most healthful liquid refreshments, that you will find to be far less expensive than the commercially produced variety and most important of all, freshly made fruit and vegetable juices contain life supporting enzymes. All forms of commercial drinks are deficient in enzyme activity and without enzymes, the body metabolism will degenerate, leading the way to overweight conditions, regular sickness and a general lack of physical and mental energy. When taken regularly, home made fruit and vegetable juices will restore your body metabolism to a state of maximum efficiency.

CHLOROPHYL – LIQUID LIFE

Both a juice extractor and a blender are the best investment for your health and they could easily replace the kitchen stove and oven routine that so many people use for the preparation of those tasty lifeless meals. Your health is dependant on the life elements from the plant kingdom and not from the destructive influence of heat and cooking. A well balanced diet should supply over 70% raw foods and with the assistance of both a juicer and blender, the taste of those 'raw foods' can be greatly enhanced to assist you in obtaining delicious drinks and complete meals.

For those people who may hesitate to get accustomed to a new experience of freshly made juices, it would be of benefit to realize the following points: all forms of cooked foods are deficient in enzymes, freshly made juices will provide a balance in restoring those essential enzymes. Preparation time for a fruit or vegetable juice is far less than a cup of coffee, you will have more time and far more effective stimulation from a freshly made juice than from a cup of coffee. The expense of a freshly made fruit or vegetable juice is on average, less than half the price of a commercially prepared fruit juice. Freshly made juices will supply a major portion of the essential daily nutrients: calcium, phosphorus, potassium, sulphur, chlorine, sodium, fluorine, magnesium, iron, manganese, silicon, copper, iodine, vitamins: A, C, E, B1, B2, B3, B5, B6, B15, biotin, choline, folic acid p.a.b.a. and vitamins: K, U and P. All of those nutrients are obtainable from a combination of fruit and vegetable juices and compared to any vitamin or mineral tablet, freshly made juices are far more effective, due to the 'balanced supply' of associated nutrients and the abundance of enzymes. Also, compared to the expense of vitamin or mineral tablets, freshly made juices (fruit juice in the morning, vegetable juice for lunch and a blended fruit drink for an evening treat) will ensure that you obtain not only the essential daily mineral and vitamin requirements but also a main portion of your daily carbohydrate — energy supply and a good amount of protein, depending on the type of juices obtained, in fact, it is possible to obtain all your daily protein requirements from a combination of carrot, lettuce and parsley juice without overloading the body with excess fluid. Other types of blended drinks such as a combination of apple juice, banana, almonds and tahini will supply excellent amounts of protein, two glasses will supply your daily protein requirements.

The illustration on the right shows the chemical composition of Chlorophyl and Hemin-whole blood. The remarkable similarity between the two life-liquids, one from plants, the other from humans, gives us the opportunity to directly improve the quality of our blood and by obtaining regular amounts of Chlorophyl foods and drinks, our health and lives will be based on the best nutrition – Chlorophyl.

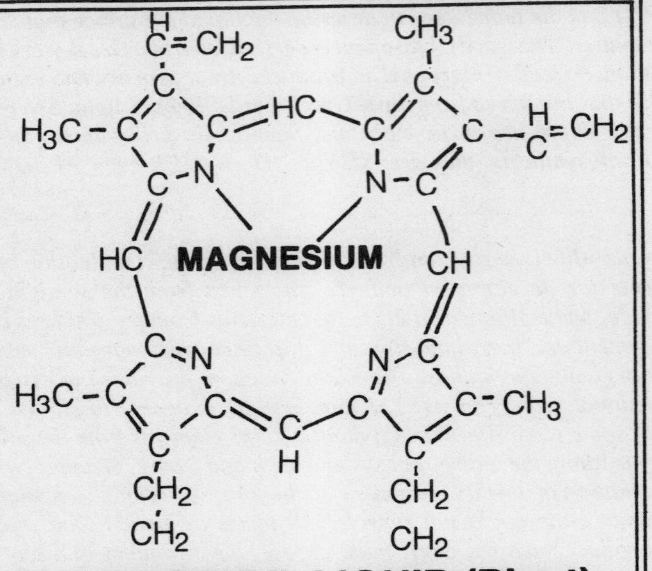

CHLOROPHYL LIQUID (Plant)

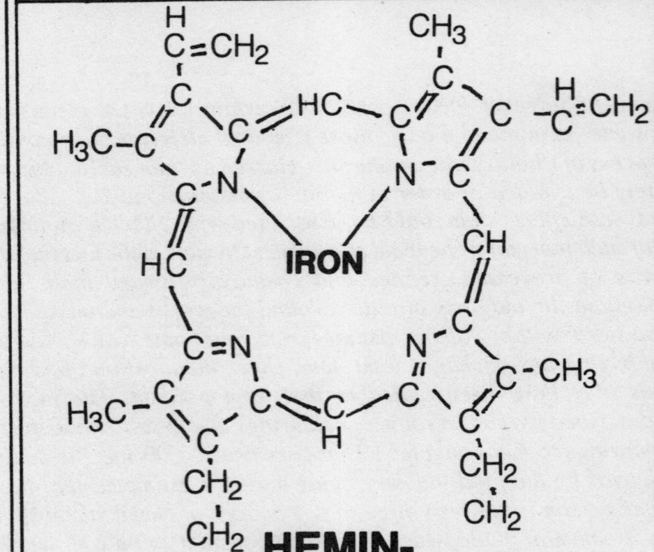

MAGNESIUM

HEMIN- WHOLE BLOOD (Human)

IRON

VEGETABLES NUTRIENT COMPOSITION CHART

ALL AMOUNTS ARE FOR 100 Gramms Aprox.	CALORIES	CARBOHYDRATES	PROTEIN	FAT	CALCIUM	PHOSPHORUS	POTASSIUM	IRON	SODIUM	MAGNESIUM	COPPER	MANGANESE	ZINC	A.	C.	E.	B1	B2	B3	B5	B6	BIOTIN	FOLIC ACID
Asparagus	26	5.1	2.5	.2	22	63	281	1.0	2.2	20	.11	.19	.98	915	33	1.9	.18	.20	.15	.15	.17	.50	.06
Beetroot	43	10	.07	1.6	16	34	349	.67	60	23	.22	.95	.05	22	10	na.	.03	.05	na.	.15	.05	na.	.09
Green Beans	30	7	.18	2.0	56	42	250	.7	6	30	.24	.40	.3	600	18	.08	.07	.10	.4	.16	.06	na.	.04
Broccoli	32	5.9	3.6	.3	103	78	382	1.1	15	24	.03	.15	.2	2500	113	na.	.1	.23	.9	1.1	.19	na.	.06
Brussel Sprouts	45	8.3	4.9	.4	36	80	390	1.5	14	29	.05	.27	.38	550	102	1	.1	.16	.9	.72	.23	.4	.07
Cabbage Cooked	20	4.2	.2	1.1	43	20	160	.27	14	15	.09	na.	.4	130	.32	na.	.04	.04	.27	na.	na.	na.	.01
Carrots raw	42	9.7	1.1	.2	37		341	.7	47	23	.15	.1	.4	11,000	8	.45	.06	.05	.6	.28	.15	2	.03
Cauliflower	28	5.2	2.7	.2	25	56	295	1.1	13	24	.15	.17	.37	80	69	.15	.11	.1	.8	.64	.21	1.5	.05
Chives	30	6	2	tr	70	40	250	2	tr	30	.11	na.	na.	5,800	60	na.	.08	.13	1	na.	.18	na.	na.
Celery	16	3.9	.08	.08	39	29	340	.38	126	21	.14	.16	.13	266	9	.47	.03	.03	.3	.43	.06	.10	.01
Cucumber	15	3.5	.8	.09	25	27	160	1.1	5.8	11	.08	.14	.21	250	11	8.2	.03	.04	.18	.24	.04	.09	.01
Garlic	96	128	6.4	1.2	32	192	512	1	32	32	.25	na.	1	20	.32	na.	.32	.1	.1	na.	na.	na.	.01
Lettuce	15	2.6	1.3	.18	36	26	280	2.0	9	9	.15	.7	.5	1000	7	.40	.05	.05	.38	.2	.05	.68	.04
Leek	52	11	2.2	.3	52	50	347	1.1	5	23	.09		na.	40	17	1	.11	.06	.5	.12	.2	1.4	na.
Onions	37	8.9	1.7	.15	27	36	160	.54	10	12	.15	.36	.36	42	10	.26	.03	.04	.18	.13	.13	.91	.02
Parsley	43	8.5	3.6	1.5	203	63	726	6.1	45	40	.48	.93	na.	8,500	171	na.	1.1	na.		.30	.16	.4	.11
Peas	98	16	7.3	.48	31	140	370	2.3	2.7	41	.27		9	750	31	2.5	.42	.16	3.4	.89	.17	na.	.02
Pepper-Capsicum	22	4.7	1.2	.16	8.6	22	212	.7	12	18	.16	na.	.06	425	127	na.	.07	.07	.5	.23	.26	na.	.02
Potatoes raw	76	17	2.2	.13	7.5	53	407	.6	3.3	na.	na.	na.	na.	tr	20	na.	.10	.04	1.0	.06	na.	na.	1.6
Pumpkin	33	7.8	1.0	.28	25		240	.4	2	32	.1	.2	na.	6,344	5	na.	.03	.05	.6	.04	.05	na.	.01
Radish	19	4.2	.9	.1	35	26	180	.6	16	14	.13	.05	.26	10	32	na.	.03	.02	.4	.18	.06	na.	.02
Watercress	21	3.3	2.4	.3	159	57	297	1.8	54	19	.1	.56	na.	5,160	84	na.	.09	.18	.9	.32	.13	.42	.05
Eggplant-cooked	19	5.8	1	.2	11	21	150	.6	1	14	.1	.11	na.	10	3	na.	.05	.04	.05	.2	.06	na.	.01
Parsnips	76	17	1.7	.5	50	77	541	.7	12	32	.1	.2	na.	30	16	na.	.08	.09	.2	.6	.09	.1	.06
Kale	38	6	4.2	.8	179	73	318	2.2	75	37	.09	.5	.26	8,900	125	8	.16	.26	2	1	.3	.5	.06
Lotus root	69	15	2.8	.1	4	81	290	.6	11	7	1	.05	.9	0	2	.58	.14	.01	2.9	1.5	na.	11	.01
Artichoke	44	9.9	2.8	.2	51	69	301	1.1	30	na.	.2	.36	.35	150	8	na.	.07	.04	.7	na.	na.	na.	.05
Collards	40	7.2	3.6	.7	203	63	401	1	43	57	na.	na.	na.	6,500	92	na.	.2	.31	1.7	.2	.06	na.	.1
Dandelion greens	45	9.2	2.7	.7	187	66	397	3.1	76	36	.15	.3	na.	14,000	35	na.	.19	.26	na.	na.	na.	na.	na.
Spinach	26	4.5	3.4	.3	100	54	500	3.2	75	80	.60	.8	1	8,900	56	2.5	.11	.2	.5	.30	.25	7	.21

CHAPTER THREE

PROTEIN

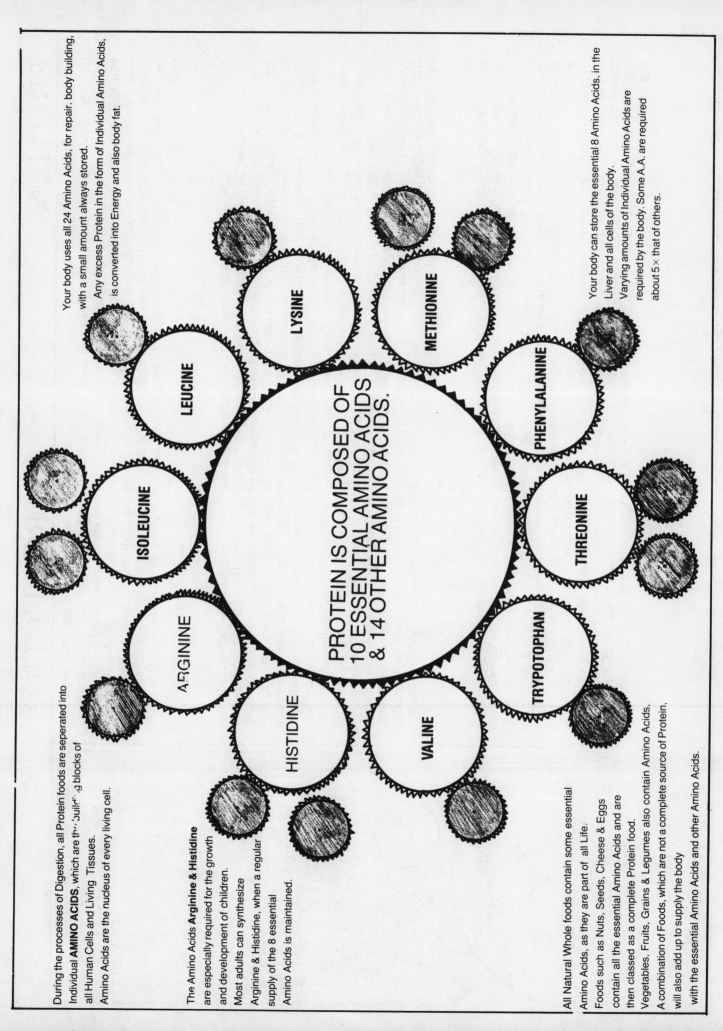

During the processes of Digestion, all Protein foods are seperated into Individual **AMINO ACIDS,** which are the building blocks of all Human Cells and Living Tissues.
Amino Acids are the nucleus of every living cell.

The Amino Acids **Arginine & Histidine** are especially required for the growth and development of children.
Most adults can synthesize Arginine & Histidine, when a regular supply of the 8 essential Amino Acids is maintained.

All Natural Whole foods contain some essential Amino Acids, as they are part of all Life.
Foods such as Nuts, Seeds, Cheese & Eggs contain all the essential Amino Acids and are then classed as a complete Protein food.
Vegetables, Fruits, Grains & Legumes also contain Amino Acids, which are not a complete source of Protein, will also add up to supply the body with the essential Amino Acids and other Amino Acids.

Your body uses all 24 Amino Acids, for repair, body building, with a small amount always stored.
Any excess Protein in the form of Individual Amino Acids, is converted into Energy and also body fat.

Your body can store the essential 8 Amino Acids, in the Liver and all cells of the body.
Varying amounts of Individual Amino Acids are required by the body. Some A.A. are required about $5\times$ that of others.

PROTEIN IS COMPOSED OF 10 ESSENTIAL AMINO ACIDS & 14 OTHER AMINO ACIDS.

LYSINE

METHIONINE

LEUCINE

PHENYLALANINE

ISOLEUCINE

THREONINE

ARGININE

TRYPOTOPHAN

HISTIDINE

VALINE

81

PROTEIN

INTRODUCTION

PROTEIN was first discovered in the late 1830's and at that time it was described as being the most important food substance, the name 'protein' was given and that is derived from a Greek word meaning primary or 'to take first place'. Since that time, scientists have discovered that the large protein molecule is made up from numerous smaller elements and these have been termed AMINO ACIDS. The word amino is given to describe a nitrogen-containing compound — 'amine', also the word amino is used to describe a base or alkali substance. A protein molecule is made up from both alkali and acid elements. The nitrogen contained within a protein molecule is required to combine both the acid and alkali elements together and that enables the formation or building of body cells, tissues, organs and complete living creatures. Half the dry matter of an adult human is made up from amino acids.

AMINO ACIDS are the foundation of all protein, Amino Acids are composed from the following elements: carbon, hydrogen, oxygen and nitrogen, some Amino Acid structures also contain sulphur, phosphorus and iron. The main difference between a protein and a carbohydrate molecule is the presence of nitrogen within the protein molecule, carbohydrates contain only carbon, hydrogen and oxygen. All protein and carbohydrates are formed by the plant kingdom, proteins (amino acids) are developed by the following process: certain microbes (soil living bacteria) absorb nitrogen from the atmosphere, converting it into a form that plants can use, all amino acids require nitrogen for their development. The atmosphere is composed of 80% nitrogen. In combination with the energy from the sun, water and atmosphere, plants have the ability to transform those elements from the soil into all forms of human food: amino acids, glucose, fatty acids, minerals and vitamins. All animals must rely on plant life for their nutrition. When food is obtained directly from plants, it is termed primary produce, food that is obtained from animal origin is termed secondary produce, the animal converts those plant elements into a concentrated store of nutrients, mainly proteins (amino acids) and Lipids (fats and oils), the carbohydrate food group is obtained directly from plant source: fruits, vegetables, whole grains and legumes, they contain all three main food groups: carbohydrates, proteins and lipids. Some plants such as grains and legumes store good amounts of both amino acids and carbohydrates, fruits and vegetables store mainly carbohydrates and a minimum amount of protein. All foods contain amino acids and carbohydrates, they are the basis of plant life.

ESSENTIAL AMINO ACIDS are those required for the maintenance of human life and they must be supplied with the diet. For adults, there are 8 essential amino acids, children need 10 amino acids to be supplied with their diet, all the essential amino acids are obtainable from the following food groups: whole grains, legumes, nuts, seeds, eggs, cheese, dairy products, meat, poultry and fish. On the following pages there is a list of all the essential amino acids and their associated bodily functions. Apart from the essential amino acids, there are another 14 amino acids and these can be prepared by the body when all the 8 essential amino acids are supplied with the diet. All concentrated protein foods will supply both the essential amino acids and a fair range of the other 14 amino acids. The following is a list of all the essential amino acids: ISOLEUCINE, LEUCINE, LYSINE, METHIONINE, PHENYLALANINE, THREONINE, TRYPTOPHAN, and VALINE. For infants, the amino acid HISTIDINE is also essential. The other non-essential amino acids are manufactured by the body, where the essential amino acids are obtained from the diet. The non-essential amino acids are: GLYCINE, GLUTAMIC ACID, ARGININE, ASPARTIC ACID, PROLINE, ALANINE, SERINE, TYROSINE, CYSTEINE, ASPARAGINE, GLUTAMINE, HYDROXYPROLINE and CITRULLINE.

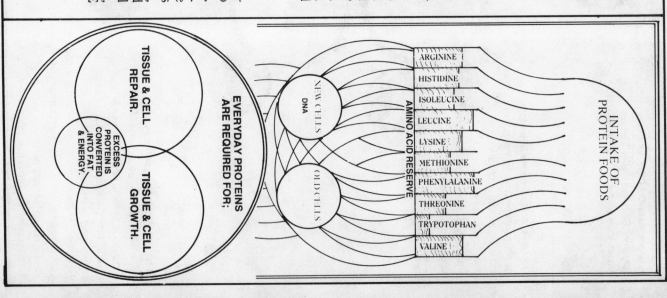

ESSENTIAL AMINO ACIDS

PROTEIN

TRYPOTOPHAN: $C_{11}H_{12}N_2O_2$
- required for healthy skin and hair condition.
- promotes growth of cells and body tissues.
- assists in the production of gastric juices.
- regulates sleep and mood patterns.
- transfer of chemical messages (seratonin) from the brain to the pituitary gland.
- nourishes and promotes optic system functions.
- assists in blood coagulation – clotting.

TRYPOTOPHAN NATURAL FOOD SOURCE:
avocado, banana, dates, figs, grapefruit, oranges, papaya, peach, pear, persimmon, pineapple, strawberry, tomato.
ALL VEGETABLES.
ALL GRAINS. ALL LEGUMES.
ALL NUTS except pistachio. ALL SEEDS.

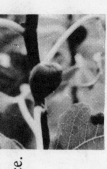

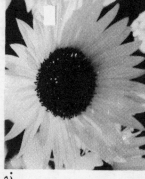

VALINE: $C_5H_{11}NO_2$
- required for glandular functions.
- essential for the nervous system.
- required for normal growth of cells.

VALINE NATURAL FOOD SOURCE:
apple, apricot, dates, figs, peach, pear, persimmon, strawberries, tomato.
ALL VEGETABLES except celery and lettuce.
ALL GRAINS. ALL LEGUMES.
ALL NUTS. ALL SEEDS.

THREONINE: $C_4H_9NO_3$
- works in combination with other amino acids to improve nutrient absorption.
- required for new cell development.

THREONINE NATURAL FOOD SOURCE:
apple, apricot, dates, figs, peach, pear, persimmon, strawberry, tomato.
ALL VEGETABLES except celery and lettuce.
ALL GRAINS. ALL LEGUMES.
ALL NUTS. ALL SEEDS.

LEUCINE: $C_6H_{13}NO_2$
- compliments the functions of isoleucine.
- required for blood development.
- regulates digestion and metabolism.
- assists the functions of the glandular system.

LEUCINE NATURAL FOOD SOURCE:
apple, apricot, dates, figs, peach, pear, persimmon, strawberry, tomato.
ALL VEGETABLES except celery, lettuce and radish.
ALL GRAINS. ALL LEGUMES.
ALL NUTS. ALL SEEDS.

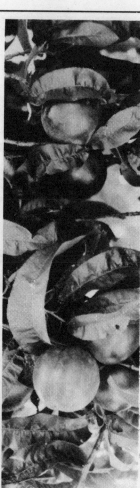

PHENYLALANINE $C_9H_{11}NO_2$
- essential for production of adrenalin.
- promotes vitamin C absorption.
- assists the secretion of thyroxine – hormone.
- assists the functions of the kidneys and gall bladder, elimination of waste.
- assists in the formation of skin and hair pigment and hormone – melanin.

PHENYLALANINE NATURAL FOOD SOURCE:
apple, apricot, dates, figs, peach, pear, persimmon, strawberry, tomato.
ALL VEGETABLES except celery, lettuce and radish.
ALL GRAINS. ALL LEGUMES.
ALL NUTS. ALL SEEDS.

ESSENTIAL AMINO ACIDS

METHIONINE: $C_5H_{11}NO_2$
– controls fat levels of the blood.
– required for blood – haemoglobin development.
– is the main limiting amino acid, very few foods supply sufficient amounts of methinone.
– promotes digestion and metabolism of fats.

METHIONINE NATURAL FOOD SOURCE:
apple, apricot, avocado, banana, cantaloupe, dates, figs, oranges, papaya, peach, pear, persimmon, pineapple, strawberry, tomato.
ALL VEGETABLES.
ALL GRAINS. ALL LEGUMES.
ALL NUTS. ALL SEEDS.

HISTIDINE: $C_6H_9N_3O_2$
– essential for growth of children.
– required in the formation of glycogen.
– a vital component of blood.
– helps to control the mucus levels of the respiratory and digestive system.

HISTIDINE NATURAL FOOD SOURCE:
apple, pineapple, papaya.
ALL VEGETABLES except celery, radish and turnips.
ALL GRAINS. ALL LEGUMES.
ALL NUTS. ALL SEEDS.

ARGININE: $C_6H_{14}N_2O_2$
– essential for growth of children.
– assists in nitrogen elimination.
– required for muscle contraction.
– controls body cell degenerations.
– required for cell reproduction.

ARGININE NATURAL FOOD SOURCE:
apple, apricot, peach, strawberry, berries, pineapple, tomato.
ALL VEGETABLES except celery and turnips.
ALL GRAINS. ALL LEGUMES.
ALL NUTS. ALL SEEDS.

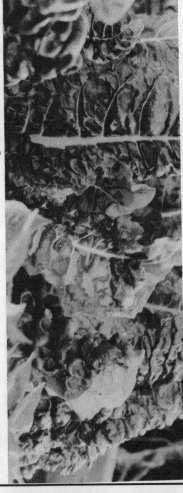

ISOLEUCINE: $C_6H_{13}NO_2$
– required for blood development.
– assists digestion and metabolism.
– maintains correct nitrogen levels.
– regulates the functions of the thymus, spleen and pituitary gland.
– essential for growth.

ISOLEUCINE NATURAL FOOD SOURCE:
apple, apricot, dates, figs, peach, pear, persimmon, strawberry, tomato.
ALL VEGETABLES except celery, lettuce and radish.
ALL GRAINS. ALL LEGUMES.
ALL NUTS. ALL SEEDS.

LYSINE: $C_6H_{14}N_4O_2$
– assists digestion and storage of fats.
– regulates the pineal and mammary glands.
– controls acid-alkaline blood levels.
– essential for all amino acid assimilation.
– regulates the functions of the gall bladder.

LYSINE NATURAL FOOD SOURCE:
apple, apricot, avocado, banana, cantaloupe, dates, figs, grapefruit, oranges, papaya, peach, pear, persimmon, pineapple, strawberry, tomato.
ALL VEGETABLES except mushrooms.
ALL GRAINS. ALL LEGUMES.
ALL NUTS. ALL SEEDS.

DIGESTION

PROTEIN

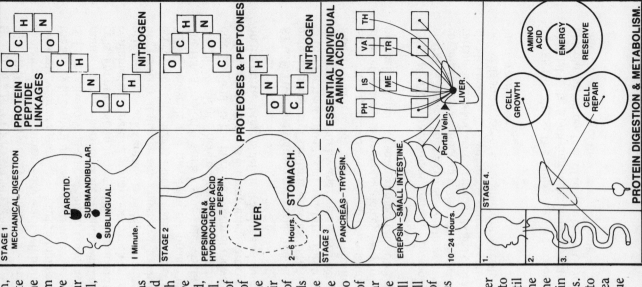

STAGE ONE: Protein foods (all foods) are initially prepared into smaller particles by Mechanical Digestion — mouth, teeth, jaws, tongue and the salivary secretions, all work together to convert a solid mass of food into a semi-liquid mass. Adequate chewing of concentrated protein foods (meat, poultry, nuts and seeds) is essential, as 'the stomach has no teeth'. Only the smallest particles of food that enter the stomach will receive proper attention, larger particles will only obtain a minimum preparation around the outside portion of the food mass. Proper chewing of food is the first and most important digestive process and the only one time that you have complete control. From now on, chew your food properly and you will do your stomach a great favour, your digestive health will improve and you can obtain over twice the food value from the same meal, if you chew more often. Relax and enjoy more.

STAGE TWO: Food passes from the mouth to the stomach by a series of involuntary muscular movements known as Peristalsis, that takes place within the Oesophagus, a muscular tube with an average length of 20-25 cm. When a concentrated protein food enters the stomach, special digestive enzymes will be prepared by the multitude of cells within the stomach lining. There are two main protein digestive enzymes, they are Pepsinogen and Gastric Hydrochloric acid. These two digestive enzymes take at least half an hour to become effective, they also require a considerable amount of energy to be produced, that often shows as a temporary spell of inactivity after eating a concentrated protein food, especially a meat or poultry meal. When the two enzymes combine, the hydrochloric acid acts as a catalyst upon the pepsinogen, converting it into the form of Pepsin, the main enzyme produced by the stomach for the conversion of proteins — 'peptide linkages' into the form of 'proteoses and peptones' (see illustration). This process of protein conversion can take up to six hours preparation within the stomach and for some people that means they have had a satisfying meal. To the contrary, for all that effort to obtain their daily protein requirements and with the numerous disadvantages associated with the toxic residue from the digestion of meat, the body could not be satisfied, only exhausted (see pp. 114–116 for details). Other protein foods such as nuts and seeds require only a minimum amount of preparation within the stomach, they also require less concentrated amounts of the protein digestive enzyme — pepsin and they supply an abundance of essential nutrients to enhance the digestion of the protein foods. Animal protein foods (meat, poultry, cheese, eggs and fish) are termed as pre-formed proteins and they have to be re-converted into the form of living protein, that requires enzymes, the body must supply these enzymes from the intake of living foods (fresh fruits, vegetables, sprouted seeds, grains and legumes). To be sure of obtaining positive health, the regular meat eater must intake an abundant supply of live foods, otherwise the body metabolism will become sluggish, leading the way to overweight conditions and lack of physical and mental energy. Another common mistake that so many people are well adjusted to is the combining of excess liquid with their protein meals, that is most detrimental as those excess liquids will dilute the essential protein digestive enzymes, leading the way to very poor protein preparation and during the next stage of protein conversion — absorption, those poorly prepared protein elements will enter the bloodstream and cause numerous health risks.

STAGE THREE: After the protein (proteoses and peptide linkages) leave the stomach, they travel slowly into the upper section of the small intestine. At this stage, two new enzymes assist in the conversion of proteoses and peptide linkages into the form of 'short-chain peptides'. The liver produces an alkaline liquid termed Bile, that is stored in the gall bladder until required for protein conversion. The pancreas produces the enzyme — Trypsin, both enzymes, Bile and Trypsin convert the proteoses and peptides into short-chain peptides. The final stage of protein conversion to take place within the small intestine is performed along the Jejunum and Illeum, the tail end of the small intestine. The enzyme produced here is called — Erepsin and this completes the digestive cycle by converting the short-chain peptides into the form of water-soluble Amino Acids. These Amino acids are then absorbed through the walls of the small intestine, enter the bloodstream and are transported to the liver, via the portal vein. The liver removes the Nitrogen containing portion from the Amino acids, converting it into urea and that is taken to the kidneys and excreted with the urine. Amino acids are now free to perform the vital functions of tissue and cell development and repair and also to maintain a specific Amino acid balance, controlled mainly by the liver.

D.N.A. - R.N.A.   PROTEIN

DEVELOPMENT OF NEW CELLS:

STAGE ONE: During every moment of life, your body replaces old cells and builds new cells. Numerous billions of cells are contained in the human body, each cell being formed from a combination of nutrients: proteins, carbohydrates, lipids, minerals, vitamins and water. Apart from those main nutrients, there are special molecules known as hormones, they have the ability to control the rate of activity around and within the cell's activity such as the adrenalin hormone, others like the pituitary hormones control growth over a few years and numerous other hormones are produced within the body, all having their unique bodily functions and relationship with body cells. For new cells to be formed there must be a suitable balance and supply of Protein — (amino acids), these amino acids are contained in all natural primary foods such as: fruits, vegetables, grains, legumes, nuts and seeds, and concentrated amounts of these amino acids are also available from animal produce: meat, poultry, eggs, cheese and fish. Cells are the simple form of life, however, it still remains a mystery as to what initiates a cell to develop into a complete form of life. Within the structure of every living cell there is a secret code, that is stored in the so-called D.N.A. molecule (deoxyribonucleic acid). Every cell has a D.N.A. molecule and they have the unique ability of issuing instructions for the reproduction of identical new cells. The D.N.A. molecule sends it's messages via the R.N.A. (ribonucleic acid) to the outer boundaries of the cell — (cytoplasm) — (see illustration.) There is a constant flow of nutrients around the outer boundaries of cells, those nutrients are products of digestion and via the intricate system of the veins, arteries and capillaries, nutrients are transported throughout the entire body. If a persons diet is deficient in any particular nutrient, cells may be unable to form as nature planned, the result depends on the nutrient that is deficient and the amount of time with that particular deficiency.

STAGE TWO: Individual amino acids and all other nutrients (glucose, fatty acids, minerals and vitamins) combine at the outer boundaries of a cell and when the D.N.A. requests a particular nutrient, the R.N.A. messanger will assist in the transfer of that nutrient into the cell structure. This transfer of nutrients is extremely intricate and when you consider that it occurs every moment of your life and millions of times per day, you may be inclined to respect your body in a more nutritious way. All food that enters the body should be obtained directly from the natural source, those chemically formulated foods, preservatives, refined foods and other unnatural ingredients that are manufactured and combined with man-made foods will all be considered as poor nutrition by every living cell of the body. The nutrients that are supplied by natural whole foods are precisely balanced to ensure proper cell nutrition.

CELL NUTRITION: Carbohydrates are composed of carbon, hydrogen and oxygen as well as glucose, minerals and vitamins, energy is formed when a cell absorbs those carbohydrate nutrients and then arranges the exact ingredient mixture to create combustion or burning up of the carbohydrate fuel, that is called oxidation and the waste products of that combustion are carbon dioxide and water. Lipids (fats and oils) are also composed of carbon, hydrogen and oxygen as well as fatty acids, these are also used as fuel within the structure of the cell. Proteins (amino acids) provide the building material to assist growth of new cells and repair or replacement of old cells. All three main groups: Carbohydrates, Proteins and Lipids are required for the life of a cell.

TYPES OF CELLS: The human body is composed from six main groups of cells, they are: Nerve cells, Blood cells, Muscle cells, Skeletal cells, Epithelium cells and Connective cells (see illustration.) All of the six main groups of cells require slightly different nutrition, they all require carbon, hydrogen and oxygen as well as glucose, amino acids and fatty acids but they need different amounts of these essential minerals and vitamins. Natural foods are the only source of every nutrient.

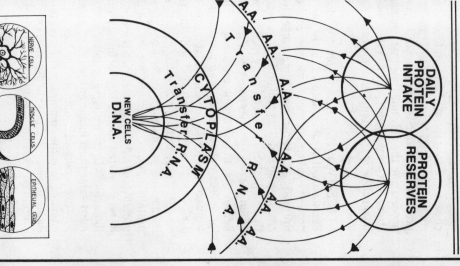

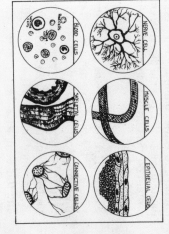

PROTEIN % CONTENT. — Chart One

Food	Protein %	Food	Protein %
Barley	12	Human milk	1
Buckwheat flour	11	Goat milk	3
Corn flour	8	Cows milk	3
Pearl Millet	11	Evaporated milk	7
Oats	14	Buttermilk	3
Rice-brown	7	Dry non-fat milk	35
Rye flour	12	Camembert	17
Sorghum	11	Cheddar cheese	25
Wheat	14	Cottage cheese	17
Wheat germ	25	Cream cheese	9
Black Gram	23	Parmesan	36
Broad beans	25	Swiss	26
Chick peas	20	Eggs	12
Cowpeas	22	Egg white	10
Pinto beans	23	Egg yolk	16
Lentils	25	Sirloin steak	17
Lupine beans	32	Lamb	18
Mung beans	24	Pork	14
Peanuts	26	Ham	15
Kidney bean	22	Bacon	9
Soya beans	34	Rabbit	21
Soya flour	44	Chicken	21
Almonds	18	Duck	21
Brazil	14	Porterhouse	16
Cashew	18	Sausage	14
Hazel	12	Salami	23
Walnuts	15	Cod	22
Pumpkin seeds	30	Flounder	28
Safflower seeds	42	Haddock	24
Sesame seeds	19	Turkey	24
Sunflower seeds	23	Beef	18
Brewers yeast	46	Coconut meal	20

Chart Two — ESSENTIAL AMINO ACIDS

Food	TRY.	LEU.	LYS.	MET.	PHA.	ISL.	VAL.	THR.
barley	160	889	433	184	661	545	643	433
corn	61	1296	288	186	454	462	510	389
millet	248	1746	383	270	506	635	682	456
oats	183	1065	521	209	758	733	845	470
RICE	82	646	296	135	377	352	524	294
rye	137	813	494	191	571	515	631	448
wheat	173	939	384	214	691	607	648	403
chick pea	170	1538	1434	276	1012	1195	1025	739
kidney bean	214	1985	1715	233	1275	1312	1401	1002
lentils	216	1760	1528	180	1104	1316	1360	896
lima	195	1722	1378	331	1222	1199	1298	980
soya bean	526	2946	2414	513	1889	2054	2005	1504
almonds	176	1454	582	259	1146	873	1124	610
brazil	187	1129	443	941	617	593	823	422
cashew	471	1522	792	353	946	1222	1592	737
hazel	211	939	417	139	537	853	934	415
pecan	138	773	435	153	564	553	525	389
pistachio	0	1520	1080	370	1090	880	1340	610
walnuts	175	1228	441	306	767	767	974	589
pumpkin seed	560	2437	1411	577	1749	1737	1679	933
sesame seed	331	1679	583	637	1457	951	885	707
sunflower seed	343	1736	868	443	1220	1276	1354	911
cheddar	341	2437	1834	650	1340	1685	1794	929
egg	211	1126	819	401	739	850	950	637
milk	49	344	272	86	170	233	240	162
yoghurt	37	336	282	78	180	214	255	160
tuna	290	2178	2556	842	1074	1481	1554	1249
beef porterhouse	192	1343	1433	407	674	858	911	724
chicken	250	1490	1810	537	811	1088	1012	877
lamb	233	1394	1457	432	732	923	887	824
turkey	0	1836	2173	664	960	1260	1187	1014
wheat germ	265	1708	1534	404	908	1177	1364	1343

NET PROTEIN UTILIZATION: (N.P.U.%).

30 — Lentils.
36 — Mung bean sprouts.
38 — Other Legumes: navy, pea bean, white bean.
39 — Gluten flour.
42 — Black bean.
43 — Peanut, Peanut butter, Chick pea.
45 — Turnip greens, Collards, Whole wheat bread, Cow peas, Mustard greens.
47 — Peas.
48 — Broad bean.
50 — Spinach, Chard, Brazil nut, Walnut, Pignolia nuts, Spaghetti.
52 — Lima bean.
53 — Green peas.
54 — Kale.
55 — Millet, Wheat bran.
56 — Soya sprouts.
58 — Sunflower seeds, Cashews, Rye.
60 — Pumpkin seeds, Bulgur, Squash seeds, Triticale, Wheat, Brussel sprouts, Barley, Potato.
61 — Soya beans, Soya grits, Soya flour.
65 — Tofu, Chicken, Lamb.
66 — Oatmeal.
67 — Wheat germ, Pork, Porterhouse.
69 — Sardines.
70 — Rice, Parmesan cheese, Swiss cheese, Camembert, Edam, Cheddar cheese.
72 — Corn-cob.
75 — Cottage cheese, Tigers milk.
80 — Fish.
82 — Milk – non fat, Milk, Yoghurt.
83 — Egg white.
94 — Egg.

Chart Three

PROTEIN FOOD NUTRIENT CHARTS

Chart One: page 87, left side.
PROTEIN % CONTENT. The foods listed are evaluated by comparing the proportion of Protein with the food, in comparison to the supply of other nutrients: carbohydrates, lipids, minerals, vitamins and water content. The foods with amounts over 30 are to be considered as concentrated protein sources, most foods are valued at between 15-25% protein content and with such foods-drinks as milk, they have a high water content and therefore show a low level of protein % in comparison to the other foods.

Chart Two: page 87, centre.
AVAILABLE ESSENTIAL AMINO ACIDS. As explained on pages 81-86, the body requires a certain pattern of essential amino acids, this chart gives the amount of those essential amino acids obtainable from a wide variety of protein foods. By referring to Chart 5—page 88, you can calculate the amount of protein required in relation to your body weight—kg., and then refer to Chart 2, and select a food group to see the amount of protein obtainable from a 100 gram—3.5 ozs. serve of that food. If one or a few amino acids are undersupplied by that food (limiting amino acids,) you may improve the 'protein availability' by combining another food, which has a better supply of the limiting amino acids (refer to pages 42 and 98 for details).

Chart Three: page 87, right side.
NET PROTEIN UTILIZATION—N.P.U. %. This chart lists the % of usable Protein, based on the individual amino acid requirements in comparison to the supply of amino acids obtainable from those foods listed. The best N.P.U. % is obtainable from eggs, as the pattern of amino acids supplied by eggs is very similar to human protein-amino requirements. Such foods as lentils and mung bean sprouts may provide adequate amounts of most essential amino acids, but, if even one amino acid is low—termed 'limiting amino acid', the N.P.U. % will be greatly reduced.

Chart Four: page 88, top right.
There are 8 vertical blocks, each one represents an amino acid in proportion to human protein requirements. The amino acid—tryptophan is required least and as can be seen from chart 2, most foods supply less amounts of tryptophan in comparison to other amino acids. The supply of essential amino acids obtainable from various foods will often supply similar amounts, in comparison to the amounts required and represented by this chart.

Chart Five: page 88, lower right.
This chart was prepared from information supplied by the American Academy of Sciences—recommended dietary allowance (daily). The top horizontal column lists body weight in kilograms and the vertical column represents milligrams of individual amino acids required for 1 gram of body weight. For example, if your body weight is 70 kg., you would require 210 mg. of tryptophan daily and 700 mg. of methionine etc. By referring your body weight and the required amount of amino acids—mg. to chart 2, you can evaluate the protein potential of the associated food.

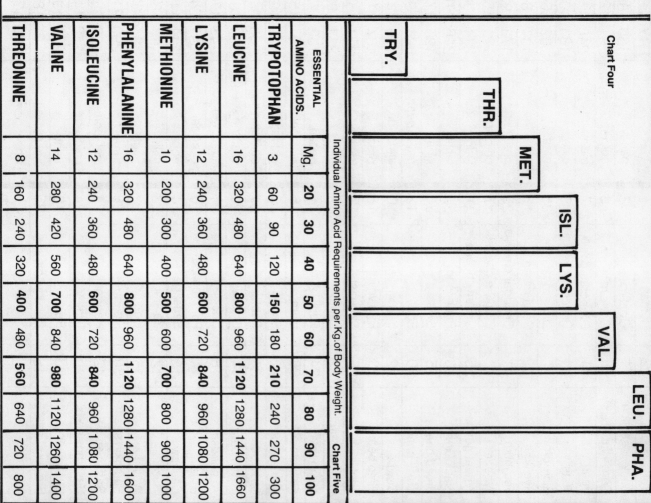

Chart Four

TRY. | THR. | MET. | ISL. | LYS. | VAL. | LEU. | PHA.

Chart Five

ESSENTIAL AMINO ACIDS.	Individual Amino Acid Requirements per Kg. of Body Weight.								
	Mg.	20	30	40	50	60	70	80	90	100
TRYPTOPHAN	3	60	90	120	150	180	210	240	270	300
LEUCINE	16	320	480	640	800	960	1120	1280	1440	1660
LYSINE	12	240	360	480	600	720	840	960	1080	1200
METHIONINE	10	200	300	400	500	600	700	800	900	1000
PHENYLALANINE	16	320	480	640	800	960	1120	1280	1440	1600
ISOLEUCINE	12	240	360	480	600	720	840	960	1080	1200
VALINE	14	280	420	560	700	840	980	1120	1260	1400
THREONINE	8	160	240	320	400	480	560	640	720	800

SOYA BEANS

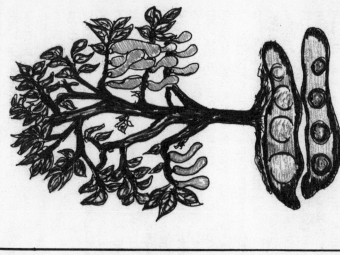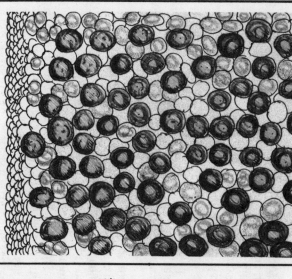

SOYA BEANS have provided people with excellent nutrition for over 4,000 years, the Soya Bean plant is a native of China and it is now cultivated throughout many parts of the world, especially America from where Soya Beans are exported world wide. The Soya Bean provides numerous nutritional benefits and possibly the best recognized of these is the excellent supply of protein. Soya Beans are the most economic source of protein, they supply over twice the protein value of beef, over 3 times that of cheese or eggs and more than 12 times the protein value of cows milk. Apart from supplying over twice the protein value of beef, they are also four times less expensive, weight for weight. The regular meat-eater may hesitate even to consider using Soya Beans as an alternative to meat, however, when properly prepared, Soya meals will delight the taste buds and quite easily satisfy daily protein requirements as well as supplying an excellent range of minerals a very low fat content and most important, they are an alkaline forming food. One of the great disadvantages of meat-protein is due to the highly acid forming reaction that occurs after digestion of such food. At least 75% of the daily diet should be based around alkaline forming foods: fruits, vegetables, some grains, legumes nuts and seeds. All processed and refined foods are highly acid forming. Maximum health potential can only be maintained when the diet is based on at least 75% alkaline forming foods daily. Another great advantage of Soya protein is due to the excellent supply of unsaturated fats, especially linoleic acid – 54% one of the essential fatty acids (see pages 123 and 135 for details). A regular meat-eater would obtain generous benefits from the 'occasional' Soya protein meal, animal proteins are very rich in saturated fats and very low in lecithin content. Soya Beans are one of the best natural sources of lecithin, they are often used to prepare commercial lecithin supplements (see page 126 for details). Soya Beans are an excellent source of all the main minerals and one not only promotes their digestion but provides the body with a correct balance of active nutrients. The calcium content of Soya Beans is over 20 times that contained in top quality beef, calcium foods are essential for growth and development of children/teenagers and they also promote smooth functioning of the heart muscles and protect against the development of virus infections. Soya Beans supply over 10 times the potassium compared to cheese or eggs, potassium foods promote repair of damaged liver tissues and protect against hardening of the arteries. Soya Beans supply over 3 times the amount of phosphorus compared to chicken, phosphorus foods are essential for healthy skin, hair and teeth, and for maintenance and repair of the nervous system. Soya beans are an excellent source of the mineral iron, they supply over 5 times the iron content of cheese, twice the iron content of eggs and meat, iron foods protect against blood disease, virus infection and influenza. A good supply of iron foods is most important for women, especially expectant mothers and adolescents. Soya beans provide one of the most easily assimilated forms of the mineral iron. Other nutrients also well supplied with Soya Beans are: sodium – promotes digestion, chlorine and sulphur – essential for elimination of waste matter, silicon – healthy hair and skin, vitamins: A – promotes digestion of fats and protects against virus infections, B1 – healthy nerves, B2 – healthy skin, B3 – promotes digestion. A Soya meal is one sure way to satisfy your body.

SOYA BEAN PREPARATION:

Soya bean preparation is easy, if you have never tried to prepare a Soya meal, there are a few points to help you obtain the best results. After purchasing a packet of Soya beans, place two cups of dried Soya beans into a large wooden bowl, add 4 cups of water and leave to soak for no more than 6 hours, then rinse the beans in a collander or large sieve, place in water-bowl again and leave for about six hours. This initial pre-soaking of the Soya beans will improve their digestion and greatly reduce cooking time and your fuel bill. You can continue to soak the beans, with a rinse every six-eight hours, after the initial soaking and that will soften the beans so that they need only 5 minutes cooking. After three days of soaking and rinsing the beans, they will have enlarged nearly double their original size. It is a good idea to prepare a large quantity of Soya beans at a time, as they can be kept for up to two weeks in the fridge, after the cooking, and whenever you need a quick protein meal, the Soya beans will be ready. During the soaking and rinsing of the Soya beans, you will notice that the outer-skin of the beans will be separated and usually most of that will float to the top of the water bowl, just skim them off, using a ladle or sieve. To cook the Soya beans, place in a large cooking pot, add some miso-soya bean paste, soya sauce or one of your favourite spices and bring the Soya beans to the boil, be careful to watch the cooking pot to avoid foaming of the beans and loss of water. Allow to boil for no more than 5 minutes, then turn stove off and let the Soya beans cool, then rinse them again and drain off all water. The Soya beans can then be used or stored in the fridge, ready to use any time you need a quick and easy to prepare Soya meal

Prepare for a Soya meal today.

SOYA PRODUCTS

SOYA PRODUCTS: There are two types of Soya Beans: the edible bean and the commercial field variety. The majority of Soya products are produced from the commercial field variety, some of these products have been used for thousands of years and others have been developed only recently. Both the Chinese and Japanese have used Soya products long before the Western world even heard the name Soya.

TRADITIONAL SOYA PRODUCTS:

TOFU: developed by the Chinese, it is prepared from ground Soya Beans and then powdered gypsum is added to promote a curdle effect, it can be eaten as such or fermented to produce Tofu-cheese

MISO: used by the Japanese for over 2,000 years, it is prepared from fermented Soya Beans, cooked rice and sea salt. Miso preparation is a very lengthy process, the mixture is placed in large wooden vats and slowly fermented with the organism: aspergillus oryzae. Miso is available at most natural food stores. It supplies excellent amounts of protein and can be suitably combined to enhance soups, spreads, gravies or diluted and mixed with a salad dressing.

HAMANATTO: developed in Korea, it is made from steamed Soya Beans, roasted wheat and then fermented. The mixture is poured into large wooden buckets and placed in the sun, salt and ginger are also added. This process takes about one year and then the mixture is placed on wooden trays and allowed to dry. Hamanatto supplies excellent amounts of protein and it combines well with most cooked meals.

TEMPEH: developed in Indonesia, it is prepared from fermented Soya Beans and then wrapped in banana leaves, the result is a cheese with a very strong distinct taste.

NATTO: developed by Buddhist monks over 2,000 years ago. The process includes cooked Soya Beans, innoculating them with 'bacillus subtilis', the mixture is then wrapped in thin sheets of pinewood and allowed to ferment for a few days.

SOYA SAUCE: the most widely used Soya product, it is prepared from cooked Soya Beans mixed with roasted wheat and then impregnated with the ferment — 'aspergillus oryzae'. The mixture is placed into wooden vats, salt is added and allowed to ferment for a minimum six months, sometimes five years. The mixture is then strained and the liquid placed in glass. Soya sauce or Soy sauce as it is commonly called combines very well with savoury rice dishes, salad dressings, gravies and any cooked meal that you would otherwise use salt with, also try Soya sauce with alfalfa-mung bean sprouts.

TAMARI: a similar product to Soya sauce, fermented for at least 3 years, it will enhance the taste of rice dishes, fresh garden salad or many other cooked meals. Tamari is available at most natural food stores, try the taste sometime, use as an excellent substitute for table salt. Fermented foods promote digestion and health.

SOYA MILK: an excellent substitute for either powdered or pasturized cows milk. Soya milk is prepared from pre-soaked, ground Soya Beans. The mixture is then boiled and strained and re-boiled. Commercial Soya milk is available in a dry powdered form. Compared to cows milk, Soya milk is not mucus forming, far richer in the mineral iron and more compatible with human digestion. The taste is different to cows milk, try a half-half combination and you will obtain the best of both taste and nutrients.

SOYA GRITS: an essential food for every kitchen, Soya grits are prepared from cracked Soya Beans, the one advantage over the beans is that they require far less cooking time, less than half an hour moderate heat. Soya grits will enhance the protein value of all meals, small amounts could be served as a side dish mixed with steamed vegetables or combined with any soup, casserole, bean loaf or cooked mung beans.

SOYA FLOUR: an excellent source of complete protein, there are three types of Soya flour; full-fat — 20% fat content, medium-fat — 5% or the popular fat-free Soya flour. Soya flour contains no gluten, producing a very compact home made bread. In combination with wheat, rye or triticale flour, Soya flour could be used in the following proportions: 3 cups wheat (rye or triticale) with half a cup of Soya flour, that will produce a light bread with an exceptional protein content. Make sure your kitchen is always stocked with some Soya flour and Soya oil (see page 135 for details).

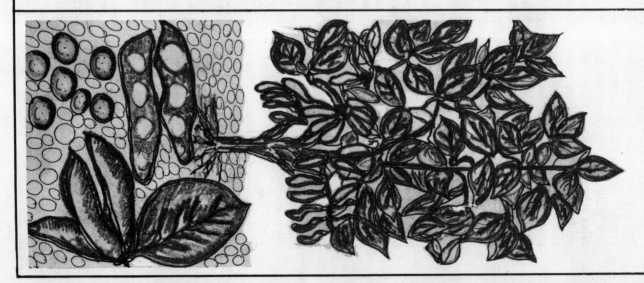

SOYA BEAN – PROTEIN RECIPES

SOYA BEAN BURGERS:

INGREDIENTS: 2 cups of cooked Soya beans, ½ cup of cooked brown rice, 1 cup of toasted sesame seeds, 2 free-range eggs – beaten, ½ cup of whole wheat flour or medium fat Soya flour, 1 cup of grated natural cheese, 1 tbl.sp. Soya sauce, 2 tbl.sp. wheat germ, ¼ cup of leek-onions chopped and sauteéd.

METHOD: Mix together: Soya beans – rice – sesame seeds and eggs. Slowly mix in all other ingredients and form small hand-size Soya burgers, these may be stored on a flat dish and placed in the fridge. To cook, place four small burgers into a frypan – oiled, allow 5 minutes each side – medium heat. These Soya burgers can then be placed into the oven, whilst preparing more. To serve: place one Soya burger inside two slices of whole grain bread or bread roll, add lettuce, beetroot, capsicum and parsley for a most rewarding complete protein meal. Three medium sized Soya burgers will provide approx. 40% of your daily protein requirements, have them at your next bar-b-que, Soya burgers are one of the natural alternatives!

SOYA BEAN APPLE and APRICOT PIE:

INGREDIENTS: 1 cup of cooked – ground Soya beans, 1 granny smith apple – prepared into 12 cuts, 4 ripe apricots – cut in quarter pieces, 2 free-range eggs – beaten, 1 cup of prepared Soya milk, 1 tsp. cinnamon, 3 tsp. tahini-sesame paste, ¼ cup of pure honey, ¼ cup of sultanas.

PASTRY: INGREDIENTS: 1 cup of whole wheat flour or medium fat Soya flour, ½ cup of 'better-butter', ¼ cup of wheat germ flakes, 1 tsp. veg. salt, 2 tsp. honey, 2 tsp. tahini, . cups of water – add ½ cup of Soya milk powder and mix in blender.

PASTRY PREPARATION: Combine flour, wheat germ, veg. salt, in large wooden bowl, slowly add and mix – small pieces of better-butter, tahini, honey and diluted Soya milk – water. Mix all ingredients for Pastry together and knead into a large ball, knead briskly and gently. Place the pastry-ball into the refrigerator for 1 hour or longer. Prepare a lightly floured chopping board, take pastry dough from the fridge and using a rolling pin, spread an even surface – ¼ cm. thick and carefully place over a pie plate, cut excess pastry away.

FRUIT PIE PREPARATION: Slightly cook apple pieces – 5 minutes low heat, combine together: cooked – ground Soya beans, eggs – beaten, tahini, honey and sultanas – cinnamon. Pour these ingredients into the pie plate and arrange pieces of apricot and apple around the top of the mixture, add extra wheat germ if the mixture is too moist. Place in a pre-heated oven – 400°F. for 30 minutes, serve straight from the oven or allow to cool and the Soya Fruit Pie will be ready when you are, the taste is worth preparing for. Serve with fresh cream or tahini ice cream. A complete protein meal anytime, try it this week.

SOYA MAYONNAISE:

INGREDIENTS: 1 cup of cold pressed Soya oil, 1 free-range egg, 2 tbl.sp. cider vinegar, ½ tsp. veg. salt, ½ tsp. mustard powder.

METHOD: Place ¼ cup of Soya oil and all other ingredients into a blender – 30 seconds low speed, slowly add more Soya oil. This Soya mayonnaise will last for two weeks in glass, stored in the fridge, you can make sufficient to share with friends.

SOYA DRINK IDEAS — hot and cold

MILKSHAKE: 2 cups of water, 4 tbl.sp. Soya milk powder, 2 tsp. Carob chocolate, 2 tsp. tahini. Place all ingredients into a blender for 30 seconds medium speed, add more Soya milk powder for a 'thick shake'. Serve in a chilled glass for summer.

SOYA BEAN VEGETABLE SOUP:

INGREDIENTS: 1 cup of cooked Soya beans – slightly mashed, 1 cup of freshly chopped celery, 1 cup of diced carrots, 1 cup of broccoli – cauliflower – leek, ½ cup of mixed parsley and onions, 3 cups of vegetable stock or water, 1 tbl.sp. miso-Soya paste, 1 tsp. of your favourite spice: thyme, marjoram, sage, oregano, etc., 3 tbl.sp. Soya sauce and ½ cup of cooked brown rice.

METHOD: Place Soya beans – cooked into a saucepan, add 2 cups of water-vegetable stock, bring to the boil and then simmer. Mix in: miso, cooked rice, freshly prepared vegetables and 1 cup of water, allow to simmer for 5 minutes, reduce to low heat, add parsley – onions, spices and Soya sauce, leave on low heat for 20 minutes and serve with whole grain bread, an ideal quick to serve meal and an excellent source of protein, minerals and vitamins. Soya bean soup can also be stored in the fridge for over a week, try it soon.

SOYA BEAN BREAKFAST IDEAS:

INGREDIENTS: 1 cup of cooked Soya grits, 1 cup of whole grain: oats, rice, barley, millet or wheat sprouts. ¼ cup dry Soya milk powder, 2 cups of water, 2 tbl.sp. tahini, 2 tbl.sp. wheat germ, 2 tbl.sp. coconut pieces – grated, 1 grated apple, ¼ cup of sultanas, any one of the following fruits as extras: 2 apricots, 1 peach, 1 pear — sliced.

METHOD: Place 1 cup of water and 1 cup of cooked Soya grits into a saucepan, bring to the boil and turn onto low heat, mix in Soya milk powder and 1 cup of water, add 1 cup of any whole grain, and leave on low heat for 15 minutes, then add, sultanas and coconut pieces. Stir all ingredients, then leave to cook for another 5 minutes. Prepare grated apple – fruits, place into a breakfast bowl and serve cooked mixture on top, add tahini or extra Soya milk and any other freshly prepared seasonal fruits. The basic Soya-whole grain mixture can be stored in the fridge for up to two weeks, ready for any breakfast, just remember the fruits, they are an excellent substitute for sugar, especially sultanas! One medium-serve bowl of this breakfast will provide over ¼ of your daily protein requirements and a valuable supply of energy. Note: for rice, allow an extra 10 minutes on low heat.

NUTS

INTRODUCTION

Nuts provide numerous nutritional benefits and throughout the following pages there is a descriptive evaluation of the main benefits associated with the most common varieties; Almond, Brazil, Cashew, Hazel, Pecan, Pistachio and Walnut. On page 98 there is also a nutrient composition chart with which you may compare a variety of other Nuts: chestnut, coconut, hickory, macadamia and pine nuts. Generally speaking, Nuts are the best primary source of complete protein, all essential life supporting amino acids are generously supplied by the Nut kingdom (see page 97 for details). Nuts could easily replace all other foods for protein value and requirements. Nut protein has supported human life for thousands of years and when other foods were in short supply, the people who carefully stored a supply of Nuts would have truly appreciated the life supporting ability from a diet of Nuts. As we are fortunate these days to have a wide variety of foods to choose from, the value of nuts has increased and for many people they are an expensive food item and unfortunately avoided for that reason. When you consider the number of years and energy that goes into the development of Nut trees and their preparation for market sales, you may also appreciate their value and cost in comparison to a variety of other protein foods. At first glance, a packet of cashews, almonds or brazil nuts may seem to be over-priced, that depends on the place of purchase and the number of price alterations since the original time of harvest, when after all, they are supplied by Nature and with no price tag attached. The initial reaction after seeing the price of Nuts may deter you from their purchase but when combined correctly, Nut protein is better value than the usual alternative of a piece of meat, poultry or fish, all depending of course on your accessibility to such produce (see page 97 for information on the economy of Nuts). Apart from their capacity to provide top quality protein, Nuts are usually obtained in the raw state and for this reason they are not affected by cooking which can destroy a considerable amount of protein value and other essential nutrients. The general custom of serving cooked meat, poultry and fish has a detrimental effect on the availability of protein — amino acids and the minerals and vitamins. When obtained raw, Nuts supply generous amounts of easily assimilated protein, minerals and vitamins and an excellent supply of essential unsaturated fatty acids. All animal foods supply an abundance of saturated fatty acids in comparison to the essential unsaturated fats and with a regular intake of such saturated animal produce, various health problems may develop and one of the most obvious is an overweight condition. Saturated fats are not easily used by the body, they must first be re-converted by the liver into the form of unsaturated fats and for that to take place, certain nutrients that are not supplied by the animal produce must be obtained. Nuts supply all the essential nutrients for utilization of their fat content and because those fats are unsaturated, they can be readily used by the body. Over half of the food value of Nuts is composed of unsaturated fats and these provide a very satisfying effect on the appetite as well as providing an excellent source of energy, one serving of 150 grams of mixed Nuts will provide an average of only 900 calories and that is one third of the daily calorie allowance for men between the ages of 20 – 50 and with such a serving, all the daily protein requirements are obtained. When properly combined, a mixture of almonds, brazil and cashew nuts will supply all the daily protein and still not exceed the recommended daily fat intake. As fruits, vegetables and some grains and legumes have a very low fat content, you could easily obtain an excellent variety of nourishing meals when using Nuts as the main daily protein provider, that is the basic idea of a well balanced diet. Some Nuts such as the macadamia and pecan are exceptionally high in fat content and therefore they could only be relied upon for a small portion of their protein with the average diet, for people in a very cold climate, those nuts could be a most valuable food as the body requires a greater portion of fats to generate heat. Apart from the excellent supply of protein and unsaturated fats, Nuts provide an abundance of the main minerals especially calcium, phosphorus, potassium, iron and magnesium, with each particular variety of Nut having certain dominant nutrients and by reading through the following pages, you will obtain information about the combination of minerals supplied and the associated benefits from a regular use of those Nuts. Another great benefit obtained from Nuts is the abundance of B group vitamins and with some Nuts, they supply excellent amounts of vitamin E and good amounts of vitamin A. Both the mineral and vitamin content of Nuts is far superior to that of animal produce. Proper combination of Nuts is very important and for the best value, Nuts should be eaten alone and definitely not combined with animal proteins as they both require completely different types of preparation within the stomach. If they are combined, both food groups will receive incorrect preparation and that results in poor food value, various digestive problems and a waste of valuable digestive energy. A combination of Nuts will make an ideal lunchtime protein meal and easily provide the majority of daily protein requirements with other protein being obtained from either a whole grain breakfast meal or a legume and vegetable evening meal. Nuts are an essential food group when you intend to have a well balanced diet.

ALMONDS

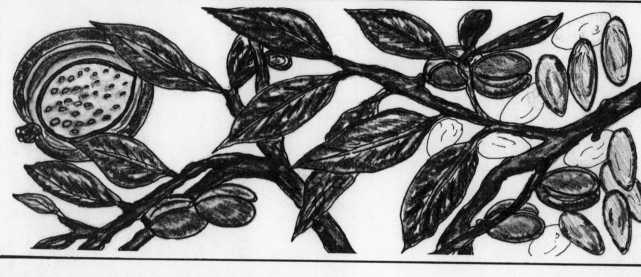

Almonds have supported human life for thousands of years and during times of famine, the Almond nut was one of the few survivors and providers of nutrition. There are two main types of Almonds: the bitter almond and the sweet almond, only the sweet almond is worth eating or prepared into almond paste, almond oil, almond butter or marzipan, all are delicious and most nourishing ways to enjoy the treasure of nutrients supplied with Almonds. When obtained fresh, direct from the shell, Almonds are one of the most nourishing and palatable foods and there are so many associated benefits such as: magnesium, Almonds are an excellent source of this mineral, it promotes a most beneficial alkaline effect, 75% of the daily diet should be based on alkaline foods. Almonds are the most alkaline of all nuts, that alone is a major benefit. Taken regularly, one handfull of Almonds per day is an optimum way to ensure proper nerve functioning, nerve transmission and correct muscular and glandular activity. Both alcohol and cigarettes deplete magnesium reserves. Almonds also provide a correct balance of the mineral phosphorus, that is essential for mental ability and digestion of fats, proteins and carbohydrates. Almonds are the best nut-source of calcium – the main mineral of bones and essential for healthy heart functioning. Almonds are one of the richest food-source of vitamin E – also essential for heart and muscle vitality and for effective blood circulation, promoting the life of body cells and repair of damaged skin tissue. Almonds also provide the essential B group vitamins and they are especially rich in Niacin-B3, that is essential for healthy skin, hair and nerves. Apart from the abundant supply of minerals and vitamins (see nutrient chart for more details), Almonds are an excellent source of Protein, they supply over 18% complete protein and when combined with brazil and cashew nuts, their protein availability – N.P.U., improves over 25%, therefore with 150 grams of mixed almonds, brazil and cashews, a person weighing 70kg. can obtain all their daily protein requirements. Other combinations such as Almond butter: mix 100 grams of Almonds with ½ cup of tahini-sesame paste, will provide a delicious substitute for butter and an excellent source of complete well-balanced protein. Remember to buy some unshelled Almonds next time you see some, compared to their nutritional benefits, they are an inexpensive food. Crack open a few Almonds during one of those 'nerve-shattering' television programs or buy a packet of freshly shelled Almonds for your next hectic lunch break or whilst travelling in the car. Almonds and fruit are the best take-away foods, they are food and medicine for the whole body.

ALMOND MILK: COMPLETE PROTEIN MEAL: DRINK:

INGREDIENTS: 1 cup full of raw-shelled Almonds, 2 tbl.sp. Sesame seeds, 2 tbl.sp. Soya milk or dry low fat milk, 3 cups water.

METHOD: Place 2 cups of water into a blender, add Almonds, sesame seeds, 2 tbl.sp. Soya milk or dry low fat milk, 30 seconds, then add more water.

This recipe will combine well with the morning whole grain breakfast, hot or cold Carob-chocolate drink and numerous other natural recipes. The mixture can be stored in glass and kept for up to one week in the fridge, ready to serve you with an abundance of nutrients and a most rewarding taste. Try some Almond milk today. To prepare Almond-butter, use 1 cup full of Almonds, ½ cup of sesame seeds and 1 cup of water. Place in the blender for one minute, medium speed, slowly pour Almonds into the blender, the sesame seeds can be put in first with the water. Almond butter has very good keeping qualities and it tastes excellent especially when combined with home made fruit-bread or use it for a side dish when serving fresh fruits, a natural fruit-dip.

	Carb.	Calo.	Fat	Cal.	Phos.	Mag.	TRY.	LEU.	LYS.	MET.	PHA.	ISL.	VAL.	TRY.
R.D.A. 80 kg. person.	345	2300	76	800	800	325	240	1280	960	800	1280	960	1120	720
Almonds-100 gram.	19	598	52	228	512	272	176	1454	582	259	1146	873	1124	610
Egg whole-100 gram.	1	164	11	54	206	12	211	1126	819	401	739	850	950	637
Almond- milk-100 gr.	19	594	51	461	537	249	214	1510	582	354	1224	928	1064	634
Almond Brazil Cashew	19	604	55	150	324	254	278	1368	606	517	903	896	1179	589

NOTE: All amounts are for 100 gram edible portions.

BRAZIL NUTS

Brazil nuts have been a popular food since the early 1600's and today they are exported worldwide, mainly from Brazil where a Brazil tree often grows to a height of over 40 metres. The nut is stored inside a large fruit-shell which contains around 10 individual Brazil nuts and these have a very hard shell, you need a heavy duty nut-cracker to open them and when you do, there are numerous nutritional benefits that you can expect and without any doubt the main one is related to the valuable supply of protein and especially the remarkable supply of the amino acid — methionine. Brazil nuts are the best natural source of this precious protein and especially the valuable supply of the amino acid. Nearly all protein foods are deficient in the amino acid — methionine and that considerably lowers the real protein potential of many foods. Brazil nuts are one of the few foods that have no limiting amino acids, although they are low in the amino acid — lysine, as most nuts are, except cashews and pistachio nuts. Brazil nuts supply over 90% of the required methionine amounts, most foods supply around 30% and that greatly reduces protein value. Nuts should not be combined with animal proteins or concentrated starch foods, they are best combined with other nuts and such fruits as apples, pears or peaches. Try a complete nut-protein meal this week, serve equal portions of Brazil, almonds and cashews and one fruit, that combination will give you very well balanced protein and with 100 grams of such, a person weighing 60kg. can obtain all his daily protein requirement as well as an abundance of essential minerals and vitamins (see page 98 for details) and still have the chance to enjoy over 2,000 calories of other natural produce. Brazil nuts give you the opportunity to obtain the most valuable protein meals.

	Carb.	Calo.	Fat	Cal.	Phos.	Iron.	TRY.	LEU.	LYS.	MET.	PHA.	ISL.	VAL.	TR
Brazil 100 gram.	10	654	66	187	690	3.4	187	1129	443	941	617	593	823	422
R.D.A. 60 kg. person	345	2300		800	800	15	180	960	720	600	960	720	840	560
120 gram: Alm Br + C	19	604	55	150	324	3.9	332	1641	727	620	1083	1075	1414	706

CASHEW NUTS

Cashew nuts originated from Brazil, the name cashew is derived from a south American Indian word — 'acaju'. Cashew nuts are often the most expensive of all nuts and that may deter many people from obtaining the following unique cashew benefits: In comparison to other nuts, Cashews have the lowest fat content and a greater concentration of the essential amino acids especially tryptophan, isoleucine and valine, all of which are supplied in amounts above the required daily allowance (see chart p. 97) per 100 gram portion and when combined with other nuts, the Cashew provides an excellent protein balance, especially with almonds and brazil nuts. When eaten alone, Cashews are an expensive protein food, that is due to their limiting supply of the amino acids methionine and phenylalanine, by combining both brazil and almonds with Cashews, you will obtain excellent protein value. With 150 grams of those mixed nuts, a person weighing 75kg. can obtain all his daily protein requirement plus an excellent source of essential main minerals (see page 98 for details) and a very low calorie count of less than one third the daily calorie allowance. Next time you have the chance to buy some Cashews, also invest in equal amounts of almonds and brazil nuts and discover the satisfying taste and positive protein value, no need for plates and cutlery. Only the best kitchen will always keep stock of nut-protein. A diet of nuts, fresh fruits and vegetables is the optimum health restoring diet, try it at least once a week and more often during those hot summer months, relax and enjoy the best health with nuts.

		Iron	Mag.	B1	B2	B3	TRY.	LEU.	LYS.	MET	PHA.	ISL.	VAL.	TR
R.D.A. 75 kg. person	3900	15	325	1.3	1.5	16	225	1200	900	750	1200	900	1050	680
150 gram: Alm Br + C	651	3.9	254	.5	.4	2.3	417	2052	909	775	1354	1344	1768	883
Cashew 100 gram	464	3.7	265	.4	.2	1.7	471	1522	792	353	946	1222	1592	737

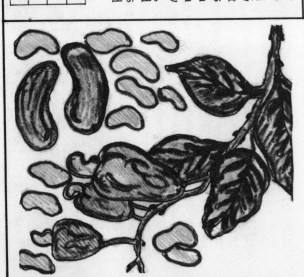

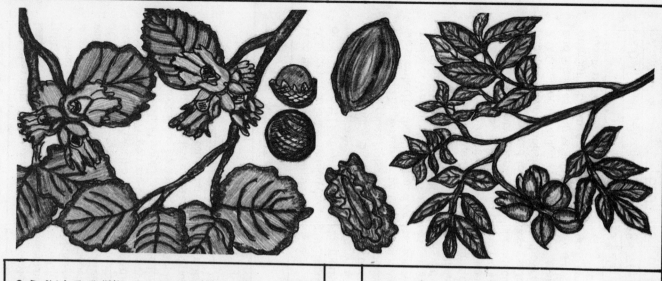

HAZEL NUTS

Hazel nuts are a member of the Corylus family of trees and depending on their country of cultivation, Hazel nuts may also be termed as Filberts or Cob nuts, they all have a slightly different taste, appearance and nutritional qualities. Generally speaking, Hazel nuts are one of the best food-source of vitamin E, they supply over 20 mg. per 100 gram portion, they are equal best with the almond nut for vitamin E – a handfull of Hazel nuts is the most beneficial substitute for any vitamin E capsule. Hazel nuts are one of the best nut-source of the essential unsaturated fatty acid – Linoleic acid, that in combination with vitamin E is vital for healthy arteries, regulation of cholesterol levels and prevention of heart disease. Hazel nuts are an excellent food for maintenance of healthy blood and development of muscle cells due to a generous supply of the following nutrients: iron, copper and manganese, these are the three main blood minerals. Hazel nuts are the best nut-source of manganese – blood development, nerve nourishment and maintenance of sex-hormone production. Hazel nuts are also a very good source of zinc – the mineral that is required for the breakdown of alcohol, it also promotes carbohydrate digestion and is a vital component of insulin. One of the less-known minerals: selenium is also very well supplied with Hazel nuts, selenium works in combination with vitamin E to promote normal body growth, preservation of skin tissue and contributes to fertility. Hazel nuts are the best nut-source of vitamin A – healthy skin, promotes protein digestion and assists in the building of strong bones and teeth. Hazel nuts also supply ample amounts of calcium and potassium (see chart for details). All of the basic B group vitamins are well supplied especially B5 and B6. The protein value of Hazel nuts is low compared to other nuts and in order to obtain very good protein value, combine Hazel nuts with cashews and brazil nuts and a few almonds. Hazel nuts are an abundant supplier of so many minerals and vitamins that it would seem like magic if they were abundant in protein.

	Calories	Carb.	Fat	Cal.	Phos.	Iron.	Mag.	Potassium	vit. E	B1.	B2.	B3.	B5.	B6.
R.D.A. average.	2300	345	76	800	800	14	325	3900	13	1.2	1.2	16	8	2.0
Hazel nuts - 100 gram	634	16	63	214	341	3.5	235	720	25	.46	.55	.9	1.1	.5

PECAN NUTS

Pecan nuts are obtained from the Carya family of trees and another member is the Hickory nut, both are grown extensively throughout the U.S.A. and the Pecan nut is exported world wide, the Hickory nut is a local speciality. Pecan nuts are often overrated in regards to their nutritional content, in comparison to all other nuts, Pecans are the lowest in protein value due to a poor supply of the essential amino acids (see chart p. 97). The Pecan nut looks similar to the walnut but apart from that Pecans supply about 25% less protein value and compared to the almond, cashew or brazil nut, over 30% less protein value. The range of minerals supplied by the Pecan nut is generally 25% less than other nuts and with the vitamins, Pecans supply an abundance of vitamin A, very little vitamin E and a good range of the basic B group vitamins. There are no outstanding nutrient values associated with the Pecan, they are best regarded as a good all-round food, their only advantage may be the cost. Pecan nuts are generally valued at about half the price of almonds and brazil nuts, depending on the time and place of purchase. At certain times of the year, you will find that the cost of nuts is cheaper than other times, then you could invest in a bulk buy of your favourites and when well stored, nuts will retain their freshness and nutrient content especially if they are kept in their shell and stored in a cool place. Pecan nuts have a very high fat content, equal to macadamia nuts and for those people who need to add on extra weight, Pecan nuts would be an excellent choice. It would be best not to combine Pecans with other nuts as you will lower the overall protein value of that meal. Eat Pecan nuts alone and you will obtain good food value.

100 gram edible portions.	Calo.	Carb.	Fat	B1.	B2.	B3.	TRY.	LEU.	LYS.	MET.	PHA.	ISL.	VAL.	TR
R.D.A. 70 kg. person	2300	345	76	1.3	1.5	16	210	1120	840	700	1120	840	980	640
Hazel nuts	634	16	63	.46	.5	.9	211	939	417	139	537	853	934	415
Pecan nuts	687	15	70	.9	.12	.9	138	773	435	153	564	553	525	389

PISTACHIO

Pistachio nuts have grown throughout the Mediterranean regions for thousands of years, mainly in the areas of Greece, Italy, Syria, Israel and Turkey. The Pistachio nut tree is called 'pistachio vera', a small tree which bears a fruit and within the fruit, the small pistachio nut-seed is stored. Pistachio nuts are a most delicious food and they contribute the following nutrient qualities: an excellent source of the mineral potassium, the muscle mineral and essential for healthy heart muscle action, promoting blood circulation and in combination with the excellent supply of the mineral iron, also very well supplied with the Pistachio nut, promotes oxygen utilization and distribution. Pistachio nuts are one of the best natural food-source of the mineral iron — increases resistance to disease and stressful conditions, promotes protein metabolism and cleansing of the bloodstream. Pistachio nuts are natural medicine for prevention and relief of colds and in combination with the good supply of vitamin A, you can be sure of positive results. Pistachio nuts are not a complete source of protein as they lack the essential amino acid tryptophan — required for regulation of sleep and mood patterns, nourishment of the optic system and for protein digestion. To obtain a good supply of protein, always combine Pistachio nuts with Cashews and for excellent protein value, add a few brazil and almond nuts. The Pistachio nut is the best nut-source of lysine, one of the main limiting amino acids with all other nuts. Pistachio nuts are a very good source of vitamin B1 — the morale vitamin, as it promotes mental vitality. Pistachio nuts give you good taste and health.

WALNUTS

Walnuts are obtained from the 'juglans regio' fruit tree and there are two main varieties: the Black Walnut and the European Walnut which is also termed the English, French or Italian Walnut depending on the area of cultivation. The Black Walnut originated from North America and for thousands of years, the Black Walnut has provided good nutrition for the Indian tribes from that region, they relied on the Walnut for their survival. Apart from supplying only minimal amounts of calcium, the Black Walnut is superior in nutrient content when compared to the European Walnut (see nutrient chart for details). Compared to other Nuts, the Walnut supplies a good average of all the main minerals, vitamin A, B group vitamins and vitamin C. The protein content of the Black Walnut is 20%, the European Walnut is near 15%. All the essential amino acids are supplied by the Walnut and for a person weighing 50kg, they could obtain all their daily protein requirements from one cupful of Walnut pieces and compared to the cost of animal protein foods, Walnuts are very good value. In order to obtain excellent protein value, combine Walnuts with a few cashews, brazil and almond nuts and with a combination of those nuts, a person weighing 70 kg. could obtain all their daily protein requirements with one serve of 170 grams — 6 ozs. (European Walnuts). Walnuts are an excellent source of the B group vitamin — Biotin and that is essential for the conversion of unsaturated fats into the form of usable energy. All Nuts supply generous amounts of the essential fatty acids (see page 132-3) and many people avoid eating Nuts mainly because they consider them to be a fattening food. An overweight person could obtain numerous weight reducing benefits from a diet of Nuts and fresh fruits if their diet did not include any refined foods, cooked foods and sweet snack foods. For some overweight people, that may seem impossible as their pattern of eating habits totally relies on those meals. A person who obtains all their daily protein from Nuts will still have over 2,000 calories to enjoy with either fruits or vegetables and over 10 grams of Lipids (fats and oils) to enjoy a meal of grains and legumes with vegetables. The Walnut is most beneficial as it supplies an abundance of the essential fat-converting nutrient — Biotin, other Nuts supply good amounts of Biotin. The Walnut is ready to help you loose weight and obtain top quality protein.

	Calo.	Carb.	Fat	Iron.	Mag.	Biotin.	TRY.	LEU.	LYS.	MET.	PHA.	ISL.	VAL.	TR
R.D.A. 75 kg. person	230	345	15	23	225	1200	900	750	1200	900	1050	680		
Walnut 100 gram	650	15	62	3	130	37	175	1228	441	306	767	767	974	589

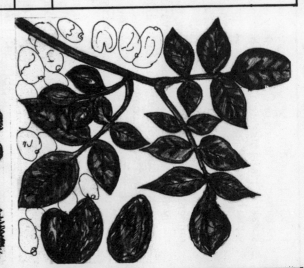

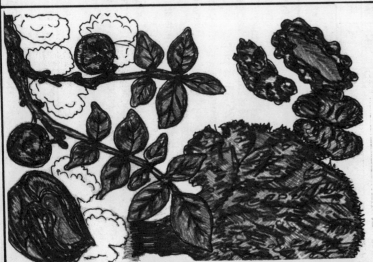

NUTS & SEEDS — NUTRIENT CHART

NUTS & SEEDS	CALORIES	CARBOHYDRATES	PROTEIN	FAT	CALCIUM	PHOSPHORUS	POTASSIUM	SODIUM	IRON	MAGNESIUM	COPPER	MANGANESE	ZINC	VIT.A	VIT.C	VIT.E	VIT.B1	VIT.B2	VIT.B3	VIT.B5	VIT.B6	BIOTIN	FOLIC ACID
Almonds	598	19	19	52	228	512	780	4.3	4.6	272	.82	1.9	na.	0	tr	15	.24	.93	3.7	.47	.10	18	.97
Brazil	654	10	14	66	187	690	710	.7	3.4	225	1.5	2.6	5	tr	10	6.5	.97	.12	1.7	.23	.17		.004
Cashews	560	29	14	47	37	372	464	15	3.7	265			4	100			.4	.27	1.7	1.3			.06
Chestnuts	190	42	2.8	1.7	27	88	453	6	1.7	41	.73	4.2			6	.5	.21	.21	6	.41	.32		
Coconut	346	9.3	3.6	35	12	95	256	22	1.7	46	.45	1.3		0	2.5	1.0	.05	.02	.5	.20	.04		.03
Hazel (Filberts)	634	16	12	63	214	341	720	2.5	3.5	235	1.2	4.2	3	108	tr	21	.46	.55	.9	1.1	.54		.07
Hickory	700	13	14	70					2.8	160	1.4				0		.55						
Macadamia	691	10	10	81	56	252			2.1					6					1.4				
Peanuts	620	22	28	53	78	440	757	5	2.4	180	.47	1.6	0	0	0	6.8	.22	.12	18	2.3	.43	36	.11
Pecans	687	15	9	70	75	300	645	tr			1.1	1.5			1.8	1.3	.9	.12	.9	1.5	.17		.02
Pinenuts	700	20	14	56	12	640			4.8					35	tr		1.2	.25	4.8				
Pistachio	594	19	18	52	133	496	980		7	160	1.1			230			.65		1.4		.06		.06
Walnuts	650	15	15	62	98	380	450	2	3	130	1.3	1.8	2	30	2	1.5	.3	.13	.9	.9	.7	37	.06
Safflower seeds	615	12	19	59	na.	620											1.1	.40	2.2				
Sesame seeds	582	21	18	49	1160	612	725	60	10.5	181	1.9			30		.41	.98	.24	5.4	5.4	.1		.19
Sunflower seeds	560	20	24	47	120	837	920	30	7.1	38	2.1			50		3.1	1.9	.23	5.4	5.4			
Pumpkin seed	554	15	29	45	50	1144			11:2					70			:24	:19	2:4				

NOTE: All amounts are for 100 gram edible portions.

LIST OF COMMON FOOD ADDITIVES: PACKAGED FOODS and DRINKS, CANNED and BOTTLED PROCESSED FOODS.
Acidifiers, Acidulants, Aerating agents, Alkalies, Antibiotics, Antibrowning agents, Anticaking agents, Antifirming agents, Antifoaming agents, Antimould agents, Antimycotic agents, Antioxidants, Antirope agents, Antisticking agents, Antistaling agents, Artificial colours, Artificial sweeteners, Bleaching agents, Bodying agents, Bread emulsifiers, Bread improvers, Buffering agents, Buffers, Carriers, Chelating agents, Clarifiers, Coating agents, Crisping agents, Crystalline inhibitors, Crystallization modifiers, Crumb-firming agents, Curing agents, Defoaming agents, Dough conditioners, Dusting agents, Emulsifiers, Extenders, Fillers, Fining agents, Firming agents, Fixatives, Flavour enhancers, Foaming agents, Food colours, Food dyes, Freshness preservers, Fumigants, Fungicides, Glazing agents, Humectants, Hydroscopic agents, Leavening agents, Lubricating agents, Maturing agents, Moisture-retaining agents, Mould inhibitors, Neutralizers, Nonutritive sweeteners, Oleoresins, Preservatives, Propellants, Release agents, Sequestrants, Softeners, Solvents, Stabilizers, Washing agents.

PROTEIN ALTERNATIVES — ESSENTIAL AMINO ACIDS

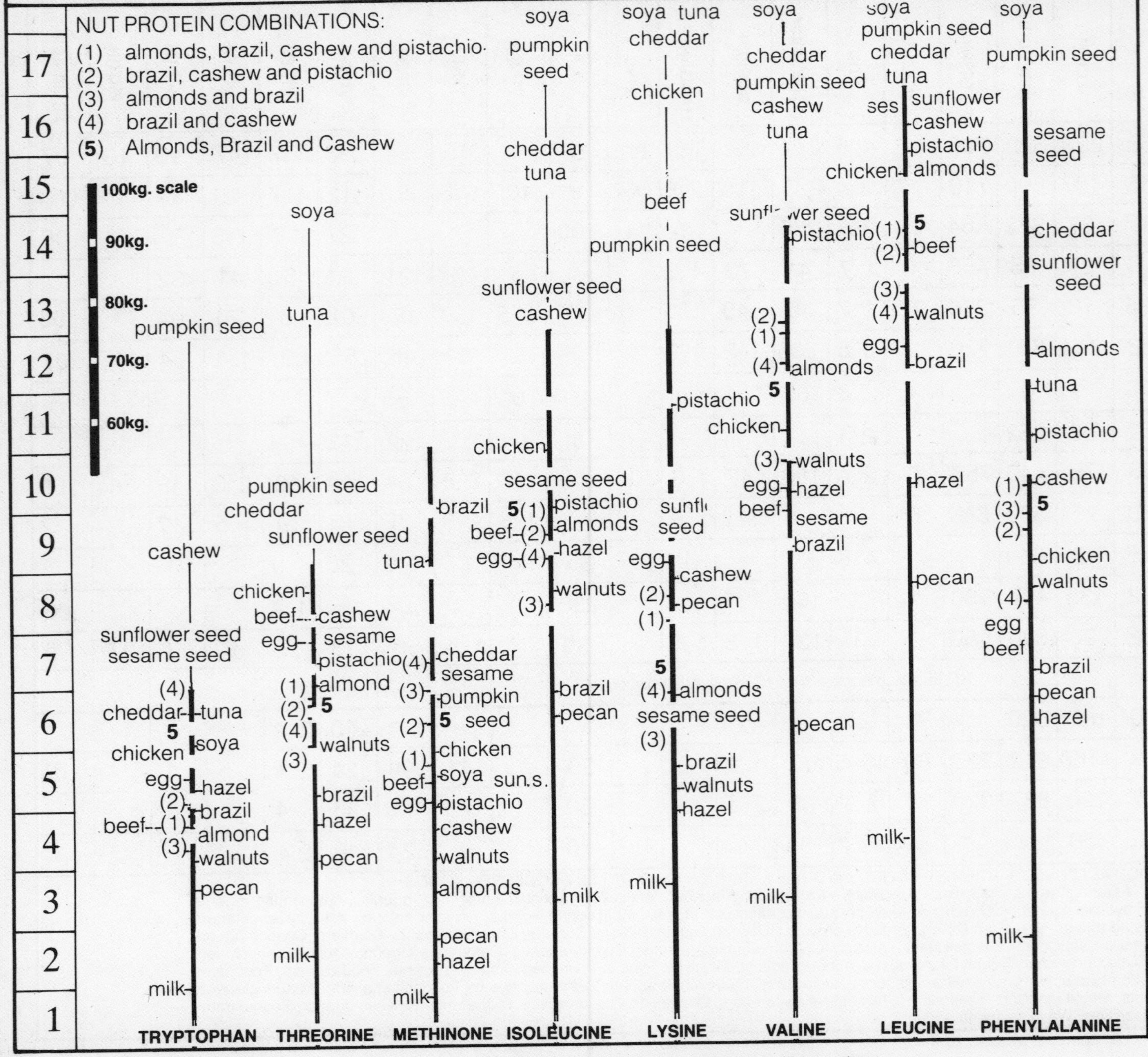

The chart on the left: shows the varying amounts of Protein — amino acids obtainable from the following foods: Nuts — almonds, brazil, cashew, hazel, pecan, pistachio and walnut. Soya beans, chicken, beef, cheddar cheese, tuna fish, eggs and milk-cows. There are also 5 important Nut-combinations, they are of great benefit as they supply a substantial amount of protein availability — N.P.U.', amount of protein or 'limiting amino acids'. The chart is based on the recommended daily protein requirements (Food and Nutrition board, National Academy of Sciences, U.S.A.). The measure for the amino acid — Tryptophan — TRY., has been doubled, it should actually show the amount of 3 — (300), the line has been doubled to provide a better visual display. All other amino acids: THR. — Threorine, MET. — Methinone, ISL. — Isoleucine, LYS. — Lysine, VAL. — Valine, LEU. — Leucine, PHA. — Phenylalanine, are displayed in amounts (dark line) equivalent to the daily amino acid — protein requirements for a person weighing 100kg. To calculate your individual daily protein — amino acid requirements (see chart page 88), or visually calculate — 10% of the dark line equals 10kg, except for Tryptophan — 20% =10kg.

The numbers on the far left: 1-17 are to be expressed in terms of: 1 =100 miligrams. For example, THR. — Threorine daily requirement for a person weighing 100kg =800 grams. All foods are given in amounts of 100gram edible portion.

NUT PROTEIN COMBINATIONS:
(1) almonds, brazil, cashew and pistachio.
(2) brazil, cashew and pistachio
(3) almonds and brazil
(4) brazil and cashew
(5) Almonds, Brazil and Cashew

100kg. scale
90kg.
80kg.
70kg.
60kg.

Scale numbers: 17, 16, 15, 14, 13, 12, 11, 10, 9, 8, 7, 6, 5, 4, 3, 2, 1

Column headers (amino acids):
TRYPTOPHAN — THREORINE — METHINONE — ISOLEUCINE — LYSINE — VALINE — LEUCINE — PHENYLALANINE

NOTE: All amounts are for 100 gram edible portions.

3.5ozs. = 100 grams approx.

PROTEIN ALTERNATIVES — ESSENTIAL AMINO ACIDS

Pages 98 and 99 will provide you with a comparison guide of 'available amino acids' (protein units), between the following food groups: Nuts, Seeds and Animal proteins. When comparing the various groups of protein foods, it is quite evident that you could obtain all your daily protein requirements from the group of Nuts and Seeds and by referring to page 42, you can also compare the availability of protein from the food groups: Grains and Legumes. A well balanced diet including only natural primary protein foods: whole grains, legumes, nuts and seeds, and not including any animal protein foods, will easily supply an abundance of minerals, vitamins and essential unsaturated fatty acids, plus, over 300 individual protein recipes (refer to chapter 7, pages 201–211, for the variety of protein recipe combinations).

When comparing the cost of primary protein foods with animal protein foods, there is little difference in the price between all primary protein foods mentioned in comparison to the group of animal protein foods. If you can afford to purchase regular supplies of meat, you could save on your weekly shopping expense by preparing the 'occasional' soya meal, nut protein lunch or seed snack, as well as a whole grain breakfast or any number of legume meals; and by obtaining regular supplies of primary protein meals, you can maintain your maximum health potential and discover the tastes and range of recipes that are enjoyed by people throughout the world, variety is the spice of life! and only natural foods can provide both the variety and the life. Prepare for primary protein today.

AVERAGE COST PER 100 Grams, edible portion
(amounts calculated: January 82, Vic. Aust.).

A1, Br + C	–	90 cents
Almonds	–	80 cents
Brazil	–	70 cents
Cashew	–	1.30 cents
Walnut	–	70 cents
Soya bean	–	15 cents
Edam cheese	–	60 cents
Rump steak	–	70 cents
Tuna-canned	–	50 cents

AMOUNT REQUIRED FOR A 70kg. MAN.
(based on R.D.A. National Academy of Sciences, U.S.A. – Adult Male).

A1, Br + C	– 150 grams
Almonds	– 180 grams
Brazil	– 210 grams
Cashew	– 200 grams
Walnut	– 250 grams
Soya bean	– 150 grams
Edam cheese	– 120 grams
Rump Steak	– 180 grams
Tuna-canned	– 100 grams

ESSENTIAL AMINO ACIDS.	Mg.	20	30	40	50	60	70	80	90
TRYPTOPHAN	3	60	90	120	150	180	210	240	270
LEUCINE	16	320	480	640	800	960	1120	1280	1440
LYSINE	12	240	360	480	600	720	840	960	1080
METHINONE	10	200	300	400	500	600	700	800	900
PHENYLANINE	16	320	480	640	800	960	1120	1280	1440
ISOLEUCINE	12	240	360	480	600	720	840	960	1080
VALINE	14	280	420	560	700	840	980	1120	1260
THREORINE	8	160	240	320	400	480	560	640	720

ESSENTIAL AMINO ACIDS

	TRY.	LEU.	LYS.	MET.	PHA.	ISL.	VAL.	THR.
soya bean	526	2946	2414	513	1889	2054	2005	1504
almonds	176	1454	582	259	1146	873	1124	610
brazil	187	1129	443	941	617	593	823	422
cashew	471	1522	792	353	946	1222	1592	737
hazel	211	939	417	139	537	853	934	415
pecan	138	773	435	153	564	553	525	389
pistachio	0	1520	1080	370	1090	880	1340	610
walnuts	175	1228	441	306	767	767	974	589
pumpkin seed	560	2437	1411	577	1749	1737	1679	933
sesame seed	331	1679	583	637	1457	951	885	707
sunflower seed	343	1736	868	443	1220	1276	1354	911

NOTE: All amounts are for 100 gram edible portions.

SEEDS — INTRODUCTION PROTEIN

Seeds are the beginning of Life. Seeds are the most compact form of Life. Seeds are the universal code for Nature. Seeds are latent life. Seeds are the guiding force behind regeneration of new life, they are the link in the chain of evolution that decides the pattern of life and they are the most valuable asset of mankind. From one Seed we can assist Nature and progressively create an infinitesimal number of the same species. The Seed you plant today will need care and attention and when fully developed, that Seed will return the favour and supply you with an abundance of food for your enjoyment and energy requirements. The world we live in may have many problems and is there anything more disastrous than to be starving from lack of food. Half the world's population live with food shortages and over one quarter of the people today have 'starvation diets'. To every problem there is a solution that will be sensible, practical and with long term benefits. World wide campaigns against hunger are very common these days and does that problem ever get solved. Would it not be just as worthwhile if every donation was backed up with constructive planning for the future by utilizing the most elementary 'gift to mankind', the Seed has the potential of a new life, a new world. For those people who are fortunate enough to purchase regular and fresh supplies of food, they may become so adapted to buying food rather than having even a small city vegetable garden. The benefits of freshly picked produce are only appreciated by a small percentage of people, so much food is left for days, sometimes weeks before it is eaten and when you consider the most delicate foods: fruit and vegetables, their taste and positive benefits can only last a few days, even though refrigeration seems to postpone their enzyme activity, they are different in taste to the freshly picked produce.

You may have experienced the satisfaction from some fresh foods, an apple or peach straight from the tree, into your hands and then the delicious taste with all those valuable living nutrients. Many foods can be grown in one season of a year, others require two seasons and most fruit and nut trees require over four years development. So many home gardens are cluttered with colourful plants but how many of those are essential for well-being. If you have any spare land, plant a fruit tree, nut tree and a basic vegetable garden, we all need some exercise and there is far greater value in planting a Seed in comparison to a running-around the local streets routine, just for exercise! Within every apple, peach, pear, apricot, cherry and various other fruits, vegetables, grains and legumes, there is a new generation, hidden in the Seed and the second generation from one Seed could supply enough Seeds to start a small orchard, vegetable garden or crop of grains and legumes. Carefully consider the possibilities of this natural development and make proper use of the land you may own, the soil is one key to Nature and the first one to be opened, the Seed is then ready to accept the invitation. The Seed will remain dormant until we give the initial spark, then Nature will continue to open the keys and show us a real desire for life. You are the one who can keep life going, it is your time to plant a seed and then, let Nature feed you.

The following pages (101–106) will describe the main benefits that are associated with the most common edible seeds: pumpkin, sesame and sunflower as well as a section on sprouting Seeds. Nearly all seeds can be used as sprouts, the most common being: alfalfa, buckwheat, chickpea, fenugreek, lentil, millet, mung, rice, rye, sesame, soya, sunflower and wheat. All whole grains and legumes are considered as Seeds, they will all sprout when placed in water and rinsed several times per day, after three to five days, they could be planted in the soil and allowed to grow, or, they could be eaten directly as a sprouted food, the benefits of which are to be discussed on pages 103–106. All Seeds contain an individual life force and with such energy, they are capable of developing into their own seed-bearing stage, a continuously blooming cycle that will assist people and with which, people must assist. Apart from sprouted Seeds, the three most common edible seeds: pumpkin, sesame and sunflower are one of the best natural source of complete protein, minerals and vitamins. When Seeds are eaten, they will provide you with their individual life-force and no other food-group is more compact and generous, one handfull of sesame seeds may contain near five hundred individual life units, their capacity to promote your health and life are second to none. A well balanced diet must include Seeds, they are the best substitute for animal protein foods and they supply all the nutrients that are available from animal proteins, except for vitamin B12, that can be obtained from a weekly intake of natural yoghurt or cheese. A vegetarian diet, when properly balanced, includes over fifty individual protein foods, both Seeds and Nuts are the most concentrated protein source with a few legumes having equal protein quality.

Seeds can be combined in numerous ways, all depending on your imagination, range of recipes and purchase of such food. If you have never tried any of the three basic Seeds: pumpkin, sesame and sunflower, you could greatly improve your health and range of recipes, it may take some time before you become well acquainted with those three basic Seeds and a variety of recipes and once you do, you can be assured that you are obtaining the best nutrition. There is nothing abnormal about eating natural foods so when you see a packet of pumpkin or sunflower seeds, even though they may look neglected in the packaged form, consider the colourful and abundant growth of their original source. Obtain a packet of pumpkin seeds, leave them in the glove-box of your car and whenever you find the travelling and city traffic irritating, chew on a few, they are an excellent protein and mineral food and with a remarkable rejuvenation ability. During winter, have some sunflower seeds instead and whenever you are confined indoors, you can obtain numerous benefits from a simple snack of sunflower seeds. Sesame seeds are one of the most versatile natural foods and an excellent source of protein, minerals and vitamins, try some tahini with a fresh garden salad or make a sesame milk shake. All of the three basic seeds are compatible with various fruits, nearly all vegetables, some grains and legumes. The variety of unique combinations would be near two hundred, try at least a few of them this year. Seeds are waiting for you.

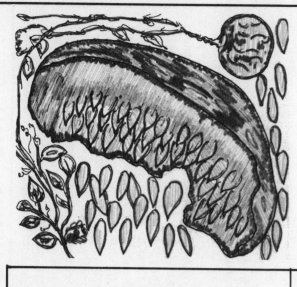

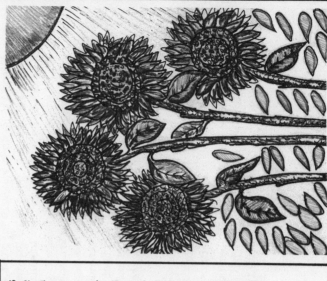

PUMPKIN SEEDS

Pumpkin seeds are one of Nature's best protein foods, they supply 30% protein and all the essential amino acids are generously supplied in a well balanced form, over 60% of the protein contained is usable – (N.P.U.). The amino acids: isoleucine, methionine, lysine and leucine are especially well supplied and compared to whole grains, legumes and various animal protein foods, Pumpkin seeds provide perfect protein. There are numerous ways to combine Pumpkin seeds for a most delicious complete meal or they can be eaten alone for an ideal, convenient and healthful snack. Dried Pumpkin seeds are available at most natural food stores and they are inexpensive and a most rewarding food, one handfull of Pumpkin seeds will supply over half your daily protein requirements and they really give you something to chew on, even a few Pumpkin seeds per day will provide a variety of benefits that most other foods, especially animal protein foods, could not and the main benefit, apart from the protein value is the remarkable revitalizing, invigorating and regenerative power of the Pumpkin seed. Regular use of Pumpkin seeds will ensure that your body metabolism obtains those essential revitalizing nutrients and also some valuable natural plant hormones which are a vital ingredient for production of the male: androgen hormone. For women, the Pumpkin seed has numerous benefits and one of these is due to the abundance of the mineral iron, over 11 mg. per 100 gram are supplied, that is over four times the amount of spinach and ten times that of chicken. The abundance of the mineral phosphorus in combination with iron will promote healthy blood development and efficient nerve and mental activity. Vitamin A and the basic B group vitamins are also well supplied and in combination with the excellent supply of protein, those vitamins and minerals will protect you against conditions of stress. If you lead a busy hectic life, Pumpkin seeds will help you to enjoy health as well. Always have a packet of Pumpkin seeds in your car and whenever the traffic is shredding your nerves, chew on a few Pumpkin seeds, the relief is natural.

SUNFLOWER SEEDS

Sunflower seeds have been used as a food source for thousands of years, both the Persians and American Indians recognized the nutritive and associated medicinal value of the Sunflower plant and seed. Many people have admired the brilliant golden face of the Sunflower plant and for those people who have eaten the seeds, they would have obtained a variety of benefits such as the excellent supply of protein, over 24% complete protein is obtained from Sunflower seeds, with a N.P.U. (usable protein) of 58%, all the essential amino acids are well balanced to ensure maximum protein value. Sunflower plants have the remarkable ability to follow the sun's direction and for this reason they are a unique food source, capable of supplying us with the sunshine vitamin – D. A regular supply of Sunflower seeds during those dark winter months is highly recommended for maintenance of maximum health potential. A lack of vitamin D can upset the metabolism of all main minerals and that alone will greatly retard the action of the glands, muscles, nerves and digestion. Apart from the unique supply of vitamin D, the Sunflower seed will also provide excellent amounts of calcium – promotes strong bone development, proper digestion and muscle growth; phosphorus – promotes mental alertness and repair of the nervous system; potassium – muscle development, energy development and healthy heart action; magnesium – nerve mineral, promotes digestion, bone growth and healthy teeth; silicon – protects against arthritis, promotes – healthy hair, skin and eyesight; iron – blood development and protection from pollution; B group vitamins: B1, B2, and B3 – essential for effective digestion, improves condition of the skin, hair and nerves, protects against stress and muscular weakness. Very few foods can provide you with such an abundance of essential life supporting nutrients and so when you regularly combine Sunflower seeds with other natural foods: fruits and vegetables for best combinations, or eat them as a snack meal, you will obtain more than just a reflection of the sun's energy.

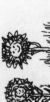

SESAME SEEDS

Sesame seeds are a traditional and extremely versatile food, they originated from the land around Turkey and Arabia where they are still regarded as the 'seed of immortality'. The nutrient benefits associated with the regular use of Sesame seeds is very impressive. If you have never tried Sesame seeds or a delicious Sesame paste-Tahini, you could discover a complete new taste sensation and find out about the multitude of ways to combine the taste and benefits of Sesame seeds with other natural foods. An excellent supply of top quality protein is available from Sesame seeds, they supply over 20% complete protein and are one of the richest source of methinone, an essential amino acid and the main 'limiting amino acid' with all animal protein foods and various grains, legumes, nuts and other seeds. A small amount of ground Sesame seeds can easily improve the value of any protein meal. Sesame seeds need to be ground or prepared into Tahini as the tiny seeds are not capable of being properly digested, unless they have obtained through chewing. Both ground and Sesame paste-tahini are available at most natural food stores, they are one of your best health investments. Sesame seeds are the best food-source of the main mineral calcium and for those people who attempt to get calcium from milk, their efforts would have more detriment than benefits. Milk and other dairy produce are mucus forming foods, Sesame seeds and Tahini are not. You could prepare a milk from Sesame seeds and when you get accustomed to the taste, the associated benefits and delicious recipes are the reward. Sesame seeds – milk and Tahini are an excellent source of vitamin E, one of the best food-sources of this vitamin with over 30 mg. per 100 gram portion of Tahini. See page 136 for more details on Tahini and Sesame oil. Another vitamin also very well supplied is vitamin T, it is often termed the 'sesame seed vitamin' and very few foods are even a good source of vitamin T: improves memory and concentration abilities and in combination with the excellent supply of phosphorus, Sesame seeds are a most nourishing brain and nerve food. Vitamin T also assists in the formation of blood plateletes and in combination with the excellent supply of the mineral iron, Sesame seeds will ensure healthy blood development and blood purifying abilities. Other nutrients also very well supplied are the minerals: potassium – assists the functions of the kidneys, promotes oxygen distribution – especially when combined with vitamin E and phosphorus, both in excellent supply from Sesame seeds. Magnesium is also abundant and that promotes protein metabolism and the absorption of all the main minerals. Very few foods supply better amounts of B group vitamins, especially B3-niacin – improves blood circulation and protects against excess cholesterol. For a person who eats regular amounts of animal proteins, Sesame seeds will provide an essential balance of revitalizing nutrients as well as an ideal protein substitute. For those people who smoke cigarettes, drink coffee and tea, they could also obtain numerous benefits that will repair the daily damage from those smokes and drinks. You could prepare a Sesame milk shake, Sesame butter, Sesame ice cream, Sesame cookies and a full range of Sesame recipes all of which provide an abundance of the before mentioned nutrients as well as an excellent source of natural lecithin – reduces blood fat levels and is essential for protection from environmental pollutants and nicotine. Sesame seeds may look very small but when compared to their abundance of benefits, they are one of the greatest natural foods.

SESAME PROTEIN MILKSHAKE: For two or three people.

INGREDIENTS: ¼ cup of Sesame paste – Tahini, ¼ cup Soya milk, 2½ cups of water, 1 tsp. Carob-chocolate powder, dash of cinnamon, optional: 1 ripe banana or 3 tsp. natural L.B.A. yoghurt.

METHOD: Place one cup of water in blender, then the Soya milk powder, Carob and Tahini, then add extra water and spice. Turn blender onto medium speed, mix for 30 seconds. The banana or yoghurt can be added last. Sesame milkshakes are very rewarding to drink, serve in a chilled glass for summer happiness.

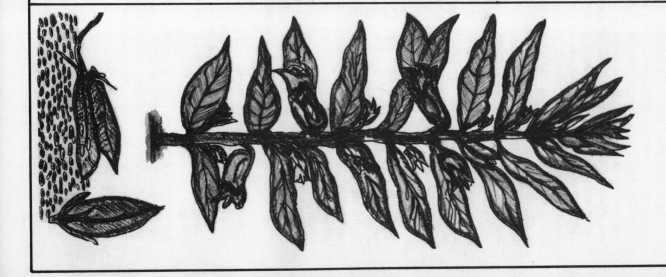

SPROUTING INTRODUCTION — ENZYMES

Sprouting seeds. grains and legumes is by no means a recent discovery. over 3.000 years ago. the Chinese discovered the potential of Sprouted foods and now. with modern methods of food analysis. the wisdom of their ways with food-sprouting is made obvious. In this era. many people are still unaware about the potential of sprouted foods and unaccustomed to the ways of preparation and combination of sprouted foods with other meals. Throughout this section on sprouting. you may discover (if not already) the methods of sprouting preparation. their associated benefits and a few basic ways to include sprouted foods with other common foods.

Sprouting is a natural development. the seed is transformed from a state of latent energy into a complete living form. with the assistance of water and air. Sprouting could be also termed 'seed-germination' and during this 'sprouting stage'. numerous changes occur in order for new life to develop. some of which provide a valuable supply of essential human nutrient requirements. As the seed begins to sprout. those elements contained in the seed are used to provide energy. the starches contained in the seed are slowly converted into natural sugars. the protein content of the seed is transformed into available amino acids and the fat content is converted into soluble compounds. all these changes during the sprouting stage improve the nutrient quality and human digestion of seeds – grains and legumes. After a few days of seed development. the most substantial contribution from that time is the 'life-rate activity' within the seed. ofter termed the 'enzyme activity'. **The human body requires regular supplies of various enzymes, some for promoting digestion (see pages 19, 85, and 125 for details), other enzymes are required for body development and repair, enzymes are the catalyst with all living development** Sprouted foods are one of the best source of living enzymes. other foods such as fresh fruits and vegetables are also a vital provider of living enzymes. Apart from fruits. vegetables and sprouted foods. there are very few foods that contain living enzymes. nearly all processed and refined foods are deficient in enzyme content. all cooked foods have very little enzyme content and without enzymes. a food cannot provide maximum nutritional benefits.

The most common enzymes that are available from sprouted foods are: AMYLASE – promotes digestion of carbohydrate foods. PROTEASE – protein digestion. LIPASE – fat digestion. COAGULASE – assists blood clotting. EMULSIN – sugar conversion. INVERTASE – sugar conversion. sprouted foods provide an excellent supply of these essential enzymes as well as their various protein. carbohydrate. lipid. mineral and vitamin content.

Sprouted foods are very economical. 1 table-spoon of alfalfa seeds may cost about 10 cents but when fully developed. there will be enough alfalfa sprouts to fill a large salad bowl. Sprouted foods provide an excellent source of Vitamin C and various B group vitamins as well as a good supply of the essential amino acids – protein and other amino acids and such vitamins as: E. G. K and U are all obtainable from a variety of sprouted foods. The mineral content of sprouted foods is based on the original source: whole grain, legume or seed, refer to pages 43, 61, 79, and 97 for details. You can start sprouting today!

Sprouted foods are a most valuable addition to the diet, especially for overweight people. A large number of overweight people have developed such a condition due to a decreasing rate of their own metabolic enzyme production and a prolonged lack of essential living enzymes from the foods eaten. As mentioned earlier. sprouted foods, fruits and fresh vegetables are the main source of enzymes and to ensure that your body metabolism remains active. regular supplies of those enzyme-foods must be eaten. otherwise the digestive system will become sluggish and if that is allowed to continue for a few years, a definite overweight condition results and to repair the body to a state of normal metabolism, the diet must include more enzyme-foods. An overweight person can obtain excellent re-generative energy from a regular supply of sprouted foods, fresh fruits and vegetables.

An overweight person's metabolism is often geared to convert food energy into body fat: because of their slowly increasing appetite. their decreasing intake of living foods – enzyme foods and last but not least. an overweight person has difficulty in exercising sufficiently. they feel they have done enough work-exercise but that is often just sufficient to cater for their 'real weight'. not the excess! Without the essential nutrients being supplied by a meal. that includes enzymes, minerals and vitamins. food cannot be converted into efficienty energy and that may cause a person to eat even more. in an effort to obtain those 'essential active nutrients'. When refined. processed and cooked foods are eaten. they are sure to lack at least some of the essential nutrients. often most. and with those active nutrients missing, an overweight condition is very likely to develop. especially for middle-age people who have maintained an enzyme-deficient diet for many years. As the excess body-fat cells all 'desire' proper nutrition. the overweight person may continue to feel hungry'. even after a large meal.

Sprouted foods have the potential to replenish your supply of enzymes and all nutrients required for efficient digestion and energy expenditure. It may take many months for a person to return to normal weight. all depending on the time the overweight condition has developed and the supply of active nutrients and well balanced meals. The most re-assuring advice is that, you can loose weight, if, you ensure that at least 30% of the foods you eat, and drinks, are made up from living foods – enzyme foods: fresh fruits and vegetables, and sprouted foods, you can eat large quantities of these foods and not add excess weight, if they are obtained in the natural state! There are hundreds of ways to combine living foods with cooked meals and numerous other ways that provide even better weight reducing abilities. On pages 201–211, there is a guide to the combination of natural foods and with practice, and determination, you can avoid all forms of processed and refined foods and greatly reduce your 'need' for heavy cooked meals, there are more than weight problems associated with those enzyme-deficient meals, the amount of chemical additives associated with refined and processed foods is enough to cause concern, apart from their price!

ALFALFA SPROUTS

Alfalfa sprouts have recently become one of the most popular foods to sprout. The name Alfalfa means 'best food', the term 'father of all foods' was given to Alfalfa by the people from Arabia, dating back before the Christian era, at first, the Arabs fed their horses with Alfalfa grass and produced one of the finest breeds, later on they realised the potential of the Alfalfa seed and began to use it in combination with their meals. Alfalfa is also known as Lucerne or Buffalo herb, they all have a very small seed which has the remarkable ability to grow extra long roots, capable of picking up the vital alkaline elements from deep in the ground, sometimes reaching 20 metres. Alfalfa sprouts contain an abundance of alkaline minerals, especially calcium — protects the body against infection and is required for proper heart functioning, iron — also protects against infection and is essential for blood development. Potassium, sodium and magnesium are also alkaline minerals and well supplied from Alfalfa sprouts, apart from the alkaline minerals, Alfalfa sprouts also supply essential acid minerals to balance, the mineral phosphorus is correctly balanced with the main mineral calcium: 2.5 calcium with 1 part phosphorus — the mineral phosphorus is required for mental development and repair of the nervous system, the mineral silicon is well supplied — promotes strong bone development, healthy hair growth and a good skin condition, apart from the excellent supply of minerals, Alfalfa sprouts also provide an excellent source of protein, the Alfalfa seed is said to contain 40% complete protein,

Alfalfa sprouts provide 5% protein, due to addition of water, the sprouts by weight give a lower level of total protein, however, all the essential amino acids are supplied. Alfalfa sprouts supply one of the widest range of vitamins, compared to any other food. Vitamin C is most abundant with mature sprouts and so are the basic B group vitamins as well as B5, B6, B15 and it is reported that traces of B12 can also be obtained, depending on the type of seeds. Some other less-known vitamins have also been traced available from Alfalfa sprouts: Vitamin K — the anti-hemorrhage vitamin, protects against continuous bleeding, Vitamin U — most beneficial for treatment of peptic ulcers, Vitamin D — is also available from mature sprouts, Vitamin A and E are also well supplied. Alfalfa sprouts are known to contain at least 8 special enzymes which promote digestion and provide new life to body cells. To write more about Alfalfa sprouts would be easy, but the main points have been described, the proof is in the eating, try combining Alfalfa sprouts with your next salad sandwich or serve as a side dish for any cooked meal, try them soon for best results. Alfalfa sprouts are easy to prepare, see page 106 for details.

LENTIL SPROUTS

Lentil sprouts are far more nutritious and easier to digest than cooked Lentils, as described in the Introduction to Sprouting — page 103 and Legumes Introduction — page 33, numerous changes occur to the legume-seed during the sprouting stage, a valuable supply of essential enzymes are formed and these not only promote digestion but also provide replenishment for the body's store of enzymes and that is vital for good health, especially as we get older. Lentil sprouts do supply a fair amount of protein and when combined with such foods as sesame seeds — tahini, rice, wheat germ or pumpkin seeds, there is a great increase in protein availability, refer to pages 37, 42, 87, and 88 for details. As with all sprouted foods Lentil sprouts provide a good source of Vitamin C and the basic B group vitamins, during the sprouting stage, these nutrients increase over twice their original nutrient value, a benefit that gives sprouted foods their remarkable energy to provide maximum health potential. Lentil sprouts can be combined with numerous types of meals: vegetable soup, home made pasties, cabbage rolls, casseroles, gravies, fresh garden salads and home made hamburgers. Lentil sprouts supply good amounts of the minerals: iron — promotes oxygen distribution to muscles, potassium — promotes growth and strong muscles, zinc — assists the production of insulin, a component of numerous digestive enzymes, the minerals calcium and phosphorus are also well supplied. Lentil sprouts are a most sustaining food, they provide long-lasting energy and when combined with a favourite recipe, Lentil sprouts will enhance the taste and nutrient quality, as well as being one of the most economical energy-foods available. The reddish-brown Lentils are the most common to use for sprouting, split Lentils will not sprout. The value of Lentil sprouts is around top-class. For details on the method for sprouting Lentils, turn to page 116.

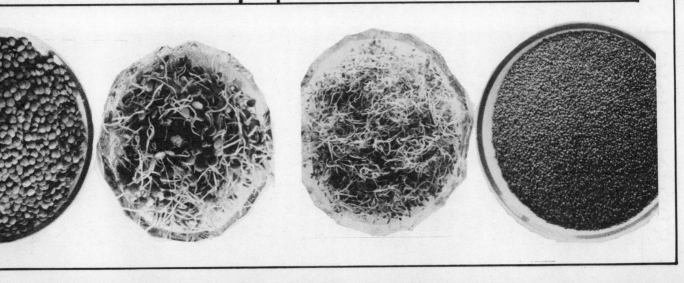

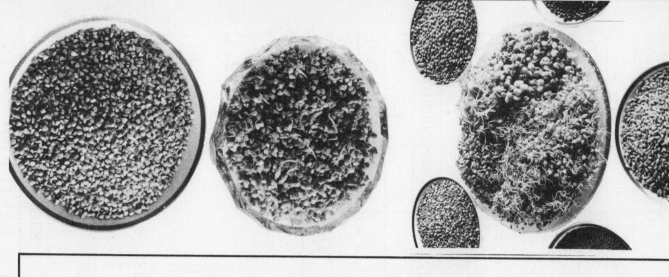

BUCKWHEAT — OTHER SPROUTS

Buckwheat sprouts are prepared from the Buckwheat seed, neither a grain or legume, Buckwheat is botanically related to rhubarb. The protein content of Buckwheat is similar to the potato, all essential amino acids are supplied and for 100 grams, Buckwheat supplies around 7 grams of protein, about half the protein content of most grains and one-third the protein content of legumes, the potato supplies about 8 grams of protein per 100 grams. Buckwheat combines well with whole grains and legumes, there are numerous recipes to try and discover such as: Buckwheat pancakes, Buckwheat – wheat bread, roasted Buckwheat and oats, Buckwheat muffins, Buckwheat noodles and Buckwheat cookies, although more expensive than whole grains and legumes, Buckwheat provides specialized nutritive value due to the abundant supply of Vitamin P — bioflavonoids, a water soluble vitamin with the following components: rutin, flavones, flavonals, hesperidin and citrin. Apart from citrus fruits, grapes, plums, blackcurrants, apricots, cherries, blackberries and rose hip, there are few other good sources of vitamin P, Buckwheat is the richest natural source of rutin. Vitamin P has numerous functions such as: it is essential for effective Vitamin C absorption and utilization, the white pulp part of citrus fruits provide a very good source of Vitamin P, the juice contains the Vitamin C and with such a combination, also supplied by Buckwheat sprouts, those two vitamins are vital for production of collagen, the intercellular substance that joins skin tissue together, providing firmness, strengthens the capillary walls and protects against infections. As Buckwheat is the best natural source of rutin, one of the bioflavonoids, it has remarkable curative abilities for cases of hardened arteries, varicose veins, poor blood circulation and certain weak heart conditions, bruising and arteriosclerosis, Buckwheat could be your best food-medicine and when sprouted, Buckwheat will also provide Vitamin C, for details on the Buckwheat sprouting method, turn to page 106. Buckwheat sprouts will also provide an excellent range of the basic B group vitamins, the mineral iron — essential for the blood, protects against peptic ulcers and increases resistance to infection. Buckwheat also provides good amounts of phosphorus and calcium. Vitamin E is also well supplied and that promotes the functions of both Vitamin P and C, both Buckwheat and Buckwheat sprouts combine well with such meals as: soups, bread, breakfast cereals, rice and vegetables, fresh garden salad, vegetable pies and party dips. Discover your favourite Buckwheat recipe and the specialized benefits.

Mung beans sprouts have retained their popularity for over 3,000 years, the Chinese discovered the method and preparation of Mung bean sprouts and today, people from around the world are discovering an important part of Chinese culture and cuisine. On page 39, a full description of the nutrient benefits associated with Mung beans is given, the Mung bean sprouts provide extra benefits such as: there is an increase in protein availability from 23 grams up to 37 grams per 100 gram portion, complete in all the essential amino acids, see pp. 42, 87, 88, 98 and 99 for details. The supply of B group vitamins is also improved during the sprouting process, especially Vitamin B1, a cupfull of Mung bean sprouts will provide 20 mg. of Vitamin C and 30 mg. — 20 I.U. of Vitamin A, plus an abundance of enzymes, all of which promote digestion and greatly improve the nutrient value compared to Mung beans — boiled, steamed or ground. There are numerous recipes for Mung beans, most are compatible with Lentils, see Lentil sprouts for recipe ideas and page 106 for Mung bean sprout preparation. Take part in a little Chinese kitchen-wisdom today, Mung bean sprouts are easy to prepare.

Other Sprouts: nearly all whole grains, legumes and seeds are suitable for sprouting, on page 106 there are details on the methods of preparation for the most common foods to sprout and by referring to the page describing the food you choose to sprout, you can read about the nutrient benefits, recipe ideas and some historical information. Most sprouts can be eaten raw, especially the whole grains and seeds, however, with the legumes, they are best slightly cooked, soya bean sprouts must be boiled for five minutes to obtain maximum protein value. Excess cooking of sprouts will destroy the valuable enzyme content and Vitamin C, the B group vitamins will also be reduced in value. Apart from the soya bean sprouts, you can obtain maximum value and taste appeal by giving the legume-sprouts either a 5 minute steam or combine them with other cooked food just before serving, also try combining sprouted grains with your breakfast cereal, mix half-half sprouted grain with cooked grain. Sprouted foods add a special life and taste when combined with cooked foods, even a table-spoon of fresh sprouts can greatly improve a cooked meal's potential, the enzymes and Vitamin C are essential for digestion and replenishment of body vitality.

SPROUTING CHARTS TIMES & METHOD

GRAINS	LEGUMES	SEEDS
BARLEY	ADZUKI	ALFALFA
BUCKWHEAT	BROAD	CABBAGE
CORN	CHICKPEA	CHIA
MILLET	KIDNEY	CLOVER
OATS	LENTILS	CRESS
RICE	LIMA	FENUGREEK
RYE	MUNG	FLAX
WHEAT	NAVY	PUMPKIN
TRITACALE	PINTO	RADISH
NUTS		SESAME
ALMONDS		SUNFLOWER

NAME	AMOUNT	days	METHOD
ALFALFA	1tbl.sp.	–3	Soak (8 hours). rinse 2× daily.
BUCKWHEAT	3tbl.sp.	–3	1st day.(rinse only, every 4 hours).
CHICKPEA	½ cup.	–5	Soak (6 hours). Rinse 3× daily.
FENUGREEK	3tbl. sp.	–3	Soak (6 hours). Rinse 3× daily.
LENTIL	½cup.	–3	Soak (6 hours). Rinse 2× daily.
MILLET	3tbl. sp.	–4	Soak (6 hours). Rinse 3× daily.
MUNG BEAN	½ cup.	–3	Soak (6 hours). Rinse 2× daily.
RICE	½ cup.	–5	Soak (6 hours). Rinse 3× daily.
SESAME	3tbl.sp.	–3	Soak (6 hours). Rinse 3× daily.
SOYA BEAN	½ cup.	–4	Soak (4 hours). Rinse 6× daily.
SUNFLOWER	½ cup.	–7	Soak (6 hours). Rinse 3× daily.
WHEAT	½ cup.	–5	Soak (6 hours). Rinse 4× daily.

Alfalfa sprouts are one of the easiest to grow, excellent for a beginner. After purchasing a packet of Alfalfa seeds, place one table-spoon of the seeds into a 1 litre glass jar, attach a fine cheese cloth lid using an elastic band. Rinse the seeds directly from the tap for less than a minute, then allow 4-6 hours for the seeds submerged in water, rinse again and drain off water. The alfalfa sprouts should be given moderate sunlight after the first shoots appear, usually 4 days, and continue to rinse — drain the sprouts every 4-10 hours. Once the Alfalfa sprouts have developed bright green shoots, they are at their maximum potential, fully of chlorophyl and vitamin C. By preparing a larger quantity of sprouts, you can place some young sprouts in the fridge, they should last 2 weeks, and whenever you need some for a combination with a meal, give them a rinse, moderate sunlight and a final rinse before serving. Alfalfa sprouts can be ready everyday for many meals.

Buckwheat sprouts require special attention, place 3 table-spoons of Buckwheat seeds into a 1 litre glass jar, attach cheese cloth with an elastic band and then rinse the seeds for about 20 seconds, directly from the tap, allow no more than 2 hours submerged in water, then rinse and drain every 4-8 hours for 3 days, the sprouts should develop a stem and leaves about 1 cm long. Place extra Buckwheat sprouts in the fridge, until required for use, then rinse and give moderate sunlight, rinse again before serving. Buckwheat sprouts are well worth preparing.

Lentil sprouts, Mung sprouts, Chickpea, Soya, Oats and Wheat sprouts are all similar when preparing for sprouting as well as those packets of mixed seeds and legumes. See chart for details on times and amounts. Place the required amount of the seeds-grains into a 1 litre jar, attach a cheese cloth lid, using an elastic band, rinse directly from the tap and allow to soak for the recommended time. By using warm water for rinsing and soaking, the sprouting time will be reduced. keep the sprouts in a dark position. After 3-6 days the sprouts will be ready to combine with other meals, or, then can be stored in the fridge for up to 2 weeks. always rinse before serving. Once the 'art of sprouting' becomes practised, you can develop your own techniques, you may want sprouts but because of your occupation, you have little time to prepare them, you could place them in the fridge when you are away and continue to grow them, taking from the fridge, and placing in a warm position overnight or anytime. Sprouted foods will help you survive with health.

MILK

Milk is the first natural food, mother's milk is the perfect food for development of contented and healthy children and depending on the duration of breast feeding, and the health of the mother, a child will obtain all the essential nutrients to assist the early, vital stages of body development. A contented baby needs a contented mother, and a healthy mother, able to provide more than just the nutrients from her Milk, at this early stage, a baby lives from the total sharing of goodness. The supply of Milk from the mother will last usually up to 12 months, sometimes longer and more often than not, these days, mother's milk has become more of a temporary food, for even less than 3 months. As the mother's milk is the best food for babies, special care should be taken by the mother to ensure that she also obtains the best foods: natural foods. There are a few other, very important elements supplied by mother's milk, such as bacillus bifidus, a natural bacteria that protects the child from other bacteria and it also assists digestion of the milk-sugar: lactose (see page 20).

As the child is weened off mother's milk, the use of cow's milk and other milks are usually given as the next main food. For those children who obtain both a supply of mother's milk and other milk, for some time, the natural bacteria provided by the mother's milk will assist digestion of the other milk, until such time that no more mother's milk is available. From that time onwards, the new milk-food will start supplying it's own bacteria and for some children, a milk-allergy develops, due to a deficiency of the digestive enzyme: lactose, provided by the other milk, causing difficulty in digestion of the milk-sugar: lactose. Cultural trends in this deficiency are common, some countries have for many centuries used cow's milk or other milk: goats, buffalo, camel or sheep, and therefore developed the capacity to digest milk.

Milk has played an important role in human survival and in parts of India, for example, the cow is given special importance and care. Within the developing digestive system of children, a very important 'temporary digestive enzyme' is produced, called rennin (see pp. 83 and 157). On average, this digestive enzyme will remain within the child's digestive system, until the first full set of teeth are developed, usually around the age of seven. Slowly, from that time onwards, the ability of a child to digest milk, depends greatly on their total health and their body ability to adapt to a new system of Milk digestion. The special enzyme, rennin, is required to convert the caseinogen content of Milk into the form of casein. In comparison to human milk, cow's milk contains 300% more caseinogen, the function of this substance is mainly to assist in the production of the hormone: thyroxine, used by the thyroid gland to control the general metabolism, nervous system, glandular system, mental development and growth rate. As cow's milk contains greater quantities of caseinogen, and it is designed for calves, which have a growth rate 4 times that of human children, numerous physical and possible mental imbalances can occur from the excessive consumption of cow's milk.

With regard to the calcium content of cow's milk, see nutrient chart page 117, there is a good supply of calcium obtainable from Milk and especially cheese. During the early stages of growth, calcium provides the strength to the bone structure (see pages 142–143), however, when comparing other calcium foods, cow's milk is not considered as an excellent source, due to the numerous other associated problems mentioned earlier.

Because of the basic similarities between mother's milk and cow's milk, e.g.: milk-sugar content and appearance, it has become common for children to be greatly encouraged to drink Milk, and even for adults it continues to provide some place in the diet. When considering nutritional benefits, cow's milk does provide some of the essential daily nutrient requirements, they can be considered advantageous, however, when comparing other types of Milk, numerous other benefits are also provided and without the ill-effects of excess casein content, harmful bacteria, digestive problems and a few more to be mentioned shortly. Such other Milks that can be highly recommended for adults, and older children can be prepared from nuts, seeds or legumes. These primary Milk preparations will provide a better compatability for human digestion, greater supply of essential daily nutrients and when properly prepared, a delicious and rewarding taste. Soya milk is very popular throughout the world, see pp. 89–91. Sesame milk, see page 102, Almond milk, see page 93, Coconut milk, see page 133, these four primary Milks are greatly recommended for teenagers and adults, as an alternative to cow's milk. The use of goat milk has also become popular, and even though it is usually harder to obtain than cow's milk, for those people who can get a regular supply, goat's milk is far more compatible for human digestion and development, compared to cow's milk.

When considering the mass milk market today, compared to the one farm one cow tradition era, numerous other detrimental factors can be added to the list, for cow's milk. A cow will make great effort to obtain the best possible feed, large areas of country-side have to be fenced against their desire for other feeding grounds, some cows have excellent quality pastures, while others are raised on the bare minimum. The supply of Milk to the city areas is often gathered from various local country areas and depending on the climate and supply of proper pasture, the city milk will vary from different sources. In the city areas, many people obtain pasteurised and homogenised milk and the main purpose of these two processes it to make Milk uniform and capable of better storage, both of which occur as well as a few detrimental factors.

The process of pasteurisation is intended to kill harmful bacteria that may be present in the Milk, however, not all bacteria are destroyed. Pasteurised milk is heated to 145°F for 30 minutes or sometimes, 161°F for 15 seconds, neither of these two treatments will completely destroy all bacteria, and unfortunately, 'friendly natural bacteria' are also destroyed, leaving a possible harmful bacteria, that may develop and contaminate the entire supply of Milk, that may happen rarely as the Milk is quickly packaged and distributed, refrigerated and consumed. By the time the Milk has reached the final destination, in the digestive system, those 'other bacteria' may be ready to destroy the natural bacteria content within the intestines, and depending on your body resistance: health, and use of such Milk produce, the harmful bacteria can either win or lose. The common cold has a great alliance with 'harmful bacteria' and if your resistance is low, and such Milk consumed, the 'bacteria-battle' may lead to another defeat, and one of those 'common colds'!

MILK & CHEESE

In those parts of the world where fresh cow's milk is obtainable, it is also common to boil the Milk, just before serving, and that will destroy harmful bacteria and can promote digestion of the Milk as well as reducing the 'mucus content' especially when diluted with water. The cup of coffee or tea with Milk, a very common combination, will assist in diluting the mucus producing properties of the Milk. Dairy produce foods: milk, cheese, butter and cream, are the most likely of all foods to promote 'a build-up of 'mucus residue', and at a time of the common cold, those excess mucus toxins are forced to be eliminated, causing regular release of mucus from the nose and mouth. At such time, it is greatly advised to restrict the intake of dairy produce foods, with the exception of a small amount of natural yoghurt. Such foods as fresh fruits and vegetables, nuts and seeds will assist in a rapid recovery to health, in times of the common cold, and always.

Milk is a meal maker, the breakfast cereal is lost without Milk, the lunchtime milkshake, the evening cups of coffee or tea with Milk, they are 'standard additions' to the diet, especially in Australia and America. This regular dependancy on Milk is based on the original life-promoting ability of mother's milk and that continued attachment to Milk, may last a life-time. Milk may provide reassurance to the body, especially when the majority of other foods and drinks are based on processed foods, and in such cases, Milk consumption is often excessive. Both the combination of the processed diet with the pasteurised milk, can provide only a very limited proportion of any essential human nutrients: minerals, vitamins and enzymes, and with such a diet, the risk of numerous 'social disorders' can develop.

To summarise the topic of Milk is as simple as to re-read the points already mentioned. Mother's milk is an excellent food for children and to substitute cow's milk exclusively, for mother's milk may develop any of the before mentioned problems. If the supply of mother's milk is supplimented with portions of cow's milk, during the latter stages of lactation, some benefits are obtainable, from freshly boiled cow's milk and if pasteurised milk is obtained, that also should be boiled, and served after allowing to cool. After the age of seven, a child should already be prepared to eat freshly prepared fruits, not canned fruits. Grated fruits and mashed vegetables are the ideal first 'earth foods' for children. Small daily amounts of Milk can also be part of the diet and around the age of fourteen, the gradual inclusion of whole grains with Milk, as well as freshly prepared fruits and vegetables will provide numerous other body building qualities. The use of soya bean milk could begin slowly from as early as the age of two, however, for many people, cow's milk is the real thing. The teenager can continue to combine milk with whole grains and gradually start to prepare the appetite for the large variety of natural foods, apart from Milk.

In those parts of the world where cow's milk has been used for generations, a special Milk-product is also consumed, to assist digestion of the Milk and to protect against harmful bacteria and subsequent illness. Yoghurt is the special Milk-product, capable of supplying valuable digestive enzymes, to assist in the digestion of Milk, and as mentioned before, the natural digestive enzyme: rennin, only lasts until around the age of seven, from then onwards, and even before, the combination of obtaining yoghurt when using dairy products, is highly recommended. See page on Yoghurt for details.

Cheese has been made for thousands of years, the origin of Cheese is thought to have developed accidently, when nomads and tribe people carried milk in containers that were made from the stomach of a milk-producing animal: cow, goat, sheep, camel or buffalo. As the nomads travelled along, the constant movement from their journey, with the effects of heat, and the contact between the milk and the animal-stomach container, produced the earliest method of milk storage: Cheese making. The special active ingredient, obtained from the animal stomach, is called rennet, and this digestive enzyme assists the calf, to digest milk from the cow. As mentioned on the page for Milk, the human child, up to the age of around seven, also produces a milk digesting enzyme.

The majority of traditional and modern methods of Cheese-making are based on the curdling effect, produced by the enzyme rennet, some Cheese is curdled by the effects of lemon juice and more recently, a vegetable rennet has been developed, it is less expensive and is greatly increasing in popularity, as a large variety of aged cheese and cottage cheese can be produced from this vegetable rennet. A special Cheese can also be mae completely from the primary source: soya bean milk, curdled with lemon juice or powdered gypsum, produces a unique Cheese called Tofu, and in China and Japan, Tofu has provided excellent nutrition for thousands of years. Tofu is prepared daily in these countries and combined with nearly all meals. The protein content of Tofu provides a major portion of the daily protein requirements for those people and many others throughout the world who have discovered the taste for Tofu. For more information about Tofu, see pages on Soya bean: 89–91.

Cheese that has been produced by the effects of rennet, will vary from country to country, depending on the type of bacteria that is formed during the Cheese-making. Today, there are over 400 individual types of Cheese, each with a different taste, texture and appearance. From Switzerland, the famous emmentalar, Swiss cheese, has unique characteristics, with holes in the cheese. From Italy, the famous mozzarella, from France, camembert and from England and U.S.A., the cheddar cheese. From all over the world different types of Cheese are produced and available in the large urban areas, from the delicatessen. In comparison to milk, Cheese provides extra benefits, firstly because it is in a pre-digested form, from the effects of rennet which greatly assist the human adult digestive system, to convert the lactose: milk-sugar, into the form of glucose: energy. Many varieties of Cheese are also given special 'friendly natural bacteria' and these will also benefit digestion of the concentrated milk product: Cheese. The two main groups of Cheese are: soft cheese and hard cheese, the main difference being in the associated water content and of course, tha taste and texture.

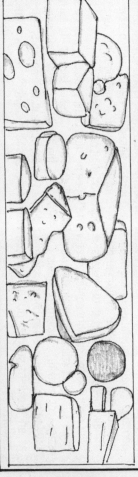

CHEESE

Cheese is an excellent source of complete protein, by referring to pages 87, 88, 98, 99 and 117, there are various charts to provide a comparison between Cheese and the other main protein foods. Cheese is a very compact protein food and one that can easily promote excess weight, as apart from the excellent supply of protein, Cheese is also the main saturated fat, animal protein food. See page 124 for details. The combination of both the excellent protein value with the saturated fat content, of Cheese, can easily promote excess weight. For an adult, weighing 70 kg., all their R.D.A. recommended daily protein allowance can be obtained from a 120 gram serve of cheddar cheese, and even though such an amount may not be eaten at the one time, when combining with the protein and fat content of other meals of the day, there may soon be an oversupply of both protein and saturated fat content, both of which assist in adding extra weight. Excess protein is likely to be converted into body fat content of other meals of the day, there may soon be an oversupply of both protein and saturated fat content, both of which assist in adding extra weight. Excess protein is likely to be converted into body fat and so the combination of both these factors as well as the lack of regular exercise, can easily promote an overweight condition. Cheese is also an excellent source of the main mineral calcium, on average, over 700 mg. per 100 gram are available from hard cheese, cottage cheese supplies around 60 mg. By referring to the nutrient evaluation chart, page 117, and comparing with the other nutrient evaluation charts, pages 43, 61, 79, and 98, you will find that, apart from sesame seeds, Cheese is the best calcium food, however, that depends on the type of Cheese, those traditional and modern 'natural cheese', free from any artificial ingredients, are well worth obtaining, in contrast, numerous types of processed cheese are also available, they should be avoided and substitutes are not worth the expense.

Another ingredient that is common with nearly all types of Cheese is salt, over 600 mg.. per 100 gram serve of hard cheese is the average and even though the R.D.A. is from 2000-6000 mg. per day, the actual salt content is in the form of sodium chloride, table salt, a substance that if taken excessively, can easily promote not only weight problems but numerous types of arterial and heart-function damage. If your diet includes regular amounts of Cheese, your added salt intake should also be considerably less and remember that processed and factory foods also supply generous amounts of added salt, as a preservative and to promote the appetite. Cheese is a good source of vitamin A, over 1000 mg. per 100 gram serve of hard cheese, in comparison to carrots, Cheese supplies one-tenth the amount of vitamin A, and in a completely different form: known as pre-formed vitamin A: retinol (see pages 174–175).

Apart from the excellent protein and calcium content of Cheese, there are only a few minor important nutrients provided, and a larger list of possible health risks. The supply of saturated fats, mentioned earlier, in combination with the high cholesterol level are the most obvious health risk factors, provided by Cheese. On page 127, the topic of cholesterol is provided plus a cholesterol chart and by referring to the page on Saturated Fats – 124, details on the possible health risk factors are given, also see Lecithin – page 126 and Digestion – page 125. The page on Milk also describes the problem of mucus, and when considering Cheese, the problem of excess mucus build-up is even more likely. The page on Yoghurt will emphasize the point that, when using dairy products, especially Cheese, the diet should also include a regular supply of natural L.B. Yoghurt. Always remember to avoid any processed cheese, the best value and variety of Cheese is obtainable from your local delicatessen, there you can discover a variety of natural Cheese, with a tradition of tastes and long established, positive reputation.

The ability of Cheese to combine with other foods, and to create new recipes is a benefit well practiced in French restaurants, local restaurants and nearly every home, and depending on the type of Cheese-combination, the benefits may be positive. A golden-green point of advice: when using Cheese regularly, also ensure that the diet provides regular amounts of fresh vegetables, the French salad and a variety of fresh fruits and freshly made juices, they will assist your body in obtaining the list of nutrients not obtainable from Cheese and they will promote cleansing and protection from the mucus, excess saturated fat content and they will provide an abundance of active enzymes. Cheese will combine very well with fresh and cooked vegetables, the simple whole grain bread and natural-traditional Cheese, grated Cheese with cooked legumes and whole grains, these are the basic recommended Cheese combinations.

Various other Cheese combinations are with animal products: the omlette, quiche or cheesecake are very common and so it must be mentioned that each animal protein food, requires a different type and time of digestion, a combination of Cheese with other animal produce does provide a very sustaining-stomach feeling, however, apart from that 'desire', the digestion of both the Cheese with the other animal produce, will retard protein digestion, reduce protein value and promote the common overweight condition. Such cheese-animal produce combinations may have regular attraction to your diet, and if you are overweight, those meals may have slowly developed the problem, and now, to attempt to lose weight, those cheese-animal produce combinations should be greatly reduced from the diet and mind, natural foods provide all the best recipes, see pp. 201–213 for recipe ideas.

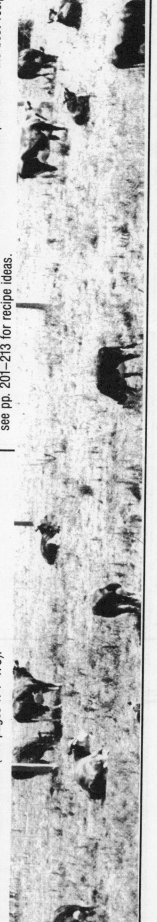

YOGHURT

Yoghurt has a long-proven history, dating back thousands of years, possibly just after the domestication of farm animals. During the early 1900s, and up to this present day, research into the nutritional quality of Yoghurt has provided very encouraging results that are also backed up from generations of people throughout the world, especially: Turkey, Balkans' regions. Greece, Egypt, Arabia, Algeria, India, China and today, more people throughout the world obtain the benefits that only Yoghurt can provide. Yoghurt can be prepared from cow's milk, goat's milk, buffalo milk, sheep milk and soya milk. The main ingredient that is common with all types of milk is lactose, often called 'milk-sugar' (see page 20), this is converted by the digestive system, into the form of glucose: energy. Yoghurt also contains lactose as well as the very important 'lactic acid enzymes', these are formed with the assistance of special bacteria. The two most common natural bacteria are: lactobacillus acidophillus, and lactobacillus bulgaricus, both are closely related, however, the L.B. acidophillus has proven to be the most effective in maintaining a correct and prolonged supply of natural bacteria within the digestive system. The word 'bacteria' may concern some people and so it must be pointed out that, even without Yoghurt, various types of bacteria will be obtained from other animal produce: meat, cheese, milk, eggs, poultry, fish and seafood as well as processed and chemically loaded foods. The bacteria that is formed from these foods can produce some harmful effects, if allowed to accumulate, and to prevent accumulation, the use of natural L.B.A. Yoghurt is highly recommended. Natural Yoghurt will destroy harmful bacteria with a 'friendly bacteria', containing valuable antibiotic qualities which provide cleansing, a healthy digestive system and improved absorption of nutrients as well as a self-generating supply of essential B group vitamins.

Apart from those foods mentioned above, various other forms of bacteria and chemical elements may enter the digestive system, via the intake of foods or drinks, chemical sprays, fertilizers, preservatives, pollution, nicotene, alcohol, see page 107 for a list of common food additives, each of these individual additives that enter the digestive system may also contain harmful bacteria and when contained within the warm environment of the small intestine and colon, these bacteria can rapidly spread and be absorbed into the bloodstream, from the area of the small intestine. It is common that antibiotics are prescribed to destroy those harmful bacteria, however, at the same time, any natural, desirable bacteria may also be destroyed. Natural Yoghurt provides the ultimate natural method of fighting harmful bacteria and when using L.B.A., Yoghurt especially, the 'natural penicillin' effects last up to 48 hours.

For those people who rarely think about Yoghurt, and many now consider it time to try, you should be aware that, if your digestive system is full of bacteria, accumulated food residue and toxins, the initial use of natural Yoghurt may imprt a considerable cleansing effect, resulting in distasteful odours and a slight rumbling within the intestines. It may take over a month of regular Yoghurt eating to eliminate all those 'hidden bacteria'. Start by using a small amount, and only use 'natural L.B. Yoghurt', about 2 tablespoons, everyday, and then after two weeks, every second day.

The original human food, mother's milk, also contains a natural bacteria: bacillus bifidus, and that provides the same valuable qualities obtainable from L.B. Yoghurt. After children are weened off mother's milk, the addition of other milk and dairy products that are included with the diet, need a natural bacteria to assist digestion and conversion of the lactose — milk sugar. For those people who consume regular amounts of milk and dairy products, the use of L.B. Yoghurt is highly recommended, and for anybody who has developed a polluted intestinal tract, diarrhoea, gastroenteritis or food poisoning, amounts of natural L.B. Yoghurt assist in restoring your intestinal flora. By obtaining regular amounts of natural L.B. Yoghurt, you can prevent the development of numerous common stomach and intestinal disorders and promote a radiant glow to your complexion and hidden digestive system!

Natural L.B. Yoghurt will keep in the fridge for about two weeks, always improving in natural bacteria content, until after two weeks it is advised to obtain a fresh supply. The cost of Yoghurt is very economical and when considering nutritional benefits, Yoghurt — L.B., is excellent value.

LIPIDS	MONO.	POLY	SATU	CHOLESTEROL FOODS	Amounts in milligrams per measure.
Butter	34	2	57	Butter	1tbl.sp. 35mg.
Cream	29	4	62	Cream Full	1tbl.sp. 20mg.
Camembert	29	3	63	Cheddar	1ounce. 28mg.
Edam	28	2	65	Edam	1ounce. 29mg.
Yoghurt	27	3	65	Lard	1cup. 195mg.
Milk-cows	29	4	63	Milk-Cows	1cup. 34mg.
Ice cream	29	4	63	Condensed Milk	1cup. 105mg.
Eggs	40	12	30	Crab Meat	1cup. 125mg.
Poultry	45	20	30	Lobster	1cup. 123mg.
Fish	20	50	25	Oysters	1cup. 120mg.
Beef	35	2	60	Beef	3ounces. 80mg.
Veal	40	2	40	Veal	3ounces. 86mg.
Lamb	36	3	54	Lamb	3ounces. 83mg.
Pork	40	2	40	Pork	3ounces. 76mg.
Almonds	68	19	8	Liver	3ounces. 372mg.
Cashew	58	16	20	Turkey	3ounces. 65mg.
Soya Beans	23	51	17	Brains	3ounces. 1750mg.
Sesame Seeds	38	42	14	Kidney	1cup. 1125mg.

EGGS

Eggs have a life-long tradition, dating back to over 2,000 years B.C. The variety of Eggs, from Poultry: chicken, duck and geese, have throughout time, provided a valuable contribution to Man's diet. The Chinese have for centuries, recognized the value of Eggs and they have developed special methods of preserving Eggs. For some other ancient culture, the Egg was not treated so enthusiastically, many people have been very wary of the use of Eggs, sometimes related to a superstition and other times the topic of Life, suggesting that by using Eggs, the life of a 'new bird' is destroyed. The question about the fertile or infertile Egg, has a direct relationship to both the superstition surrounding the Egg and also the topic of Life. A fertile egg is produced when the male species of the poultry, has contact with the female and the Egg, sometimes an infertile Egg is produced, but mainly, the Egg will hatch and produce a quaint-looking off-spring! That situation happens frequently on the farm, and at some times of the year, large numbers of Eggs are laid, and to prevent an over-population of little-chicks, the rooster or male poultry-partner is temporarily given an new position, away from the other birds. The Eggs that are laid while the rooster is away, will be infertile Eggs, and as they are not capable of producing a new life, those Eggs can be considered as proper to eat, especially in times of survival, in such a farm situation.

The nutrient benefits associated with the Egg are as follows: the protein content is of the highest quality, over 90% of the protein content in Eggs, is useable by the human, see pages: 87–88 for details on the protein content. Eggs are also a good source of vitamin A, over 1000 mg. per 100 gram, very similar to cheese and far less than the vegetables: carrots, pumpkin etc. The mineral iron is well supplied by Eggs, on average, less than for nuts. For more details on the mineral and vitamin content of Eggs, see page 117 and compare the availability of nutrients from Eggs with fresh fruits, vegetables, whole grains, legumes, nuts and seeds and discover how good an Egg is! As with all natural foods, there is always some outstanding nutrient or ingredient; with each food and for Eggs, the level of cholesterol is already obvious! By referring to pages 126–127, the topic of cholesterol and lecithin is given more thoroughly. From two standard eggs, the level of cholesterol is about 350-400mg., and in association with the cholesterol, it is lucky or naturally wise that Eggs also supply lecithin, over 3,500. The supply of lecithin from Eggs, has a major controlling effect on the problem of possible cholesterol accumula-tions and it is only when the Egg is cooked in oil or served with bacon or other saturated food that the real problem of cholesterol accumulation may occur. Eggs should not be avoided because of their cholesterol level, however, by ensuring that no more than six eggs a week are obtained, as well as a regular supply of fresh fruits, vegetables, whole grains, legumes, nuts and seeds and exercise, you can maintain very good health. The method of preparing Eggs is also important, for best results and benefits, slowly boil the Egg, starting with cold water, once it boils, allow 2-3 minutes on a slight simmer.

NET PROTEIN UTILIZATION:

70 – Rice, Parmesan cheese, Swiss cheese, Camembert, Edam, Cheddar cheese. **(N.P.U.%).**
72 – Corn-cob.
75 – Cottagecheese, Tigers milk.
80 – Fish.
82 – Milk – non fat, Milk, Yoghurt
83 – Egg white.
94 – Egg.

The value of Eggs is best recognized and practiced in combination with cooking, the Egg provides a versatile ability to produce a large range of delicious and healthful recipes, especially when combined with primary produce. When combining Eggs with animal produce, the benefits of the Egg are at stake! Firstly because of their different require-ments for digestion and often because an excess protein intake occurs, at the one meal, leading to an imbalance of essential active carbohydrates which are vital for proper and efficient protein digestion and metabolism, and for their energy. Avoid eating more than two Eggs at the one meal and always allow a few hours after eating Eggs, before attempting to eat fruits or concentrated protein foods; nuts, seeds and animal produce. You could combine a variety of fresh vegetables or lightly cooked vegetables with the Egg meal, and preferably have a freshly made juice before eating the Egg. Another valuable addition when using Eggs is lecithin, always remember to add at least a half-teaspoon per Egg, lecithin combines very well with any cooked meal and for Eggs, lecithin is an essential companion!

By referring to the page on chicken, you will notice great emphasis on the value of obtaining 'free-range' poultry produce. Unfortunately, in many city areas, free-range Eggs are not available, most people have to eat 'factory-bred-eggs', they are available everywhere, thousands of them and to suggest again the problem of harsh-treatment given to factory-birds, may just slip your mind, however, the problem is there, the Eggs are produced in factory conditions: no sunlight, artificial food and no exercise, that's the diet of the bird who makes 'factory-eggs'. Ask any farmer about the difference, the memories may be there, as even in country regions, a free-range Egg is often hard to get hold of. In times like that, it is best to avoid Eggs, have the occasional one if it seems essential, especially when preparing a natural meal that provides numerous protective elements against the possible effects of chemicals and the lowered nutrient value of the factory-egg. For many people, it would be possible to have a couple of chickens to free-range on their land and by providing extra food left-overs, you can be sure that the Egg will be worth eating. A fresh, free-range Egg is worth the weight of a golden egg, in nutritional terms. The use of raw Eggs is not recommended, even though the occasional taste is not harmful. Raw egg-white contains avilin, a substance that can inhibit the absorption of biotin, a B group vitamin, see page 194. The factory may continue to produce Eggs, but only a free-range, contented bird can provide a 'natural golden egg'!

PROTEIN SOURCE	HCL.RANGE.	TIME (STOMACH)
MEAT.	2	5-6 hours
POULTRY.	2-3	4-6
CHEESE.	3-4	4
FISH.	3.5	3
EGGS.	2-3.5	2
NUTS.	4-5.5	2
SEEDS.	4-5.5	2

POULTRY

Poultry animals such as the Chicken, Duck, Turkey and Geese have been domesticated for thousands of years. Around the years 2000 B.C., chickens were first recorded to be kept as farm animals, and at about the same time, cooking pots were first used in China. Until only recently, chickens were raised on the farm, where they would wander around freely, choosing a variety of plant and insect life, as the food supply. That free-raising of chickens is also termed free-range and in contrast, there are the factory bred and fed chickens. When considering not only the nutritional value but also some more intricate methods of evaluation the free-range chickens are without doubt, superior in quality, before they are killed and even after. The life of a free-range chicken differs greatly from the factory bred version, the lifespan of a factory chicken is not only short but considerably cruel, even though, those birds may be born and bred for the cage! In some cases, factory-chickens never see or feel sunlight, they are raised under artificial lighting and heating conditions and their diet includes mainly artificial food. Large factories, containing over 10,000 chickens at one time, and the purpose: to feed a nation, or at least a number of them. From the time that the chicken is first raised, in the factory, until the time it may reach your dinner plate or take-away food shop; the number of cruel, detrimental and disgusting treatments that are applied to the chicken, in the factory, provides not only reason to discourage such food consumption but also question about the long-term effects of eating such produce. Back on the farm, some people may raise twenty chickens, for sales to local people, however, if those birds were not in good condition, the local people would hesitate to buy. In the city, a completely different situation occurs, the people who buy the chicken are greatly encouraged by the availability of a delicious, taste-stimulating aroma, from freshly roasted chicken and that may quickly promote the appetite and provide a regular source of convenient and satisfying food, even though those chickens have lived a miserable life!

With regard to the nutritional content of a free-range chicken, or other poultry, in comparison to a factory-fed and bred chicken, the basic nutrient composition does not vary considerably, except in the case of eggs. However, as the factory-fed chicken depends on a diet containing pellets, chemical additives, special hormone injections, no sunlight, little exercise and a totally terrifying environment, the accumulation of chemicals and other numerous additives to their diet, and no fresh food, can produce a build-up of harmful substances within the flesh of the factory-chicken and those chemicals can also be transfered into human cells, after eating such produce. When considering factory chicken in terms of their total contents, their can be no appraisal of the 'product', in nutritional terms or otherwise.

Chicken raised on a free-range and prepared in the proper manner, can be considered as a valuable addition to the diet, especially in times when there is a shortage of other natural foods. The supply of complete protein from free-range chickens is possibly the main benefit, even though, their eggs are also a complete and more suitable source. Other poultry, such as Turkey, Duck and Geese, all have one common deficiency, in regards to protein. The essential amino acid: tryptophan is not supplied with such poultry, and therefore they are not a complete-protein food. See pages 82, 87, 88, 98, 99 and 117 for details on protein requirements and availability from these foods and for comparisons with other, more suitable protein foods. By referring page 98, animal produce nutrient chart, to pages 43, 61, 79 and 97, you can compare the availability of numerous other essential nutrients supplied by fresh fruits, vegetables, whole grains, legumes, nuts and seeds with those supplied by chicken or other poultry and discover that for the best nutrition, chicken or poultry is less than average nutritional value.

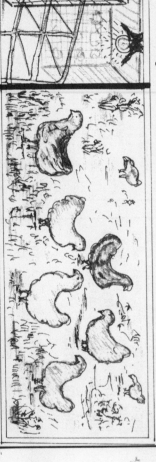

"Laugh with Health", don't just Quack!

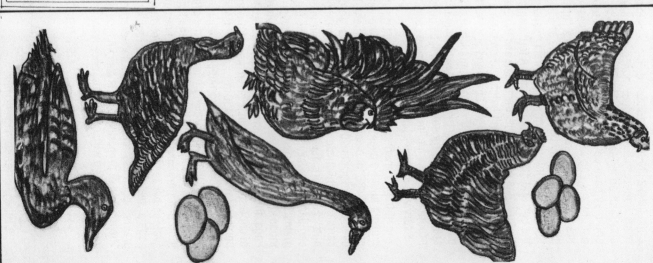

FISH

SEAFOOD

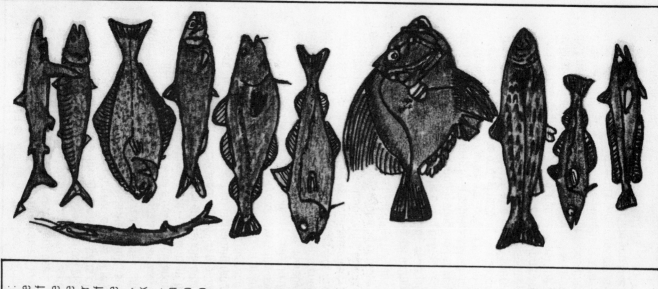

Fish is defined as: 'animal living in water. vertebrate cold-blooded animal having gills'. There are three main types of Fish: saltwater. freshwater and shellfish (including crustacea). Fish have developed from the very beginning to time and they have provided valuable clues as to the origin of Man. based on theories that Man emerged from the sea and slowly. over millions of years. developed the ability to move on land. The Fish population. throughout the world. exceeds the number of people and the varieties of Fish are greater than the number of nationalities. For about 10,000 years. Fish have been obtained by Man and in the early stages. primitive hooks and nets were used to catch Fish. and that tradition continues in some parts of the world today. For some countries. Fish is a staple food and every day fresh Fish are caught. prepared and served with local 'earth-foods'. The art of catching a Fish involves patience. determination and knowledge and once the Fish is caught. the reward of nutrients will make the effort very worthwhile. If the Fish is eaten the same day. The difference between fresh Fish (caught that day) and other Fish. refrigerated. frozen or canned is a vital guideline for the return of positive benefits. Some methods of preserving Fish. date back thousands of years. smoked Fish and dried Fish were commonly used. when the supply of fresh Fish was not caught. Unfortunately. for many people. they have no time to go Fishing and they rely on other fishermen to get a supply. usually the Fish are over a day old. kept under light refrigeration and by the time it reaches a big city market. the Fish requires special cooking to promote digestion. using added fats. spices. salt and in some cases. the Fish is covered in batter. to promote digestion and to disguise the product. When Fish is obtained fresh (less than one day old) the benefits are numerous and depending on the delay. type of additives. method of cooking and the appetite. the Fish will gradually decrease in benefits and increase in nutritional hazards.

Fish (saltwater and freshwater) are an excellent source of complete protein, on average the protein % content is 24, see pp. 87–88 for details. The (N.P.U.) net protein utilization of Fish is 80% and both these figures are far greater than for meat. When comparing tuna with beef, for example a 70 kg. person would require 100 grams of tuna-fish to obtain the R.D.A. recommended daily allowance and for beef, 180 grams are required, nearly double the amount for tuna-fish, refer to pages 98–99 for details. The cost of Fish is usually more than for meat, depending on your accessibility to such produce. The high protein value and the minimal amount of excess amino acids, from Fish, is a major benefit, when compared to meat. Excess protein: amino acids, are mainly converted into toxins, body-fat or eliminated. Fish does provide saturated fats but in comparison to meat, the difference is about 1:5, see page 117 for details.

Some seafood, especially crayfish, caviar, oysters, crab-meat and lobsters contain a high level of cholesterol, see page 127 for cholesterol chart. These foods are generally higher in cholesterol than beef. Fish (fresh water) have similar protein value to deep-sea Fish and they are similar in nutrient composition, see page 117 for full details on nutrient composition of various Fish and compare with the range of other natural foods, see pp. 43, 61, 79 and 97 for nutrient charts. The protein content of Fish is without doubt, the most valuable contribution. In Australia and America, the use of Fish is minimal, compared to meat and when considering that people eat meat for protein, they would obtain numerous benefits by obtaining a regular supply of fresh Fish, instead of meat. For overweight people, the use of fresh Fish, instead of animal produce would greatly assist in weight control, especially when the Fish is baked and use of added fats kept to a minimum. Freshly caught and then fire-backed Fish is well worth the effort of a few hours fishing, ask any fisherman about the taste of fresh Fish compared to canned fish, batter fish or un-frozen fish, discover for yourself the benefits of fresh Fish, at least once a lifetime!

Kelp is a sea-food, it has been used for thousands of years by Man and it is said to be the 'first crop', in ancient Roman, Greek and Chinese times. Kelp was renowned for its virtues and even today, the Irish, Welsh, Chinese and Japanese take part in a little more of the benefits of sea-life. Kelp is dominant in nearly all essential human nutrients, see food charts pages 158–161 and 184–186 for details. The chemical composition of human blood is said to be very similar to sea-water and by obtaining sea-food, the balance of nutrients is most suitable for effective absorption. Sea-food provides an abundance of iodine, see page 154 for details. The strong taste of Kelp is due to the abundance of nutrients, and when properly prepared and served, a Kelp meal will provide good protein value, nearly all minerals and vitamins, and for total vegetarians, Kelp supplies the essential vitamin B12, very few foods apart from animals products, supply this vitamin, see page 192 for details. Kelp and sea-food are at this stage, just beginning to be recognized as a suitable food. Kelp is food for the future!

MEAT

Meat is described as 'animal flesh as food, excluding fish and poultry'. Man has domesticated sheep and goats for over 10,000 years and the origin of the cow, from archaeological evidence, seems to be related to a wild animal known as the 'bos primigenius', a long-horned, dark coloured, seven foot beast. The last known survivor of that species was recorded in Poland, in the early 1600's. All types of domesticated cattle are related to 'bos primigenius', even though the variety of cattle today, provide a more refined looking animal, in some cases, a most placid-looking animal of the countryside. By the year 2,500B.C., there were several distinct breeds of cattle throughout many parts of the world and with each breed, Man has played a vital role, with generations of assistance. Such common, domesticated cattle, some are specially designed, by Man, to produce good quality, high yielding milk supplies, others are primarily grazed for their supply of flesh, commonly termed Meat.

Before the times of domestic animals, Man was a hunter, living from a variety of animals and also some fruits, nuts and other plant-life. In those times, Man's desire to kill another animal was directly related to 'basic survival needs': food and clothing. Even today, in some parts of the world, people hunt for their food and collect other plant-life. In other parts of the world, an excess supply of milk and meat products and various other foods occurs, due to increased farming production, specializing in one range of produce and various other methods which promote the efficiency of animals, the soil, plant-life and Man's capacity to control the system, using machinery and an increasing range of chemicals. In comparison to the hunting days, for basic survival needs, a complete new system for obtaining both milk and meat, and most other products, prevails today, especially in Australia, America and parts of Europe and the United Kingdom. In these places, and many others, many people obtain their meat and products from a local shop, supermarket or city store, very few people are maintaining the traditional and personal involvement with the production of food for their family and other local people. In this era, Man is capable of obtaining not only a wide range of foods to cultivate, but also technological assistance in doing so, thereby greatly improving on the 'struggles that our ancestors survived with', in order to obtain a 'farm survival lifestyle'. When considering the food product: Meat, in terms of the 'city lifestyle', the question of survival is no longer apparent, some people may never experience the various processes that convert a living animal, into the form of Meat, and if they did, their 'new views' about the matter may differ greatly. The basic survival-need for Meat has vanished from the eyes of the general public, the mass-slaughtering of animals, for Meat, is not essential for human survival and because the 'basic survival need' is missing, the mass-slaughtering of those cows becomes more a tragedy than a necessity! The importance of human life is guided greatly by the way we treat other humans and animals.

If people realize the cruel and detrimental methods of Meat production, and continue to eat such produce, the sincerity of their actions can hardly be recommended, especially when they encourage children to take part. The farm provides the ideal environment to take part in the eating of Meat, especially when other foods are limited, due to climatic conditions and crop failure. One cow could provide a long-lasting food supply for a large family, especially now that refrigeration is available and before those days, people would share their supply of Meat, to local people, who in turn would provide another product, sounds simple and so it is; until the numbers increase so greatly that no one knows where that Meat came from, and very few people make any effort to be interested, the 'routine of buying meat' has become so integrated that a definite dependency on the Meat product has developed. The alternative foods to Meat, as a protein source, are numerous; by referring to pages 22–106, the variety of complete protein foods and other essential foods are described and evaluated for their protein value: see pages 41, 83, 84, 98 and 99 for exact details. As there is such a large variety of 'primary produce' available in most places, the 'need' for any animal produce should be greatly restricted. Why kill an animal, when you can obtain a direct supply from a primary source! Well, most people don't kill the animal so they couldn't answer, they just keep on eating Meat, sometimes the answer is, "it tastes good and it keeps me going", that may be right but there are more foods than Meat to eat, and they taste good and keep you going also, the difference is a question of life, if Meat is mass-slaughtered, the vital respect for animal life and consequently, human life, dwindles. How can you 'live' when you take part regularly in some mass-killing of animals? The answer is for every individual to decide and to slowly make steps in understanding that the 'action you take, also provides a reaction'. If you take part in the eating of mass-produced Meat, there are some other important factors to consider, apart from the very important main point: 'Meat for survival' and not just for convenience!

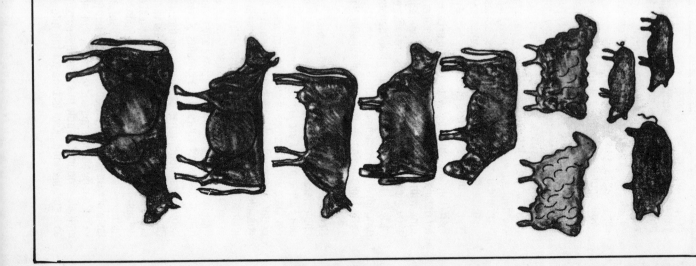

MEAT

The absence of carbohydrate content, with Meat, is also another possible detrimental factor. Without carbohydrates, protein digestion could not occur effectively and as the Meat may fill over half the plate, the supply of essential carbohydrate-companion foods, are often pushed to the side. Various forms of intestinal disorders develop from such a diet, usually later in life, and the distress of those ailments is nothing worth practising for, especially regularly. The best foods to combine with Meat are fresh leafy vegetables, some steamed vegetables and possibly small portions of whole grain bread. Fresh vegetables will provide essential enzymes, nutrients and cellulose roughage: vital for elimination of toxic waste, and with Meat, toxic waste is abundant. The substance: uric acid, is a by-product of protein digestion and from Meat, uric acid levels are especially high, often more than can be eliminated. For those people who maintain a regular Meat diet, more than one meat-meal per day, the accumulation of uric acid and other toxins can quickly promote a poor state of health. By allowing at least two days between meat-meals, you body will be able to disperse a majority of excess toxins, via the excretory organs and by ensuring that regular supplies of fresh fruits, vegetables, juices, natural yoghurt are maintained, the risk of excess toxins will be kept to a minimum.

Often directly after a meat-meal, a serve of sweet food or other is served, that common overloading of the stomach, with a mixture of completely different foods, can produce various problems, even though, those sweets are hard to resist. As protein digestion starts in the stomach, and the enzyme required is composed of hydrochloric acid, the flood of sweets after the Meat meal will greatly reduce the capacity of the protein digestive enzymes, to prepare the Meat for later stages of conversion and absorption. The result is initially soothing to the stomach, but later in the small intestine, the problem of poorly prepared protein starts to build-up. A majority of the protein value is unprepared, some is absorbed, but the real value of the Meat is not obtained, so once again, a person may resort to another in-between meal, to get what they missed before and in many cases, a meat-eater may consume large quantities of Meat, in order to obtain a daily supply of protein.

It takes more time to get protein from Meat than from any other food, see pages 85 and 116 for details. The decomposition of the animal flesh, within the human digestive system, leads to the formation of uric acid and toxic by-products, these can be slowly eliminated by the liver and kidneys, but with Meat, the amount of toxic residue that can build-up, within the 11 metre digestive tract is often more than can be satisfactorily eliminated. When considering the 'total surface 'area' of the small intestine (approx. size of an Olympic swimming pool), it becomes easier to understand that the absorption of toxic waste, bacteria, uric acid and other chemicals can enter the bloodstream and travel to body-cells. Accumulations of adrenalin, from Meat, can pass into the bloodstream and stimulate not only the adrenal glands, but indirectly, in combination with the high rate of uric acid deposits, from Meat, cause an over-stimulation of the thyroid gland: which controls general metabolism of the body, and that imparts the feeling of strength, however, it is only temporary and soon after, the body feels weak, due to a depletion of glandular strength and on the long-term; the undersupply of essential nutrients, from Meat, may lead to degeneration of the: glandular system, nervous system and circulatory system, unless an abundance of natural whole foods is obtained.

The adult human digestive system is over 10 metres long and in comparison to other (carnivorous animals: meat eaters), their digestive system is on average: 2 metres. This extra 8 metres of digestive system, in humans, is a vital indication of our original 'expected food source' (see page 44 for details). Within the last few metres of the small intestine, the build-up of toxic waste can still be absorbed, into the bloodstream, whereas with carnivorous animals, they would have already eliminated the waste products and associated toxins. When these toxins enter the lower intestine (colon), such residue as: phenols and ptomaines, produce a paralyzing effect on the muscles of the colon, and that can lead to constipation, disruption of the elimination and on long term, colon cancer may also develop. To ensure that your body does not absorb an excess amount of toxins; serve a small-portion of Meat combined with an abundance of fresh produce: vegetables are best. Avoid eating Meat regularly: allow at least 36 hours for elimination of the toxins and avoid eating Meat at breakfast time and later in the evening just before sleeping. Always obtain regular supplies of fresh fruits, vegetables, juices, natural yoghurt, whole grains, legumes, nuts and seeds, and discover the foods that Nature has provided without problems. A young-adult is often far more capable of proper Meat digestion and elimination, due to an active metabolism, but if you have overweight problems, the Meat eating will not help in any way. The degeneration of metabolic-energy, caused by a regular, prolonged Meat diet is a main factor when considering overweight conditions. See enzymes, pp. 103 and 157, for details. The combination of saturated fats and cholesterol, with Meat, is another 'hidden problem' and by referring to pages 124–127, these topics are provided in detail.

One of the main nutrient deficiencies with Meat is the lack of calcium, one of the main minerals and as it is designed for bone structure and development (see pp. 142–143), the supply from animal flesh is only minimal, and by regular consumption of meat, the calcium levels of the body are under-supplied considerably in comparison to the phosphorus content, the balance should be 2.5 parts calcium with one part phosphorus. Meat provides one part calcium to 20 parts phosphorus, definitely an imbalance which can upset the delicate balance of these two main minerals with numerous other essential nutrients.

By the time Meat is stored, prepared and cooked, the supply of essential nutrients obtainable, also diminishes, and to protect against any nutrient deficiency, the diet must include a variety of more dominant-nutrient foods. Because a piece of Meat is only a small part of the entire animal: cow, sheep, pig, the ability to obtain a wide range of nutrients is not possible from such a portion of the animal. In contrast, whole grains, legumes, nuts, seeds, vegetables, and fruits, all provide a complete life, able to regenerate into new life. Meat does not provide this valuable life-promoting asset, only a fraction of life is obtained from a piece of meat, and for humans, a fraction is not enough. When including other animal products: milk, cheese and eggs, they provide a better range of nutrients, as they are a complete food, however, some essential nutrients are only obtainable from primary produce: chlorophyl, enzymes, vitamin c, vitamin k, vitamin u, vitamin p and various other vitamins and minerals are best obtained from primary foods, as explained throughout this book.

MEAT

Meat does not supply an excellent source of protein. By referring to pages 87, 88, 98 and 99, you can see "how much protein meat supplies", and by comparing with 'primary protein foods', the value of meat protein will become obvious. Unfortunately, some people have relied on the protein content of Meat since childhood, and for this dietary trend to change, there must be suitable alternatives and in most places, there are numerous 'primary protein alternatives', refer to pp. 41 and 81-106 and chapter seven for details. Primary protein foods provide the variety of life! Meat meals are the product of an animal's death. By referring to the nutrient chart, page 117, a list of all main minerals and vitamins, obtainable from various types of meat are provided, by comparing to the other nutrient charts, pages 43, 61, 79 and 97, the supply of essential nutrients obtainable from 'primary foods' are given and in all cases, primary foods: fruits, vegetables, grains, legumes, nuts and seeds all provide a far better range and most important, a better balance of essential nutrients.

ESSENTIAL AMINO ACIDS

	TRY.	LEU.	LYS.	MET.	PHA.	ISL.	VAL.	THR.
soya bean	526	2946	2414	513	1889	2054	2005	1504
almonds	176	1454	582	259	1146	873	1124	610
brazil	187	1129	443	941	617	593	823	422
cashew	471	1522	792	353	946	1222	1592	737
hazel	211	939	417	139	537	853	934	415
pecan	138	773	435	153	564	553	525	389
pistachio	0	1520	1080	370	1090	880	1340	610
walnuts	175	1228	441	306	767	767	974	589
pumpkin seed	560	2437	1411	577	1749	1737	1679	933
sesame seed	331	1679	583	637	1457	951	885	707
sunflower seed	343	1736	868	443	1220	1276	1354	911
cheddar	341	2437	1834	650	1340	1685	1794	929
egg	211	1126	819	401	739	850	950	637
milk	49	344	272	86	170	233	240	162
yoghurt	37	336	282	78	180	214	255	160
tuna	290	2178	2556	842	1074	1481	1554	1249
beef porterhouse	192	1343	1433	407	674	858	911	724
chicken	250	1490	1810	537	811	1088	1012	877
lamb	233	1394	1457	432	732	923	887	824
turkey	0	1836	2173	664	960	1260	1187	1014
wheat germ	265	1708	1534	404	908	1177	1364	1343

Meat, when mass produced and marketed, often contains an abundance of chemicals, absorbed either directly from plant-life or injected into the animal during various stages of growth. By eating the flesh of an animal, you not only obtain their nutrients, but a range of chemicals, bacteria, poisons, and such types of additives, with mass produced Meat, are not just a myth; studies in the U.S.A. have shown that for example, the amount of D.D.T. that an animal absorbs into their flesh is on average — .28 parts per million (ppm), dairy products — .11 ppm., leavy vegetables and fruits — .02 ppm., whole grains — .007 ppm., legumes — .008 ppm. The vast difference in chemical content will mean that a person who eats meat, regularly; will injest considerably more DDT, over 30 times that from grains or legumes. There is not only DDT residue in Meat, other chemicals are obtained from artificial hormones, antibiotics, insectisides, tranquilizers and such, specific chemicals as: toxaphene, chlordane, stilbestrol, methoxychlor, dieldrin, lindane and aureomycin, to mention a few, have all been found present in beef. Some of these chemicals are added directly by Man, with injections, to increase growth rate of the animal, purely a business venture. At the time of an animal's death, the accumulations of those toxic chemicals in combination with the animal's own 'last minute ingredients': adrenalin, soluable food material in the bloodstream and waste products, all remain, and for a few hours after their death, cell activity slowly continues and those waste products in the bloodstream and living tissues, start producing more harmful bacteria and toxins, and cooking cannot remove all of them. The 'toxins of decay' are transferred from the animal to the meat-eater and when considering the delay in marketing, the problem increases. 'If the bacteria you breed is harmful and mean, think about the effect it has and how you feel!'

A piece of Meat may look fresh, even though, within the tissues, numerous bacteria and toxins are contained and when exposed to the warmth and lengthy digestive processes within the human body, Meat quickly grows in bacteria content and discharges those stored chemicals. By obtaining a regular supply of fresh fruits, vegetables, juices and natural yoghurt, you can greatly reduce the risk of excess toxins, bacteria and chemical build-up, within your body.

Meat eating promotes weight problems. There are numerous reasons for this develop-ment, from Meat, firstly, think about the origin of the piece of Meat, it belonged to an animal, weighing far more than any human could! And that in itself provides a different scale of nutrients, compared to human tissue requirements. A piece of lean ham will provide 25% protein content and 75% fat content, a trimmed steak will provide 65% protein and 35% fat, saturated fat; not easily used by the body and in cases of 'slow metabolism', those saturated fats are easily stored as body-fat.

In Australia and America, Meat is a 'standard food item' and even though more protein is obtained from sources other than meat; the well-developed cattle, sheep and dairy industry, flood the market with their produce, it is easy to obtain, relatively cheap and available at nearly all restaurants, hotels, take-away food shops and even the local schools. It becomes difficult to avoid contact with such a common food item and therefore it continues to be thought of as an essential part of the diet. General trends have shown that meat eating is not losing it's popularity, only it's original purpose: to maintain survival in times of other food shortages.

SECONDARY PROTEIN NUTRIENT COMPOSITION CHART

	protein	carbohydrate	calories	saturated	unsaturated	cholesterol	sodium	phosphorus	potassium	calcium	iron	magnesium	copper	manganese	zinc	vitamin a	vitamin b1	vitamin b2	vitamin b3	vitamin b5	vitamin b6	vitamin b12	biotin	folic acid	vitamin c	vitamin e	n.p.u.
cheddar cheese	26	1.4	450	23	11	115	700	570	110	810	.75	30			3.5	1190	.03	.42	13	.32	.08	.9		.02			
cottage cheese	13	2.7	106	2.9	1.5	15	420	138	88	63	.14	5	.02	.003	.38	171	.02	.17	.13	.22	.04	.46		.013			
edam	24	1.4	353	14	8.6	87	952	476	185	787	.72	28	.02	.01	3.6	910	.03	.35	.08	.28	.07	1.3					
parmesan	35	2.8	380	16	8	66	717	690	147	1120	.8	45	.3	2.6		1050	.03	.3	.26	.4	.09	.007		.01			
yoghurt – cows	3.8	5	68	2.2	1	13	50	102	170	130	.05	11			.67	130	.03	.15	.08	.4	.03	.4					
milk – cows																								.007	.05		
egg yolk	16	.6	370	10	18	1872	71	582	102	144	5.7	16	.27	.09	3.5	3420	.25	.44	.07	4.5	.31	3.8		.15		3.0	
egg – cooked	13	1	164	3.3	5.8	624	122	206	130	54	2.4	12	.03	.01	1.4	1180	.08	.26	.05	1.7	1.02	1.2		.04		1.4	
chicken	14	0	86	2	4	67				9	1.4					114	.03	.12	4.6	.8	.05	.05		.004	2.8		
duck	13	0	270	7	18	72	87	148	291	9				.03		0	.06	.18	6	.4		.4					
rabbit	19	0	131	2.6	2.8	74	35	284	310	16	1.1					34	.06	.05	10	.4			71			1.4	
turkey	34	0	180	1.3	2.8	79	93	216	420	9	1.2	14	.18			0	.06	.16	12	.67	.36			.006	0		
bacon	8.6	1.0	679	23	4	225	700	110	125	13	1.2	12	.17			0	.37	.12	2.5	.4	.16	.72	7.2			.45	
ham	13	0	250	7.4	10.7	53	47	150	213	7.7	2.1	16			2.9	0	.65	.16	3.6	.51	.3	.45	4.1	.009		.72	
lamb	15	0	258	12	8.5	61	50	128	230	9	1.2	14	.18						6								
beef	15	0	250	11	10	58	56	140	250	9	2.3	20	.11			43	.06	.12	3.6	.4	.32	1.3		.8			
veal	17	0	163	4.5	4.3	56	57	165	261	10	2.5	17	.26				.12	.22	5.4	.78	.27	1.3	5.1	.006			
herring	19	0	190	2	4	90	125	285	350	60	1	26	.32			125	.02	.13	4	1.1	.4	9			.5	2	
mackerel	21	0	210	2	6	98	160	265	400	5	1	30	.17	.02		500	.16	.3	9	.9	.7	9	2	.001		1.5	
salmon	26	0	155	2	1	36	418	309	390	210	.8	30	.07	.07		70	.03	.2	8	.5	.3	7		.001			
snapper	22		102	.26	.6	70	70	240	360	16	.8	30					.18	.02									
trout	23	0	220	2	3	60	40		530	20	1		.3	.03			.08	23	9	2.1	.7	5		.001			
tuna	28	0	127	.8	.8	63	41	190	279	16	1.6		.12			60	.04	.1	13	.32	.42	2.2	.5	.01			

CHAPTER FOUR

FATS AND OILS

MAIN FUNCTION OF LIPIDS

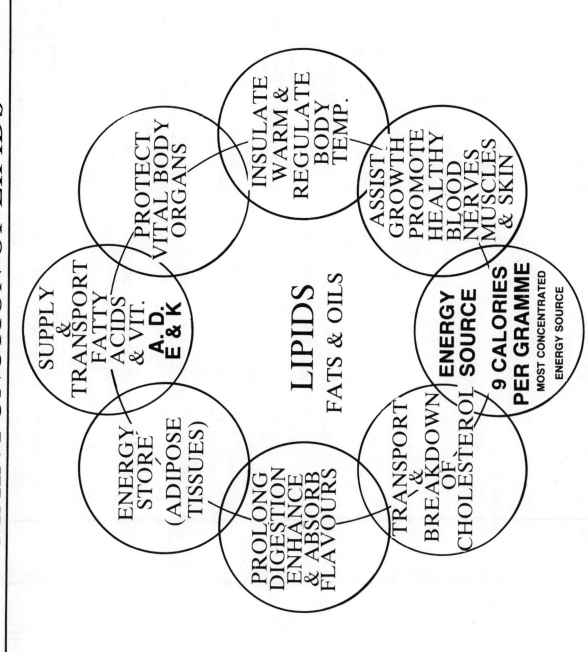

LIPIDS
FATS & OILS

- INSULATE WARM & REGULATE BODY TEMP.
- PROTECT VITAL BODY ORGANS
- ASSIST GROWTH PROMOTE HEALTHY BLOOD NERVES MUSCLES & SKIN
- SUPPLY & TRANSPORT FATTY ACIDS & VIT. **A, D, E & K**
- ENERGY SOURCE **9 CALORIES PER GRAMME** MOST CONCENTRATED ENERGY SOURCE
- ENERGY STORE (ADIPOSE TISSUES)
- PROLONG DIGESTION ENHANCE & ABSORB FLAVOURS
- TRANSPORT & BREAKDOWN OF CHOLESTEROL

NOTE: The intake of Lipids will vary with climatic conditions and type of occupation, however, for maximum nutritional benefits, the Lipid intake should not exceed 20% of the total dietary intake. Both Carbohydrates (50% daily diet) and Proteins (30-40% daily diet) are the main nutrient food groups. Those people who live in below zero climates may have a far greater Lipid intake than the recommended 20%, that extra Lipid intake is required for maintenance of body heat production.

Laugh with Health

FATS & OILS—INTRODUCTION—LIPIDS

FATS & OILS are collectively termed as LIPIDS. Fats are usually solid at room temperature and the Oils are in a liquid form. Lipids are composed of the following main Gaseous elements:

CARBON   HYDROGEN   &   OXYGEN.

LIPIDS are made up from 'chains of Carbon atoms' which have four 'links' and depending on the type of Lipid, these links are joined by a number of Hydrogen atoms. There are two main groups:

SATURATED   &   UNSATURATED LIPIDS.

A Saturated Lipid is one that has all four 'links' of the Carbon atom' connected with Hydrogen atoms. There are two main types of Unsaturated Lipids:

MONO UNSATURATED   &   POLY UNSATURATED (see pages 132–134 for details).

LIPIDS have also another chemical name: **TRIGLYCERIDES.** Over 98% of the Lipid content of food is in the form of Triglycerides and over 90% of the Lipid content of the body is in the form of TRIGLYCERIDES. Apart from the Triglycerides, Lipids are also composed of **PHOSPHOLIPIDS** and as the name implies, they contain the mineral Phosphorus. The other group of substances that are associated with Lipids are: **CHOLESTEROL and FATTY ACIDS** (see pp. 125–127).

LIPIDS are the most concentrated source of 'dietary energy' : (9 Calories per Gram). Proteins and Carbohydrates supply 4 Calories per gram. The illustration on page 119 shows the main nutrient functions of Lipids. The maximum daily intake of Lipids should not exceed 20% of the total food intake. Both Carbohydrates (50% daily diet) and Proteins (30–40%) are required for numerous functions that the Lipids are not capable of supporting (see pp. 17–21, 81–88). LIPIDS are often related to adding excess body weight. There is no doubt that the Lipids are a concentrated store of Calories (see p. 14) and there must be some restriction with their use in order to avoid obesity, however the majority of obese people have a diet that is deficient in fresh fruits and vegetables and overindulgent in processed, snack and take-away foods. The balanced diet (see illustration) is based on Natural foods only. Any food that is no longer in the 'natural state' should be avoided as there will be a deficiency of 'protective elements' that are essential for 'natural weight control' (see pp. 141–156 and 174–197 for details). With a diet of unnatural foods, the body is unable to determine how much food is required and this leads to overeating and overweight conditions, whereas with Natural foods in the 'natural state' the intake is limited, as your body is part of Nature and controlled by natural forces.

For some people, the city environment has a most distracting effect upon natural food intake. The multitude of shops that cater for the quick meal and sweet snack foods are growing in number and decreasing in their respect for customer quality. The problems that people who live in a city environment encounter often extends into an overindulgence of mass produced foods and this leads the way to regular sickness, weight problems and a general lack of physical and mental energy. There would be half as many factories and twice as many natural living activities if some people would stop eating junk foods (processed and refined to make a dime). Remember the old but accurate equation: 'every action has an equal and opposite reaction'. A. Einstein.

SATURATED LIPID

$$H-\overset{\displaystyle H}{\underset{\displaystyle H}{C}}-H$$

SATURATED LIPID

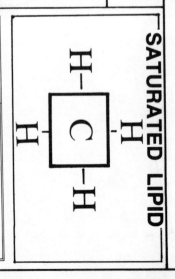

9 Calories per gram

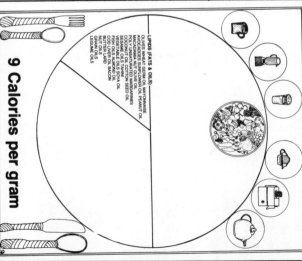

LIPIDS (FATS & OILS)
OLIVES WHEAT GERM OIL MAYONNAISE
AVOCADOES SUNFLOWER OIL PEANUT OIL
MACADAMIA NUT OLIVE OIL
POLY UNSATURATED MARGARINES
COCONUT OIL COTTON SEED OIL
SESAME OILS TAHINI
VEGETABLE OILS SOYA OIL
FISH OILS ALMOND OIL
COD LIVER OIL BACON
BUTTER LARD
NUT OILS
GRAIN OILS
LEGUME OILS

9 Calories per gram

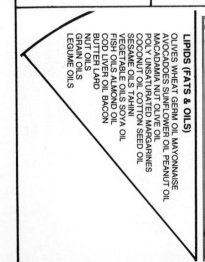

LIPIDS (FATS & OILS)
OLIVES WHEAT GERM OIL MAYONNAISE
AVOCADOES SUNFLOWER OIL PEANUT OIL
MACADAMIA NUT OLIVE OIL
POLY UNSATURATED MARGARINES
COCONUT OIL COTTON SEED OIL
SESAME OILS TAHINI
VEGETABLE OILS SOYA OIL
FISH OILS ALMOND OIL
COD LIVER OIL BACON
BUTTER LARD
NUT OILS
GRAIN OILS
LEGUME OILS

FATS & OILS—INTRODUCTION—LIPIDS

LIPIDS are essential for a healthy life. The daily intake of Lipids allows for up to 20% however the body can survive adequately with as little as a 2% Lipid intake if one essential nutrient is supplied, that is **LINOLEIC ACID** and classed as an **'essential fatty acid'**. There are two more so called essential fatty acids: **LINOLENIC and ARACHIODONIC acid.** These three essential fatty acids are often referred to as Vitamin F (see page 204 for details). All Natural whole foods contain amounts of these essential fatty acids with such food groups as: whole grains, legumes, nuts and seeds being the main source. LINOLEIC acid is a poly unsaturated Lipid (see p. 133). Most people have a daily Lipid intake that well exceeds this 2% minimum and often goes beyond the recommended 15–20% daily Lipid requirement. One of the main reasons for this over-indulgence of Lipids is due to the 'taste sensation' that 'added Lipids' can provide. Imagine a slice of bread without any added Lipids: butter, margarine, tahini, avocado etcetera. Modern food technology has utilized this 'taste sensation' aspect of Lipids to such an extent that nearly all 'snack foods' are loaded with added Lipids. Some people have great difficulty in losing weight and more often than not, they eat snack foods instead of Natural whole foods, have very little regular exercise and consume over 20% Lipid intake daily.

'the best way to keep fit and lose weight is to use Natural foods in the natural state'

LIPIDS are converted into Heat and Energy (see illustration below). After the processes of digestion have been completed (see Lipid Digestion page 138) the absorbed Lipids are then converted into the form of FATTY ACIDS and GLYCEROL. This conversion takes place primarily in the Liver. FATTY ACIDS are converted into KETONE bodies and GLYCEROL is converted in GLUCOSE. This process takes place when the body has expended extra Energy. The Energy that is produced occurs when GLUCOSE and INSULIN are converted into the form of Carbon dioxide and Water. Lipid conversion into the form of Heat-Energy is dependent on a regular supply of Carbohydrate foods: fresh fruits, vegetables, whole grains and legumes.

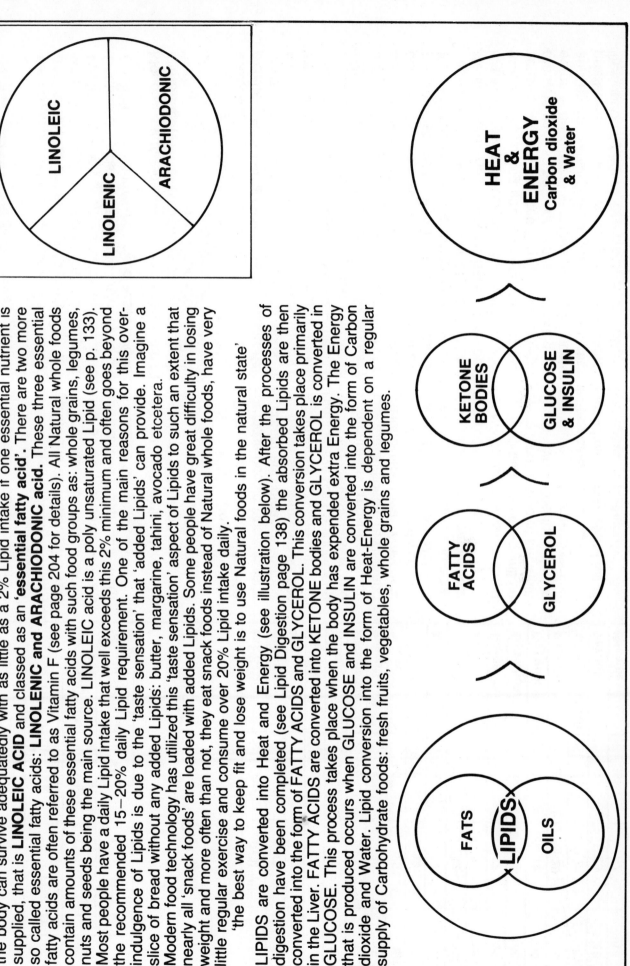

ESSENTIAL FATTY ACIDS

LINOLEIC
LINOLENIC
ARACHIODONIC

FATS — LIPIDS — OILS

FATTY ACIDS — GLYCEROL

KETONE BODIES — GLUCOSE & INSULIN

HEAT & ENERGY
Carbon dioxide & Water

MONO UNSATURATED LIPIDS

Mono Unsaturated Lipids are defined as having one double bond (or space in the fatty acid chemical chain). (see illustration). This space around the Carbon atoms allows for another element to combine with Mono unsaturated Lipids and thereby improve their digestibility. Fats in the food we eat are made up from 'fatty acid chains' and the following processes of digestion and absorption will vary with the type of fatty acids that are supplied with the meal. All natural whole foods will supply Mono unsaturated Lipids as well as Poly unsaturated and Saturated Lipids. Nuts are the main Mono unsaturated food group (see chart). Olive oil is the dominant 'cold pressed' Mono unsaturated Oil.

Mono Unsaturated Lipids do not increase the Cholesterol levels of the blood and this is important for prevention of cardiovascular disorders: high blood pressure, hardened arteries and poor blood circulation all of which are closely related to an excess consumption of Saturated Lipids (see page 124 for details).

NUTS are the best source of Mono unsaturated Lipids and they also provide an abundance of Protein and a valuable supply of Poly unsaturated Lipids that provide the 'essential fatty acids' (see page 123). For those people who regularly have 'saturated meals':meat, cheese, eggs, milk, cream and other deep fried meals it would be advisable to replace at least two of those 'saturated meals' per week with a variety of Nuts and Fruits. There are numerous ways to combine Nuts for a complete and delicious main meal. You could have per person: ½cup almonds, 1 grated apple, 1 grated pear, ½ cup of blackcurrants, raisins and sultanas and a dash of cinnamon for an easy to prepare and most beneficial main protein meal. Also try a combination of walnuts with almonds, raisins and some blackcurrants for an ideal and easy to prepare lunchtime meal. When you consider the price you pay for the average sandwich at the local sandwich bar, you could spend far less on a packet of: almonds, walnuts, pecan or hazel nuts and also have some change left for a couple of apples or some raisins and other seasonal fruits. A combination of Nuts and Fruits is the best way to promote your Health and at the same time have a delicious and most fulfilling meal. Try the natural lunch this week and discover the benefits of raw foods that are packed with life supporting and envigorating Enzymes. Any food that is cooked will be deficient in enzymes and thereby lack 'the spark of life', that is one of the main reasons why some people have overweight problems. When the food that is eaten is deficient in enzymes, the body must supply them to activate digestion and energy requirements. The older we get, the less capable our body is to produce and continually supply these enzymes. Fresh fruits and Nuts are full of life supporting enzymes.

OLEIC ACID — $C_{18}H_{34}O_2$

	LIPIDS	MONO.	POLY.	SAT.
	Almonds	68	19	8
	Brazil	33	37	25
	Cashew	58	16	20
	Hazel	77	10	7
	Macadamia	76	3	14
	Peanut	46	30	19
	Pecan	60	25	8
	Pistachio	68	13	14
	Avocado	43	12	18
	Chick pea	42	42	trace.
	Millet	33	33	33
	Margarine	58	17	22
	Egg whole	40	12	30
	Egg yolk	40	12	30
	Poultry	45	20	30
OILS:	Olive oil	76	7	11
	Peanut	47	29	18
	Sesame	38	42	14

POLY UNSATURATED LIPIDS

Poly unsaturated Lipids have four or more 'free Carbon atoms'. The illustration on the right shows a typical Poly unsaturated chemical structure where there are numerous spaces around the Carbon atom. POLY is derived from the Greek word meaning 'many'. Poly unsaturated Lipids are the most important of the three Lipid groups as they are the only source of the three ESSENTIAL FATTY ACIDS: LINOLEIC, LINOLENIC and ARACHIODONIC acid.

LINOLEIC acid is the most important of the three essential fatty acids as it cannot be produced by the body and must therefore be supplied with the diet. The other two so-called essential fatty acids can be synthesized by the body when Linoleic acid is regularly obtained with the daily diet. It has been estimated that as little as 2% of the daily diet in the form of Linoleic acid is sufficient to support all the functions of the essential fatty acids

The ESSENTIAL FATTY ACIDS are collectively termed as vitamin F. When your daily diet includes such foods as: fruits, vegetables, whole grains, legumes, nuts and seeds you will obtain adequate amounts of vitamin F as well as essential minerals and vitamins that will promote the utilization of Lipids and protect you from adding on excess weight. All foods that have been processed, refined or artificially converted are the main cause of the widespread problem of obesity. If you are overweight and have great difficulty in losing a few kg. then your diet must be out of balance. All natural foods in the natural state are protected with active nutrients: minerals and vitamins, that ensure efficient use of the food that is eaten. Throughout this book there is valuable information to help you with understanding how natural whole foods protect against obesity (see pages 14, 58, 142–156, and 174–197 for details).

Poly Unsaturated Lipids have the unique ability to lower the Cholesterol levels of the blood and this is most important for prevention of hardened arteries and heart disease both of which are attributed to excess use of the following animal produce: meat, cheese, eggs, butter and milk as well as deep fried foods, grilled foods and all other foods that have been cooked with added Lipids. It is most important to remember that the daily diet should include a wide variety of other foods apart from animal produce. Such foods as whole grains, legumes, nuts, seeds, fruits and vegetables should take the dominant role in providing your daily nutritional requirements.

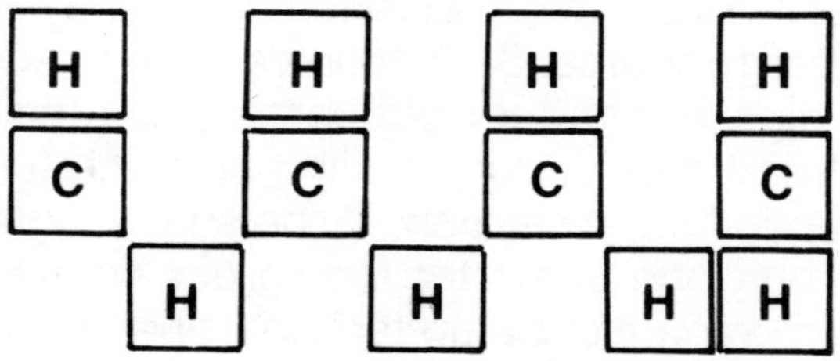

LINOLEIC ACID – $C_{18}H_{32}O_2$

LINOLENIC ACID – $C_{18}H_{30}O_2$

LIPIDS	MONO.	POLY.	SAT.
Corn Oil	28	53	10
Cottonseed Oil	21	50	25
Safflower Oil	15	72	8
Soya Beans	20	52	15
Sesame Seeds	38	42	14
Sunflower Sds	39	43	14
Sunflower Oil	19	63	13
Walnuts	18	68	8
Cornmeal	26	51	trace
Garbanzos	42	42	trace
Brazil Nuts	33	37	25
Soya Beans	23	51	17
Soya Flour	20	54	15
Tofu	24	48	24
Wheat Germ	27	46	18
Fish (average)	20	50	25

SATURATED LIPIDS

Saturated Lipids have all Carbon atoms attached to a Hydrogen atom (see illustration). Most Saturated Lipids are solid at room temperature and the more solid a Lipid is at room temperature the greater the concentration of Saturated Lipids it will contain. Saturated Lipids are the most difficult to digest and utilize as an Energy source. Such foods as: meat, eggs, cheese, butter and cream have a very high Saturated Lipid content and this will retard the digestive time of the meal and provide long lasting stomach fulfillment, that some people regularly rely upon for satisfaction. To be sure of obtaining good nutrition it is advisable to have only one Saturated food group per day. Your body is able to convert only a limited amount of Saturated Lipids per day and any excess will either be a waste or stored in the various adipose tissues of the body. Saturated Lipids are the most likely to cause overweight problems as they require complex preparation to be converted into usable Energy. Avoid combining Saturated Protein foods.

Saturated Lipids are not essential for Health. The three 'essential fatty acids' are in the form of Poly Unsaturated Lipids and as the chart shows, there is only a minimal amount of Poly Unsaturated Lipids associated with 'saturated animal produce'. The minimal amount of Poly Unsaturated Lipids that are associated with animal produce is easily converted to the form of Saturated Lipids when the particular food is cooked and this can be most detrimental when no other food with that meal contains the essential Poly Unsaturated Lipids. Regular use of Saturated foods will be a leading factor towards overweight conditions, heart disease, hardened arteries and a general lack of Energy.

Saturated Lipids are to some people the 'staple part of the diet'. Such meals as: fried eggs, bacon, grilled and roasted meat, cheese dishes, milk drinks, cream cakes and ice cream all have the ability to satisfy the appetite for an extended time, that is due to the abundance of Saturated Lipids which retard the process of digestion within the stomach and this is most detrimental for the preparation of any Protein foods that are associated with the meal. (see protein digestion p 97). To be sure of obtaining good nutrition with Saturated Lipid foods it is important to remember the following points: 1) Avoid mixing any of the following foods at the same meal: meat, cheese, eggs, yoghurt, cream or ice cream. 2) avoid having more than one Saturated meal per day. 3) always use 'cold pressed' oils for salads and cooking. 4) 30% of the daily diet should be fresh fruits. 6) Saturated Lipids are not essential for Health. Also, avoid processed and refined foods.

Fatty acid	Formula
MYRISTIC ACID —	$C_{14}H_{28}O_2$
PALMITIC ACID —	$C_{16}H_{32}O_2$
LAURIC ACID —	$C_{12}H_{24}O_2$
STEARIC ACID —	$C_{18}H_{36}O_2$

LIPIDS	MONO.	POLY.	SAT.
Butter	34	2	57
Coconut	6	2	88
Eggs	40	12	30
Camembert	29	3	63
Cottage	27	3	65
Cream	29	4	62
Tilsit	27	3	65
Gouda	28	2	64
Swiss	28	4	64
Edam	28	2	65
Yoghurt	27	3	65
Ice cream	29	4	63
Milk-cows	29	4	63
Veal	40	2	40
Lamb	36	3	54
Beef Steak	35	2	60
Pork	40	2	40

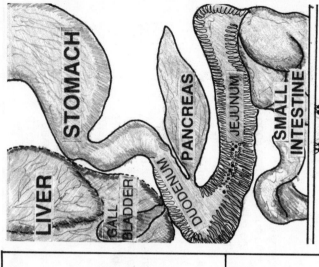

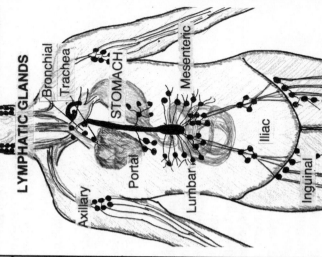

DIGESTION OF LIPIDS

LIPIDS

Stage One: After entering the Stomach, the Lipid content of the meal will have to wait until the Protein and Carbohydrate content of the meal are prepared (see pp. 19–21 and 88 for details). Protein foods: meat and eggs especially, need special preparation within the Stomach and it is at this stage that 'food combinations' are most important. Any excess Lipids (Fats & Oils) will retard the process of Protein digestion within the Stomach.
Of all the main Protein foods it is meat that is the most likely to cause digestive and other health problems when combined with excess Lipids (pp. 113–114 for details). The human digestive system is better suited to a diet of fresh fruits, vegetables, whole grains, legumes, nuts and seeds than any secondary Protein. Meat for example needs between 3 - 6 hours preparation within the Stomach depending on the type of meat and the general metabolism of the person. Any excess Lipids with the meat meal can increase this time to over 6 hours within the Stomach and by this time the meat will have started to decay. When this meat 'food chyme' passes into the Small intestine it will be absorbed by millions of 'villi' and then pass those harmful 'toxins of decay' indirectly into the bloodstream. (the Lymphatic system will be first affected). It should be remembered that Protein foods are best eaten with as little extra Lipids as possible. Such meals as fried eggs, bacon and grilled meat in particular may have a very sustaining after dinner feeling, however the benefits of such a meal will surely change to be detrimental, especially when regularly consumed.

Stage Two: After leaving the Stomach, the Lipid content of the meal will enter the Duodenum-the upper stage of the Small intestine from where a hormone known as-Cholecystokinin is secreted and this stimulates the Gall Bladder to contract thereby forcing an alkaline substance, Bile, to enter the small intestine via the Bile duct (cystic duct) (see section on Lecithin and Cholesterol, pp. 126–127). Bile is an emulsifying agent (fat dissolving) that when in combination with the enzyme Lipase that is produced by the Pancreas gland, assists in the conversion of dietary Lipids into the form of Fatty acids and Glycerol. It is at this stage that the Lipids (fatty acids and glycerol) are capable of being absorbed by the villi of the small intestine.

Stage Three: The absorption of Lipids (fatty acids and glycerol) takes place within the boundaries of the Jejunum that is also part of the small intestine. After absorption by the villi, the fatty acids and glycerol will combine with small amounts of Protein-Chylomicrons and are then ready to pass into the Lymphatic system-(the secondary circulatory system of the body), that functions as a filter of any harmful residue and bacteria before returning the fatty acids to the bloodstream. The remaining Lipids will circulate the bloodstream and with the assistance of the Liver they will be conveyed to the various fat-stores (adipose tissues) of the body or prepared by the adipose tissues into carbon dioxide and water which produces the **heat—energy.**

NOTE: The LYMPHATIC SYSTEM consists of a number of Lymphatic Glands that are situated throughout most parts of the body (see illustration). These 'lymph glands' are responsible for removal of any toxic food substances: virus, bacteria and other forms of toxic food waste that have entered the Lymphatic system after the process of digestion. When a person regularly consumes fried foods, grilled meat, processed and refined foods and has a lack of fresh fruits-(the best cleansers of the body), vegetables and other natural wholesome foods, the Lymphatic system will react and produce the more than common symptons of: fatigue, headaches, virus, chills, backache, swollen glands and the common cold. When you hear that 'a virus is going around' it is a sure sign that the people affected are having their Lymphatic system cleaned-out by the natural defense and elimination systems of the body. All forms of processed and refined foods, preservatives, food additives and other snack-foods are the main cause of a 'virus infection'. Other substances such as nicotine and environmental pollutants will also contaminate the Lymphatic system with excess toxins such as mucus. When a virus infection occurs, make sure that the diet includes at least 30% fresh fruits daily, good quality primary protein:nuts and seeds and a few glasses of freshly made fruit juice: apple, pear, orange, grape, pineapple or vegetable juice: carrot, celery and parsley.
The best medicine is natural.

LECITHIN

LIPIDS

LECITHIN is a natural substance. It is manufactured by the Liver. Lecithin has numerous functions within the body, acting as a powerful fat-dissolving agent that protects the entire body from excess accumulations of fats within the arteries. Lecithin converts Fats and Cholesterol into microscopic particles so they can readily pass through the arterial walls and be utilized by all parts of the body. The liver can produce only a limited amount of Lecithin per day and when any excess of Fats (especially saturated animal fats) are taken with the diet, the body will start to develop excess accumulations of Cholesterol and unnecessary fat particles within the bloodstream-(arteriosclerosis). Such a condition will develop if a person has a regular intake of saturated animal produce: meat, cheese, eggs, butter and other animal fats as well as having a deficiency of Natural foods: fruits, vegetables, whole grains, legumes, nuts and seeds. All processed and refined foods are lacking in Lecithin as they are subjected to heat and other processes of extraction. The best way to be assured of an adequate intake of Lecithin is to always use Natural foods in the Natural state.

LECITHIN comprise 28% of the brain matter with a healthy and mentally stable person. Modern research has discovered that with mentally retarded people the Lecithin content is often as low as 19%. The relationship between the Lecithin content of the brain and mental capacity is of great interest for some medical researchers and psychiatrists, they suggest that a regular intake of Lecithin supplements and Natural Lecithin based foods are a great preventative of nervous breakdown, mental fatigue and other forms of mental stress. During times of stress and nervousness, Lecithin that is contained in the body (especially the brain) is used up rapidly. If this Lecithin is not replaced regularly with the diet, fatigue, irritation and other forms of mental confusion may develop. Lecithin is termed as 'nature's tranquilizer'.

LECITHIN is made up from a mixture of substances that are collectively known as Phospholipids, consisting of: essential fatty acids, phosphorus and the B group vitamins: Choline and Inositol. When you obtain a regular supply of Natural foods that are a good source of Phospholipids, your body will help you by producing natural Lecithin. (see pp. 170, 204 & 208). Lecithin supplements are mainly produced fron Corn and Soya bean extraction. Lecithin supplements are obtainable in the form of pure Lecithin granules (the best value), Lecithin powders, flakes, oils and tablets. Regular use of Lecithin granules (1 tsp. per day) plus a balanced supply of Natural whole foods: fruits, vegetables, whole grains, legumes, nuts and seeds will ensure that your body will produce natural Lecithin. Everybody needs Lecithin daily. Lecithin supplements are easy to take and combine very well with most foods. Whenever you eat eggs, cheese, meat or cooked food, be sure to add a little life with some Lecithin granules. Add the Lecithin last. There are no known toxic levels of Lecithin supplementation, so be sure to have some Lecithin supplement if you have a diet of processed, unnatural foods. Natural Lecithin foods are the best value.

LECITHIN is part of the structure of every living cell of the body, especially the brain and liver. Lecithin is also part of the Endocrine gland tissues-(thyroid, parathyroid, adrenal, pituitary, sex glands, pineal, pancreas and thymus) and the muscles of the heart and kidneys. Today, the majority of processed, refined and artificial substances that some people intake, have lost all their valuable Lecithin content. A diet of Natural foods in the natural state would need no extra Lecithin supplement, however, with the marked increase of environmental pollution and other prevalent toxins, especially in the cities, an increased intake of Lecithin would be advisable. Lecithin supplements will protect your entire body from environmental toxins. Apart from that, many people are unfortunate enough to be addicted to the effects of cigarettes and some of these people also work in a highly polluted atmosphere, they will need a regular supply of natural Lecithin foods and possibly Lecithin supplements. Regular intake of alcohol, preservatives and unnatural foods will lead to a definite lack of Lecithin reserves within the body (especially the brain). Lecithin will help your body to neutralize those excess toxins. Have a tsp. daily and Laugh with Health.

CHOLESTEROL   LIPIDS

CHOLESTEROL is a waxy fat-like substance that is part of every living cell of the human body, as an essential component of cell membranes. Cholesterol is mainly produced by the Liver and Adrenal glands. Cholesterol has a similiar molecular structure to many other hormones of the human body and it is also an essential component of such hormones as: Estrogen, cortisone and testosterone. Cholesterol that is produced by the liver is also required for the nervous system as a vital part of nerve tissue. Cholesterol rich foods are not required for the production of Natural Cholesterol. Our body is capable of manufacturing all Cholesterol requirements. Within the Liver, Cholesterol is formed by a multitude of liver cells and this combines with some other secretions of the Liver: bile pigments, bile salts, mucin and water to form into an alkaline digestive fluid called Bile, that is then taken to the Gall bladder via the hepatic duct and cystic duct. The Gall bladder will store this digestive fluid—Bile, until it is required for the breakdown of Lipids: foods that contain Fats & Oils. Bile also assists the digestive action of the pancreas gland which produces three essential digestive enzymes: Lipase, Amylase and Trypsin. The Liver regulates the Cholesterol levels of the body, however this function is dependant on a regular supply of the following Minerals: Magnesium, Potassium, Manganese, Zinc and Vitamins: C, D, E, F and the B complex vitamins. The Cholesterol content of Bile fluid is comparitively minute when you consider that Bile is composed of over 90% water.

CHOLESTEROL can also be a killer. There are many factors leading to excess Cholesterol levels within the body, especially the bloodstream. Firstly, there are some foods that are very rich in Cholesterol (see chart for details), these foods should not be relied upon for good nutrition. The balanced diet does cater for a few Cholesterol foods however only in small quantities. Such foods as the Carbohydrates: fruits, vegetables, whole grains and legumes should make up 50% of the daily food intake. If you start the day with a Carbohydrate meal you will have plenty of Energy to enjoy the day. If you start the day with a Cholesterol rich food, be sure to make it the only such meal of the day. Your body produces all the Cholesterol it needs, any excess can be considered a waste product. If you regularly have more than one Cholesterol rich meal per day you will develop accumulations of Cholesterol within the bloodstream. Cholesterol should not take the place of Blood-our lifeline (see pp. 164–165 for details). Blood has better things to transport than Cholesterol. Be sure to avoid a regular intake of Cholesterol rich foods and learn to use Natural foods. Apart from the Cholesterol rich foods, your body can produce Cholesterol from Fats, Sugars or indirectly from Protein foods.

CHOLESTEROL will usually deposit in the arteries and blood vessels that have been weakened by conditions of stress, overeating, anxiety, cigarette smoking, environmental pollutants and other forms of physical exertion. To prevent excess Cholesterol accumulations within the bloodstream there are certain nutrients that assist in keeping Cholesterol soluble within the bloodstream, thereby preventing the development of hardened arteries and the following 'strokes' and 'coronary' attacks. Adequate supplies of vitamin E foods (see pp. 178–179) will protect the arterial walls from the effects of pollution, cigarette smoking and other forms of arterial stress. Vitamin E will also assist the repair of damaged blood vessels and arteries. Vitamin C foods (see pp. 176–177) are vital for protection against conditions of 'stress.' Vitamin C is required daily for a multitude of functions within the body such as for protection from the effects of toxic substances: pollution, cigarette smoking, preservatives, fluoridated water and other forms of toxic waste matter. A regular supply of Lecithin foods (see page 126) is also vital for the control of blood-Cholesterol levels. Two very important B group vitamins: Choline and Inositol are required for the production of Natural Lecithin (see pp. 195–197 for details). Also, vitamin B6 is essential for Natural Lecithin production as well as the mineral Magnesium. A prolonged deficiency of any of these nutrients can be a leading factor towards a lack of natural lecithin production as well as an excess accumulation of Cholesterol within the bloodstream. The mineral Iodine will also assist by stimulating the Thyroid gland to utilize Cholesterol. Regular exercise is one of the best ways to keep the arteries in good condition and to promote the flow of blood and utilization of excess body fats. Strenuous exercise is not advised. To sum up, there are many factors that promote the development of excess blood-Cholesterol levels. Firstly, avoid regular use of 'Cholesterol rich foods', processed and refined foods. Secondly, avoid cigarette smoking, alcohol, environmental pollutants, food preservatives, sweet refined foods and thirdly, avoid excess physical exertion, mental stress and the hectic rush to work with a stomach full of Cholesterol foods and finally, exercise regularly and learn to use Natural whole foods instead of the Cholesterol rich foods.

'Laugh with Health' and avoid being another 'heart attack statistic'.

CHOLESTEROL FOODS

Food	Measure	Amount
Butter	1tbl.sp.	35mg.
Cream ½ & ½	1tbl.sp.	6mg.
Cream Full	1tbl.sp.	20mg.
Cream Cheese	1tbl.sp.	16mg.
Camembert	1ounce.	26mg.
Cheddar	1ounce.	28mg.
Colby	1ounce.	27mg.
Edam	1ounce.	29mg.
Mozzarella	1ounce.	27mg.
Swiss	1ounce.	30mg.
Lard	1cup.	195mg.
Milk-Cows	1cup.	34mg.
Low Fat Milk	1cup.	22mg.
Condensed Milk	1cup.	105mg.
Evaporated Milk	1cup.	79mg.
Crab Meat	1cup.	125mg.
Lobster	1cup.	123mg.
Oysters	1cup.	120mg.
Beef	3ounces.	80mg.
Brains	3ounces.	1750mg.
Lamb	3ounces.	83mg.
Liver	3ounces.	372mg.
Pork	3ounces.	76mg.
Turkey	3ounces.	65mg.
Veal	3ounces.	86mg.
Chicken Heart	1cup.	335mg.
Caviar	1tbl.sp.	48mg.
Kidney	1cup.	1125mg.

Note: The above figures are approx. and a guide for comparitive purposes only.
Amounts in milligramms per measure.

BUTTER

LIPIDS

BUTTER that has been commercially produced and classed as 'salted butter' will often contain as much as 140mg. of inorganic sodium chloride per 100 grams as well as the addition of such unnecessary and harmful substances as: sodium carbonate or calcium carbonate that are added to neutralize the effect of the salt, however, all those added extras are potentially harmful when obtained regularly and over a prolonged period. Commercial Butter is often 'bleached' during processing and added colours and preservatives all add up to destroy the natural quality of Butter. If your diet is well balanced with natural whole foods and you have the occasional dab of butter to enhance a special dish there is no reason to worry about the long term effects of Butter with your diet. If your diet is or has been neglected with a regular intake of natural foods then the addition of Butter will only accumulate your 'health risk problems'. If you are not sure about the quality of the Butter you obtain, why not have a look at the factory where it may be produced and you will naturally reduce your intake without any more encouragement. There are numerous alternatives to Butter that can be used as regularly as you would use Butter and they have no synthetic chemicals added: Tahini is possibly the most versatile Butter substitute and one of the best natural foods available (see page 102 for more details). If you have never tried Tahini on bread before, try it soon and discover the taste of a unique natural food that has the capacity to completely take the place of Butter or margarine. If you eat refined bread, that is deficient in so many nutrients especially vitamin E, Tahini will supply excellent amounts of vitamin E as well as most other nutrients that are completely lacking from the daily mass produced refined bread. It may take you a while to get accustomed to using Tahini instead of Butter, so give your body a chance to adjust to a most beneficial alternative to Butter. Mix Tahini half-half with Butter if you are uncertain at first about the taste sensation of Tahini. The other alternatives to Butter are as simple as using Avocado now and again as an alternative to Tahini. By utilizing all three foods: Butter, Tahini and Avocado as part of your diet, you can be assured of adequate taste sensation as well as the abundant supply of nutrients that are associated with Tahini and Avocado. You could also improve the quality of the supermarket Butter by mixing in a blender equal portions of Butter with any of the following 'cold pressed' oils: sunflower, sesame, soya, almond or safflower oil. The result is often called 'better-butter' this is due to the added balance of essential unsaturated Lipids that are very deficient in ordinary butter and most dominant in 'cold pressed' oils. Better-Butter is easy to make and you will find that it 'spreads even better that margarine' and has numerous other Health benefits.

BUTTER is often called a Natural food and so it should be. In the last twenty years, food technology and food distribution have both upset the natural quality of Butter and now the Butter 'product' will often include unnecessary ingredients that are of 'no health benefit'. Home made butter is an excellent natural food, however, only small amounts are required and any excess can be considered a waste product and harmful for the human system. Butter that has been properly prepared is an excellent addition for the diet as it can enhance the taste of so many simple dishes. The nutritional potential of Butter is on a low scale when compared to other Natural foods and when you consider that it is taken in small quantities such as with the sandwich, Butter can only be advantageous when the associated meal is well balanced with natural whole foods: home made whole grain bread with a fresh garden salad, cookies and the occasional dab of Butter with those starch vegetables: potato, pumpkin, broccoli and some beans and peas. Depending on the type of Butter you obtain, there can be vast differences in the quality and supply of essential daily nutrients that are supplied. Modern food processing has been able to standardize the nutrient content of Butter with the addition of synthetic minerals and vitamins and with the common addition of salt, that all destroy the natural quality and potential of Butter. If you have decided that Butter is better, then be careful of the type of Butter you buy and preferably have some idea of where it was made and if any additives were used. Remember that the more Butter you use, the more exercise you will need to prevent obesity.

MARGARINE

MARGARINE was first developed in the late 1860's by a French scientist, Mege Mouries produced and patented a Margarine that was made from beef-tallow extractions and it was called 'oleo margarine'. At first, Margarine was prepared from animal source and therefore had a high Saturated Lipid content. Modern technology has developed various other alternatives to produce Margarine and now most of these are based on liquid: vegetable, seed or grain oils. The process of converting a liquid oil into a semi-solid state is called Hydrogenation and by control of the Hydrogen input, liquid oils can be made into various consistencies, depending on the amount of Hydrogenation. This new development in the manufacture of Margarine has greatly increase it's popularity and led to a decline in dairy butter sales. The controversy that continues between both manufacturing groups about the individual benefits of the two products has been left to the advertising companies and this has prompted both butter and margarine sales. The main difference between Butter and Margarine is based on the amount of Saturated Lipids compared to Unsaturated Lipids. Margarine has more unsaturated lipids as it is made from plant source and Butter has a greater saturated Lipid content as it is obtained from animal origin. Butter is termed as a natural product and Margarine has been referred to as a 'synthetic' product due to the process of Hydrogenation, that changes the original structure of Lipids into the form of a synthetic and basically incompatible substance for the body to digest and absorb and most important of all, those hydrogenated oils have a poor relationship with the structure of human cells. The most important point to remember is that neither of the two products: butter or margarine, sould be regularly relied upon and taken as if they were a 'health product'. It is a common sight to see a supermarket shopper buying large quantities of Margarine as part of their weekly food supply whereas years ago, margarine was either not available or substituted for a small amount of Butter, that was considered a luxury food and thereby restricted due to economic factors. This mass production of margarine has now spread to become a health risk problem for those people that have been convinced by advertising companies, that margarine use will protect them from heart disease. In some parts of southeastern America, where margarine consumption is highest per capita compared to butter consumption, the incidence of heart attacks is very high. This high incidence of heart attacks may sound like an isolated case however the relationship between excess consumption of margarine and heart disease is due to accumulations of fat particles within the bloodstream, that are incompatible with human cells and therefore have to be eliminated, or, be eliminated. Blood cannot be made from the limited amount of nutrients that margarine supplies. Such foods as: fresh fruits, vegetables, whole grains, legumes, nuts and seeds will supply **all** your daily Lipid requirements as well as the best form of blood building material.

MARGARINE should be considered as a waste product for the human body. The only benefit that can be associated with Margarine is that it may contain the essential fatty acids and apart from that, there are only excess calories, residue chemical substances and lack of protective elements. If you have been using margarine regularly with the diet, you can only benefit by reducing your consumption and replacing that product with **home made margarine**, that is often called better-butter. By mixing dairy butter half-half with any of the following 'cold-pressed' oils: sunflower, safflower, sesame, soya or corn oil you will obtain the most beneficial alternative to both butter and margarine and discover that it **'spreads better than margarine'**, as well as noticing that your skin condition will improve remarkably. Home made margarine is easy to prepare if you have an essential kitchen appliance, a blender, otherwise use a fork to combine the butter with the cold pressed oil. It is an excellent idea to also add some Lecithin-1tsp. per cupful of home made margarine. You can mix enough to last for several weeks of 'beneficial spreading'. The only way to be sure of the taste is to try it and as many people have already discovered, better-butter or home made margarine is the only substitute for butter and margarine. Make some this week.

FATS & OILS NUTRIENT CHART

LIPIDS;	measure 1 tbl. sp.	weight g.	calories	saturated fat g.	unsaturated fat g.	total fat g.	cholesterol mg.	calcium mg.	phosphorus mg.	potassium mg.	iron mg.	sodium mg.	magnesium mg.	copper mg.	manganese mg.	zinc mg.	vit.A. I.U.	vit.E. mg.	Vit. B1. mg.	B2 mg.	B3 mg.	B5 mg.	B6 mg.
Butter	g.	14	102	6.3	4.1	11	35	45	36	52		140	.28	.004		.01	470	.35	t	.001			t
Chicken fat	g.	14	126			14																	
Lard	g.	13	117	4.9	7.3	13	12				.129	.39	.026	.013	.039		140	.14					
Margarine -regular	g.	14		2.1	9	11		2	2	2		93		.004		.03	470	t	t	t	t		
Margarine -whipped	g.	9.4	68	1.4	6	7.6		2	2	2				.004		.03	310	.89	t	t	t		
Cod liver OILS:	g.	14	126			14	119	t					.014				11,900	3					
Corn	g.	14	126	1.4	11	14	t	t			t			.025		.025	t	10.9	t	t	t		
Cottonseed	g.	14				14	t							.025		.025		.714					
Olive	g.			1.5	11	14	t	.07	t	t	.01			.001		.025		1.8	t	t	t		
Peanut	g.	14	124	2.4	10	t	t	t						.025		.025		1.8	t				
Safflower	g.	14	124	1.1	11	14	t							.025		.025		10.5	t				
Soya bean	g.	14	124	2	9.8	14	t					t		.056		.025		7.9					
Sesame	g.	14	120	1.9	10	14	t					t		.025		.025		2.3					
Sunflower	g.	14	124	1.8	12	14	t					t						1.3					
Wheat germ	g.	14	124	2.3	8.8	14						t						21.5					
Bacon fat	14	126				14		3	2	3													t

NOTE: The figures above are all based on 1tsp measures.

LINOLEIC ACID CONTENT;

LINOLEIC ACID CONTENT;	grams
Corn oil	7
Cottonseed oil	7
Olive oil	1
Peanut oil	4
Safflower oil	10
Sesame oil	6
Soya oil	7
Better×butter (safflower oil)	5
Better -butter (soya oil)	3
Margarine (liquid)	4
Margarine (hydrogenated)	2

NOTE: These Oils all supply 124 calories.
Grams of Linoleic acid per tablespoon.

As can be seen from the above chart, Lipids supply only a limited amount of the essential nutrients. The main nutrients that are supplied are Calories, Saturated and Unsaturated Lipids, Cholesterol, Vitamin A and Vitamin E. Trace amounts of the minerals Copper and Zinc are also obtainable. **SUMMARY:** After reading through this chapter on Lipids, you will have obtained valuable information to assist you with your weekly purchase of food. It is most important to remember the following main points: 1) Always use 'cold-pressed' oils. 2) Make your own better-butter. 3) Avoid Cholesterol rich foods. 4) Be sure that your diet includes some Lecithin foods or Lecithin supplements. 5) Avoid combining excess Lipids with Protein foods. 6) The most vital Lipid nutrient is Linoleic acid. 7) Avoid processed and refined foods. 8) The average daily Lipid intake (including all Lipids supplied with whole foods) should not exceed 20% of the total dietary intake. 9) Natural whole foods are life supporting to help you live and 'Laugh with Health'.

INTRODUCTION

OILS

OILS can be extracted by various methods and the only suitable method for human consumption is when the Oil has been 'cold-drawn' or usually referred to as 'cold pressed'. This cold-pressed method is usually done with hydraulic equipment, that does not change the chemical structure of the Lipid elements thereby providing the correct balance for human digestion, absorption and metabolism. This cold-pressed or 'virgin oil' is obtained with one pressing and the remaining Oils are then extracted with the assistance of heat and various chemical solvents. The majority of Oils that are available from the local supermarket have been extracted with chemical solvents and heat processes as that is the most economic way to produce liquid Oils. Apart from the chemical solvents and the heat processes that are used to extract some Oils, there are further processing and bleaching techniques used to make the Oil clean tasting, odourless and light coloured. All those extra processing techniques are designed to get every drop of Oil from the original source, however, the amount of chemical residue that remains in those Oils is something to be avoided with caution. The only way to be sure of obtaining top quality Oil is to see the label stating 'cold pressed' Oil. You may not see that on any of the supermarket range of Oils and therefore they are not worth buying. The only Oils suitable for regular use are the 'cold-pressed' Oils, that are available at most health food stores, the price may be a little more but the quality is what you pay for. Those oils that have been extracted with heat and chemical solvents will also be deficient in certain compounds that retard oxidation of extracted Oils. Vitamin E is the dominant Lipid nutrient for prevention of rapid oxidation of extracted Oils, those heat and chemical processes will eliminate the vital vitamin E content and cause the oil to turn rancid and therefore have a limited shelf life, that is usually overcome with the addition of more preserving substances which add extra health risk problems to the already chemically loaded Oil. One of the most noticeable effects of a regular use of those chemically extracted Oils is poor skin condition. When Oil is consumed that has no vitamin E content, it has a great tendency to speed up the aging process of skin tissue and this is most noticeable around the facial areas. It is important to know that the more polyunsaturated Oils (margarine) that you consume, the greater the need for vitamin E foods in order to prevent further skin deterioration and arterial damage. Cold-pressed Oils, especially: Wheat germ oil, safflower oil, soya oil, sesame oil, corn oil and sunflower oil are the most protected with vitamin E and essential unsaturated fatty acids. The addition of 'cold-pressed' oil with the daily diet is the only safe and beneficial way to obtain the essential Lipid nutrients in a well balanced form. The following pages will provide specific details and associated benefits of individual 'cold pressed' oils: Avocado, Almond, Coconut, Corn, Olive, Peanut, Safflower, Sesame, Soya, Sunflower, Wheat germ oil as well as a section on Margarine, Butter and nutrient charts.

NOTE: The following chemical additives and preservatives may be found in any Oils that have not been extracted with the recommended 'cold pressed' method: Propyl gallate, Methyl silicone, BHT and BHA, Polyglycerides, Polysorbate 80, Oxystearic. The most common chemical solvent used to extract some Oils is Hexane, that is a derivative of crude petroleum oil refinement. This chemical solvent method of Oil extraction is said to be more efficient and economical as it retains about 99% of the Oil from the Oil from the seed, grain original source. The cold pressed method will retain about 95% of the Oil content from the original source, and most important of all, the cold pressed method will retain the original chemical structure of the Oils and thereby provide the correct balance as Nature supplied for human nutrition and health.

AVOCADO OIL

AVOCADO are the best fruit-source of natural organic Fats & Oils (Lipids). Over 20% of the total Avocado fruit is composed of Lipids and nearly half of this is Mono unsaturated Lipids with 20% Saturated and 12% Poly unsaturated. This abundance of Mono unsaturated Lipids will promote digestion of the Avocado as well as supplying the essential fatty acids and the fat soluble vitamins: A, E & K. The Avocado is one of the most sustaining natural foods and one that should regularly replace the use of butter or margarine. A ripe Avocado is an ideal substitute for either butter or margarine. Try some Avocado with toasted whole grain bread and be ready for a most fulfilling natural meal. The Avocado will need special digestion due to the abundance of natural Lipids (see Lipid digestion page 125). If you have never eaten Avocado before, try a small serve with toasted whole grain bread and you will discover the satisfying potential of the Avocado. One ripe Avocado will satisfy the appetite of 2 hungry people.

AVOCADO OIL is sometimes used as an ingredient of cosmetics, especially facial creams for normal to sensitive skin. Avocado Oil is also available in small bottles of 'cold pressed oil'. If you have sensitive skin or suffer from sunburn, try some Avocado Oil, a small amount will go a long way towards relief from sunburn as well as regeneration of delicate skin tissue. You could also apply a small amount-1tsp. of a ripe Avocado directly on the face and discover the potential of natural skin care. The expense of the Avocado may deter you at first, but the potential of this 'fruit' can only be expressed in terms of benefits. It has been analyzed that the Avocado contains at least 17 mineral elements, 11 vitamins and the best supply of natural organic Lipids. Try one.

ALMOND OIL

ALMOND OIL has been used since the Roman days as a beauty aid, one of the finest that the Roman ladies could use to moisturize their skin and to prevent the formation of wrinkles. Almond Oil is still used today as an ingredient of some exclusive facial creams. Cold pressed Almond Oil is available at some natural food stores and this can be applied directly to the skin, just as the Roman ladies did for their 'natural beauty'. A small bottle of Almond Oil will lasl longer and provide more positive benefits that most other commercial facial creams. Try some.

ALMOND OIL supplies 90% unsaturated Lipids, mainly in the form of Mono unsaturates-70%, with nearly 60% being in the form of Oleic acid, second highest next to Olive Oil. The Oleic acid content of Almond Oil is completely digestible and has the ability to improve the transfer and absorption of the fat soluble vitamins: A, D, E & K. Almond Oil also supplies 30% Linoleic acid, that is classed as a Poly unsaturated Lipid and required daily for positive health. A handful of raw Almonds will supply your body with a most nourishing food to eat as well as giving you a composition of elements that will improve your mental abilities, promote the formation of healthy skin tissue and metabolism of vitamins: A, D, E & K and protect the heart muscles and arteries from deterioration due to the effects of stress, environmental pollutants smoking and consumption of refined and processed foods and drinks, that are all deficient especially in vit.E.

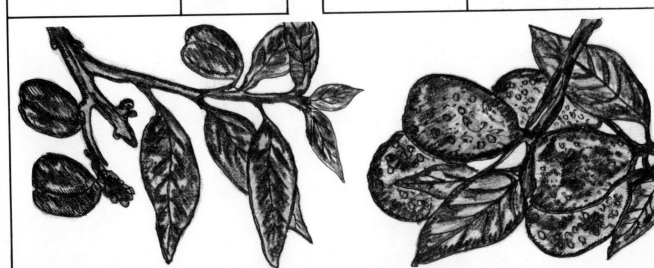

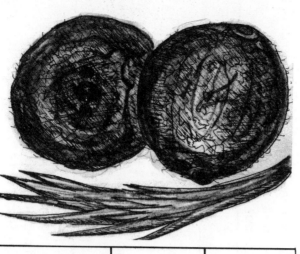

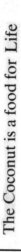

The Coconut is a food for Life

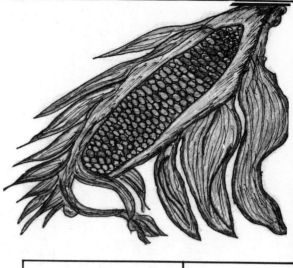

COCONUT OIL

COCONUT is the largest member of the Nut family. The origin of the Coconut can be traced back thousands of years and has often been called the 'tree that sustains Life' as the palm leaves of the Coconut will provide shelter and the Nut will supply all the essential human nutritional needs in small amounts. Coconut meat is called 'copra' and this is the most nourishing part of the Coconut. The milk of Coconut supplies valuable amounts of the minerals: Phosphorus, Calcium, Iron, Sodium, Potassium. Magnesium and a valuable supply of Vitamin C and B group vitamins: B3, B5, B6 and trace amounts of B1, B2 & B3. For some people, the Coconut is the 'staff of Life'. Discover the taste and benefits of a fresh Coconut meal. Crack one open today and see how much Coconut food your body can enjoy. A large size Coconut will serve 4 people with Health.

COCONUT OIL is available in various cosmetics, suntan creams and also soaps. The best source of Coconut oil is obtainable directly from the whole Coconut. Place all the white meat part of the Coconut in a blender and mix with a small amount of Coconut water-milk. The result is one of the finest creams for protection from sunburn and for development of a golden suntan. This home made Coconut cream is far superior to any commercial product and also less expensive.

COCONUT OIL contains over 80% Saturated Lipids, the highest primary source of Saturated Lipids. Coconut oil also supplies essential minerals and vitamins to protect you from any fat accumulation in the bloodstream. The mineral Sodium is abundant and essential for protection from blood impurities and most important of all: cleansing of the Lymphatic system.
    Take some pieces of fresh Coconut at your next lunch break.

CORN OIL

CORN OIL has been used by men and women for thousands of years. The old method of extraction retained all the essential nutrients, today there are two types of Corn Oil: one that has been obtained by the 'cold pressed' method that also retains all the essential fat soluble vitamins: A, D, & E. The other method of extraction includes the use of various chemical solvents and other chemical processes that destroy the natural quality of any Oil, thereby the benefits are no longer available. Make sure you use 'cold pressed oil' and avoid using those meals that require deep frying. Any natural Oil will be easily damaged by excess heat, due to the saturation of essential Unsaturated Lipids that are well supplied with cold pressed Corn Oil. Over 80% of the Corn Oil is in the form of Unsaturated Lipids. Corn Oil is rich in Linoleic acid—60% (see pp. 122–123).

CORN OIL combines very well with a fresh garden salad or with home made bread and cookies. Always add a small amount of lecithin granules when you use Corn Oil, especially for those cooked meals. Add the lecithin last and Health will be on your side. Corn Oil is also beneficial when used directly on the skin for treatment of eczema and other skin disorders. See section on Grains, p. 24, for recipes with 'corn on the cob' and also home made Corn bread.

OLIVE OIL

OLIVE OIL is the richest natural source of Oleic acid. On average 80% of Olive oil is in the form of Oleic acid, a mono unsaturated Lipid (see p. 122). This high concentration of Oleic acid makes Olive oil very easily digested and assimilated for use as a heat-energy source. Olives were the original provider of Man's daily Lipid requirements. In ancient times, the Hebrews used Olive oil as part of their sacred annointing oil and regarded having Olive oil as a sign of prosperity. Hippocrates, the 'father of medicine', classed Olive oil as as food-medicine. Fresh ripe Olives contain 50% organic Lipids and over 40% mineral, vitamin, carbohydrate and water content.

OLIVE OIL supplies a minimal amount of the essential fatty acid: Linoleic acid, however, as only 2% of the daily intake of food needs to be in the form of Linoleic acid and Olive oil is approx. 10% Linoleic acid, you can be assured of obtaining this essential fatty acid with regular use of Olive oil. It is a good idea to combine Olive oil half-half with any of the following 'cold pressed oils': corn, soya, safflower, sesame or sunflower. This combining of oils will provide a better range of essential fatty acids and promote the numerous functions of the essential fatty acids

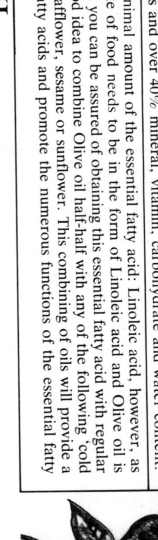

PEANUT OIL

PEANUT OIL is obtained from the Arachis Lypogae plant, that is classed as a Legume. Peanut Oil is often referred to as 'arachis'. Cold pressed Peanut Oil is composed of 80% unsaturated Lipids and 20% Saturated. The valuable supply of essential Unsaturated fatty acids is mainly in the form of Oleic acid—70% and Linoleic acid—20%. The method of Oil extraction is most important to the quality of Peanut oil. The 'cold pressed oil' is the only reliable type. Make sure you can read that on the label, otherwise you may buy an Oil that has been subjected to chemical solvents and various other heat processes that can easily destroy the quality of Peanut oil.

PEANUT BUTTER can be a most valuable addition to the diet, especially when taken in moderation and when the Peanut butter is freshly prepared. Avoid using commercial Peanut butter, they are more than likely to contain unnecessary additives and be more expensive and not as tasty. Peanut butter is an excellent food to combine with whole grain toasted bread. It is important to remember that the Peanut is an acid forming food and that the daily diet should supply only 25% acid forming foods and 75% alkaline forming foods: fruits, vegetables, some grains, legumes, nuts and seeds. When you combine Peanut butter with whole grain bread you will improve the Protein availability content of both the Peanut and the whole grain bread. This is another of the benefits of natural food combination (see section on Protein, pp. 81–91).

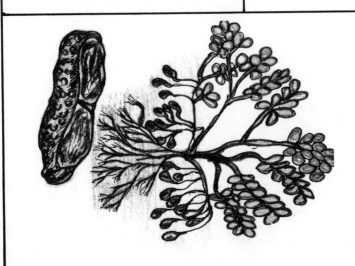
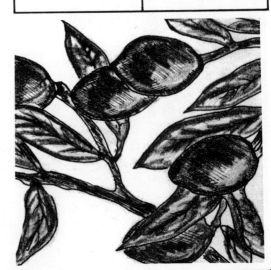

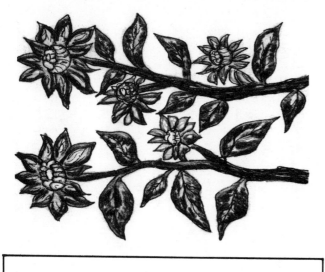

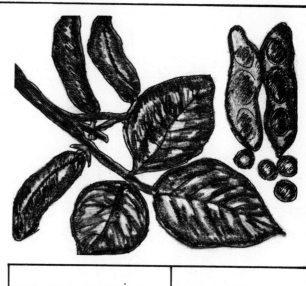

SAFFLOWER OIL

SAFFLOWER OIL is obtained from the Safflower seed, that is a member of the 'compositae' family of plants and one that ancient civilizations cultivated near the banks of the river Nile. Safflower Oil is the richest source of unsaturated Lipids, with Linoleic acid being the dominant 'fatty acid'. Nearly 90% of Safflower Oil is Unsaturated and over 70% is in the form of Linoleic acid and 20% Oleic acid. Safflower oil supplies 10 grams of Linoleic acid per tablespoon. A most common result of a Linoleic acid deficiency is dermatitis, that is also prompted by excess emotional stress and physical exhaustion. Linoleic acid is one of the essential 3 Fatty acids (see page 123 for details). This high portion of unsaturated Lipids gives Safflower oil the ability to protect you against excess blood-cholesterol, that is often caused by excess consumption of animal produce and a lack of natural whole foods such as fruits, **vegetables**, whole grains, legumes, nuts and seeds. A high blood-cholesterol level can be most detrimental to the heart muscles and the blood circulatory system. Such symptons as: arteriosclerosis, heart disease, chilblains and cramps may all be due to excess blood cholesterol levels. Be careful to avoid processed and refined foods as they are more than likely to add up an excess blood-cholesterol level. Have a snack, but have it with Nature and Natural whole foods.

SAFFLOWER OIL is available at most supermarkets so be sure to choose the 'cold pressed' Safflower Oil. A bottle of Oil should last a long time as only one tablespoon is required per day. Buy the best, buy cold pressed Safflower Oil and be sure of good value and positive Health.

SOYA OIL

SOYA OIL is a reliable source of the 3 'essential unsaturated fatty acids', with over 85% of Soya Bean Oil is made up from unsaturated Lipids with Linoleic acid being the dominant 'fatty acid' (see page 123 for details). Approx. 50% of Soya Oil is composed of Linoleic acid. Next time you buy some Oil, look around for the 'cold-pressed' Soya Oil, that has as much versatility as any other cold pressed oil plus the advantage of supplying an abundance of the essential daily Lipid nutrients. Soya Oil also supplies approx. 25% Oleic acid, that is classed as a mono unsaturated Lipid. The third essential fatty acid is Linolenic acid and approx. 10% of Soya Oil is in this form. There are so many Oils available that you may have difficulty in deciding the best type. Soya Bean Oil will be the best choice when obtained as 'cold pressed' Soya Oil. Look around for some.

SOYA BEANS are often the original source of commercially produced Lecithin (see page 126) and so when using Soya Oil in cooking or baking it would be advisable to add a little Lecithin granules (1 tsp. per person) daily. The same applies to any other Oils that are used with the diet. Lecithin granules will mix very well with nearly all types of meals and this is especially beneficial when combined with meat meals, egg meals, fried meals, home made bread, cookies and most other cooked meals. Always add the Lecithin just before serving.

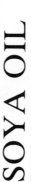

SESAME OIL

SESAME SEEDS are termed 'the queen of the oil bearing seeds'. Sesame seeds are 45% Protein and Mineral content and over 50% Lipid content. For every 500 grams of Sesame seeds you can obtain over 1 cupfull of top quality oil. Sesame oil is an excellent source of unsaturated Lipids with nearly 90% being unsaturated and 10% saturated Lipids. The extraction of Sesame oil is a simple process that requires no chemical solvents or additives as there are no husks to be removed and a top quality oil can be obtained with one cold-pressing. Sesame seeds are grown throughout many parts of the world especially Turkey, China, Africa, South-Central America, India and the southwest parts of the U.S.A. In some of these places, Sesame Oil is referred to as Gingelly oil or Benne oil. There are numerous benefits associated with a regular use of Sesame oil and Sesame seeds. The Sesame plant produces a special substance that is known as Sesamol and this is an excellent natural preservative that prevents Sesame oil from turning rancid, this is most important especially in places that have very hot weather such as Turkey from where the Sesame paste—Tahini originated. Sesame oil will last longer than other cold pressed Oils.

TAHINI is made from ground up Sesame seeds and has the same consistency as smooth peanut butter. One of the main benefits of Tahini is that it can be very easily digested and within half an hour after ingestion, Tahini can enter the bloodstream and supply valuable nutrients such as the excellent source of Vitamin E. 100 grams of Tahini will supply about 40mg. of vitamin E and in comparison to all other natural foods, Tahini can be considered as the ultimate source thereby providing numerous health benefits such as: increasing the stamina and endurance of all muscles, due to the unique ability of vitamin E, that enables both nerves and muscles to function more efficiently with the supply of Oxygen. Vitamin E also promotes the functioning of Linoleic acid (the 'essential' fatty acid, see page 123 for details) and this is most beneficial as it retard ageing of all body cells thereby helping you to preserve that youthful look and also to retain proper focusing of the eyes with the older generation. Tahini is one of the most versatile foods as it combines very well with all meals and only small amounts are required to get this excellent supply of vitamin E-the 'heart muscle vitamin'. If you have never tried Tahini, you health will surely improve when you do. Every kitchen should be stocked up with Tahini-the vitamin E food.

TAHINI and SESAME SEEDS are also an excellent Protein food. They supply over 18% complete primary protein and are especially rich in the amino acid Methinone, that is the main 'limiting amino acid' with all primary and secondary protein foods. By adding a small amount of TAHINI (1tsp. per person per meal) you can greatly increase the protein availability of any of the following foods: almonds, cashews, hazel, pecan, walnuts, soya beans, sunflower seeds, wheat germ, milk, yoghurt, whole grains and legumes. Methinone is an essential amino acid and has numerous functions such as: control of blood-fat levels and assists in fat metabolism thereby providing another form of natural weight control. Methinone also assists in blood haemoglobin development and in combination with the excellent source of the mineral Iron. Tahini can also be recommended as a food for healthy blood development (see page 102 for more details).

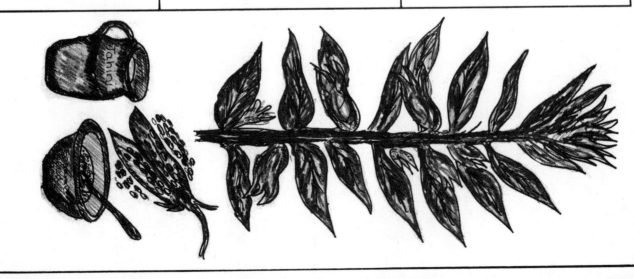

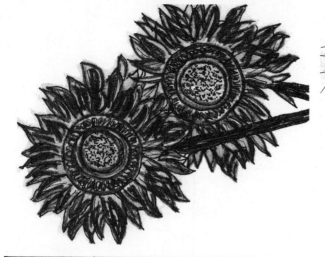

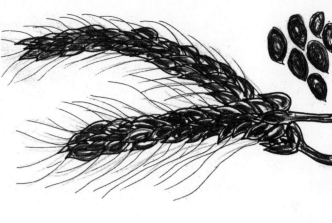

SUNFLOWER OIL

SUNFLOWER OIL is composed of approx. 90% Unsaturated Lipids and 10% Saturated Lipids. The dominant unsaturated Lipids are: Linoleic acid-60% (the essential fatty acid) and Oleic acid-30%. Sunflower Oil is obtained from Sunflower seeds, they are an excellent source of vitamin D-the 'sunshine vitamin'. Next time the winter season arrives be sure to stock up your kitchen with a bottle of 'cold pressed' Sunflower Oil and some Sunflower seeds. Vitamin D is sometimes a hard vitamin to obtain, especially if you work in the office environment all day. A lack of vitamin D can retard the growth of children as vitamin D is essential for the metabolism of the two dominant minerals of the body, that are Calcium and Phosphorus. Vitamin D is also vital for healthy skin, teeth, hair and regulation of the heart beat. Only small amounts of Sunflower Oil are required from the daily diet in order to obtain the 'essential fatty acids' and also vitamin D & E.

By using cold pressed Sunflower Oil with salads, cooking or baking, you will obtain a good supply of vitamin E, essential unsaturated fatty acids and a unique supply of vitamin D. Sunflower Oil is a wonderful assistant in promoting your 'winter health'. A handful of Sunflower seeds per day is the ultimate way to make up for those cold and dark winter months. See section on Sunflower seeds, p. 101, for more details and associated benefits of Sunflower seeds.

WHEAT GERM OIL

WHEAT GERM OIL is the most potent form of Vitamin E and was the original source from which vitamin E was discovered. The whole Wheat grain is an excellent food for your daily vitamin E requirements, however, very few people have even tasted whole wheat and have a diet that is generally deficient in vitamin E foods. 1 small bottle-200ml. of 'cold pressed' Wheat germ oil should be an essential addition with your shopping requirements especially if you eat refined white or brown bread and other refined foods, smoke cigarettes and intend to protect yourself from polluted air. By taking 1tsp. per day of cold pressed Wheat germ oil you can be assured that your arteries and heart muscles will be given adequate nutrition for protection from pollution and for every packet of cigarettes another 1tsp. can be a most advantageous addition for protection from the poisons of nicotine and the number of other poisons that are dominant in the average cigarette. Wheat germ oil should also be part of every first aid kit and used primarily for burns, skin irritations and prevention of wrinkly skin. Keep Wheat germ oil in a cool place and use whenever you have sunburn or other forms of skin damage. Wheat germ oil will penetrate deep into the skin layers and promote rapid healing by supplying more oxygen to all skin cells.

WHEAT GERM OIL when taken as a daily supplement (1 tsp. per day) will promote efficient functioning of all muscles and nerves. The vitamin E content of Wheat germ oil will improve the endurance and stamina of all muscles by promoting the flow of blood throughout all blood vessels and it also aids in supplying nourishment to the cells and strengthening of the capillary walls. If your diet is or has been deficient in vitamin E foods, be sure to get a regular supply of Wheat germ oil and vitamin E foods

CHAPTER FIVE

MINERALS

TOTAL COMMUNITY OF EARTH ELEMENTS

The Total Community of Earth Elements Chart provides a total view of all the elements and minerals obtainable on Earth. There are nine main groups, listed on the left side column. On page 140, the Total Group of Essential Minerals for human requirements are listed in a chart, designed to show the four main Gasseous Elements, Essential Minerals and Trace Minerals. The Chart on this page displays the essential minerals (bold type) and the trace minerals (medium type), to provide a view of the origin of the essential human nutrient (gasseous and mineral) requirements.

HYDROGEN HAS UNIQUE PROPERTIES. THE SUN & STARS ARE ALMOST COMPLETE HYDROGEN ENERGY.

FIRST TRANSITION METALS	Li. LITHIUM · Na. **SODIUM** · K. **POTASSIUM** · Rb. **RUBIDIUM** · Cs. CAESIUM · Fr. FRANCIUM Be. BERYLLIUM · Mg. **MAGNESIUM** · Ca. **CALCIUM** · Sr. STRONTIUM · Ba. BARIUM · Ra. RADIUM Sc. SCANDIUM · Ti. TITANIUM · V. **VANADIUM** · Cr. **CHROMIUM** · Mn. **MANGANESE**
SECOND TRANSITION METALS	Y. YTTRIUM · Zr. ZIRCONIUM · Nb. NIOBIUM · Mo. **MOLYBDENUM** · Tc. TECHNETIUM Fe. **IRON** · Co. **COBALT** · Ni. **NICKEL** · Ru. RUTHENIUM · Rh. RHODIUM
THIRD TRANSITION METALS	Hf. HAFNIUM · Ta. TANTALUM · W. TUNGSTEN · Re. RHENIUM Pd. PALLADIUM · Os. OSMIUM · Ir. IRIDIUM · Pt. PLATINUM Cu. **COPPER.** · Zn. **ZINC.** · Ag. **SILVER.** · Cd. CADMIUM. · Au. **GOLD.** · Hg. **MERCURY.**
BORON & CARBON FAMILY	B. BORON. · Al. **ALUMINIUM.** · Ga. **GALLIUM.** C. **CARBON.** · Si. **SILICON.** · Ge. **GERMANIUM.** In. INDIUM. · Tl. THALLIUM. Sn. TIN. · Pb. LEAD.
NITROGEN & OXYGEN FAMILY	N. **NITROGEN.** · P. **PHOSPHORUS.** O. **OXYGEN.** · S. **SULPHUR.** · Se. **SELENIUM.** Sb. ANTIMONY. · As. ARSENIC. · Te. TELLERIUM. · Bi. BISMUTH. · Po. POLONIUM.
HALOGENS	F. **FLUORINE.** · Cl. **CHLORINE.** · Br. BROMINE. · I. **IODINE.** · At. ASTATINE.
INERT GASSES	He. HELIUM. · Ne. NEON. · Ar. ARGON. · Kr. KRYPTON. · Xe. XENON. · Rn. RADON.
RARE EARTH METALS	La. LATHIUM. · Ce. CERIUM. · Pr. PRASEODY. · Nd. NEODYMIUM. · Pm. PROMETHIUM. · Sm. SAMARIUM. · Eu. EUROPIUM. · Gd. GADOLINIUM. Tb. TERBIUM. · Dy. DYSPROSIUM. · Ho. HOLMIUM. · Er. ERBIUM. · Tm. THULIUM. · Yb. YTTERBIUM. · Lu. LUTETIUM.
ACTINIDE METALS	Ac. ACTINIUM. · Th. THORIUM. · Pa. PROTACTIUM. · U. URANIUM. · Np. NEPTUNIUM. · Pu. PLUTONIUM. · Am. AMERICIUM. · Cm. CURIUM. Bk. BERKELIUM. · Cf. CALIFORNIUM. · Es. EINSTEINIUM. · Fm. FERMIUM. · Md. MENDELEVIUM. · No. NOBELIUM. · Lw. LAWRENCIUM.

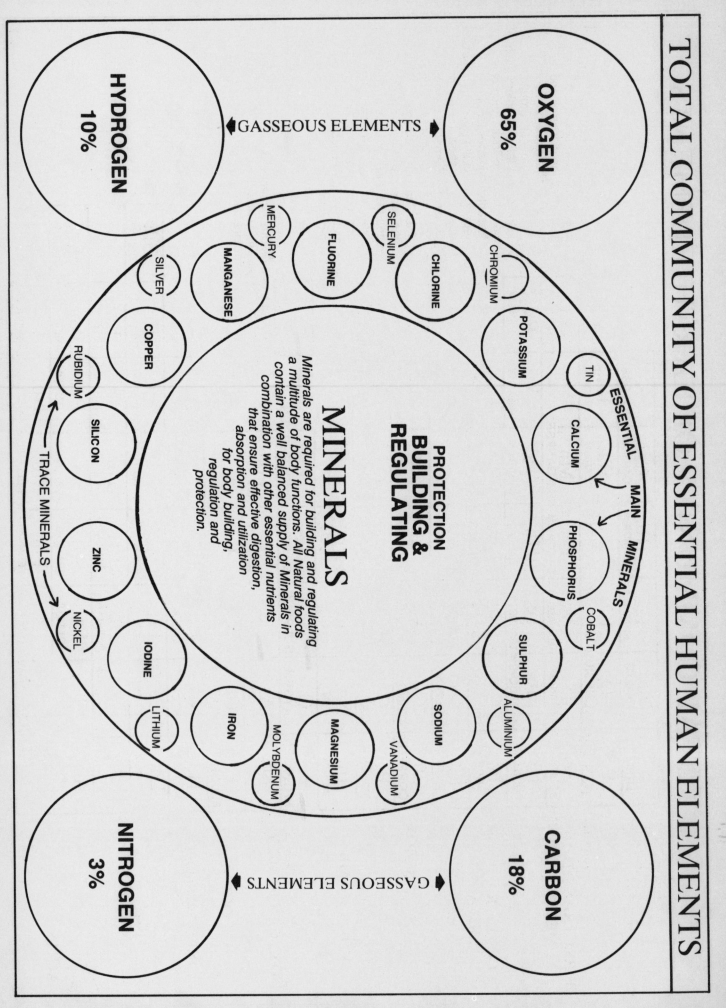

◄ GASSEOUS ELEMENTS ►

OXYGEN 65%

HYDROGEN 10%

CARBON 18%

NITROGEN 3%

◄ GASSEOUS ELEMENTS ►

ESSENTIAL

MAIN MINERALS

TRACE MINERALS

MINERALS

PROTECTION BUILDING & REGULATING

Minerals are required for building and regulating a multitude of body functions. All Natural foods contain a well balanced supply of Minerals in combination with other essential nutrients that ensure effective digestion, absorption and utilization for body building, regulation and protection.

TIN · CALCIUM · PHOSPHORUS · COBALT · SULPHUR · ALUMINIUM · SODIUM · VANADIUM · MAGNESIUM · MOLYBDENUM · IRON · LITHIUM · IODINE · NICKEL · ZINC · SILICON · RUBIDIUM · COPPER · SILVER · MANGANESE · MERCURY · FLUORINE · SELENIUM · CHROMIUM · CHLORINE · POTASSIUM

MINERALS – INTRODUCTION

A total 103 Elements have been discovered so far to be part of Nature on Earth. Many of these 103 are rare and unessential for Human requirements. The main 4 Elements are;

OXYGEN   CARBON   HYDROGEN   &   NITROGEN.

These 4 main Elements take up 96% of total body weight. The remaining 4% is composed of Mineral Elements (see diagram).

MINERALS are part of the complex of Earthly Elements and for Human requirements they are grouped into the form of **ESSENTIAL MINERALS & TRACE MINERALS.**

MINERALS are as important to the Human as a complete set of good spark plugs are for a car. Minerals culd be thought as the spark plugs and the Vitamins as the initial 'spark' that is distributed to all parts of the body. When even one Mineral is lacking from the diet, the result is felt by the entire body and the role of certain vitamins will also be inhibited which leads to even more problems such as general ill health, lack of energy, feeling of irritability, nervous disorders, muscular and mental deteoration.

MINERALS are part of every living cell of the body. They are closely integrated with one another, to perform a multitude of functions. Often 1 mineral deficiency will effect and retard the functions of various other Minerals. With Natural foods you can be sure of getting the Minerals in a Balanced form.

MINERALS of the Earth must first pass through the Living structure of plants before they are usuable for Human survival. Plants are the 'Missing Link' in providing Man with one of the Essential ingredients of Life which is Food & Nutrition. All the other 3 Main Elements (Air, Water & Sunshine) are obtainable directly: Minerals are not. Without plants, the Elements of the Soil would be directly useless without the assistance of the Plant World. When Minerals are obtained directly from Plant source (Fruits, Vegetables, Legumes, Whole Grains, Nuts and Seeds), the Mineral elements are joined in exactly the right amounts and combinations to ensure compatability with the Human system. Any refinement, processing, extraction or addition (sugar, salt & preservatives etc.) destroys the combination and places a strain on the Human system which results in a definate decline in health:(Mental & Physical.)

Foods that have been altered from the Original state are to some people the most 'satisfying' in taste, which is a result of the knowledge and application of Chemists and other Food Scientists, to have the ability to recognize and manufacture the 'most appealing tastes' which tempt the human senses into an unconscious desire for another such 'Taste Stimulation'. The supermarket is a visual display of such products which have often been so well advertised that the temptation is unbearable:-the junk food gets eaten, the 'taste stimulation' is obtained, the body metabolism disturbed, the nutrient loss leads to further complaints and often the cycle is completed with another-go at the junk-food, as an attempt to regain the 'Taste Stimulation' which is often attractive and powerful enough to 'stimulate' for a person's entire 'shortened lifespan'.

CALCIUM

— Ca — Alkaline mineral

The human body is composed of more Calcium than any other mineral. About 90% of the calcium content is contained in the bone structure, the frame of the body, the skeleton.

The total calcium content of the body is entirely renewed over a 6 year period. Every day your body makes new cells.

To obtain the right calcium intake, it is essential to eat those natural foods which contain calcium and the associated nutrients to assist calcium absorption. When the calcium reserve becomes deficient due to an inadequate supply, the mineral will be progressively withdrawn from the bones and teeth. Natural foods are always balanced.

The daily intake should be considerably increased for mothers during pregnancy, especially the last two months when the growth of the embryo accelerates rapidly. An increase should also be maintained during the following periods of lactation. When the mother's calcium reserves are deficient during these times, the child requirements will actually be withdrawn from the mother's body, resulting in loss of hair, weak bone structure and deteorating teeth conditions. Calcium foods prevent Arthritis.

Calcium foods are essential for the involuntary muscular movements of the intestines, (Peristaltic action) which aids the digestion of all foods.

Calcium foods are required for smooth functioning of the heart muscles.

Processed and refined food products are generally Calcium deficient. This is due to a lack of essential associated nutrients which assist in the absorption and utilization of the mineral Calcium. Calcium foods contain all the essential ingredients to ensure maximum benefits. Processed foods lack Enzymes .

To function efficiently, Calcium must be in combination with the minerals, Magnesium & Phosphorus and Vitamins A, C & D.

The Calcium Phosphorus balance is 2.5 parts Calcium, I part Phosphorus. A good supply of Protein assists in the absorption of Calcium from foods.

The Parathyroid glands, situated in the neck, regulate the body's storage of the mineral Calcium. If these glands are not functioning properly, the Calcium levels of the blood will be affected. Calcium foods also maintain healthy glands.

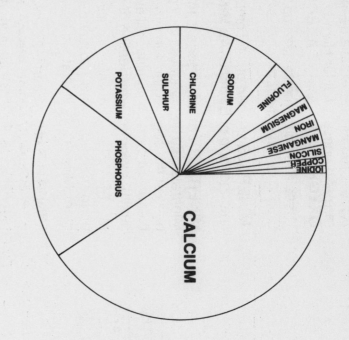

Sesame seeds, Kelp, Collard + Kale leaves Turnip greens, Almonds, Soya beans, Hazel nuts Parsley, Dandelion greens, Brazil nut, Watercress Chick pea, White bean, Pinto bean, Pistachio nut Fig (dr.), Sunflower seed, Beetroot greens Wheat bran, Mung bean, Olives, Broccoli, Broad bean English walnut, Rhubarb, Spinach, Okra, Prune (dr.) Swiss chard, Endive, Lentils, Rice bran, Cowpea Pecan nut, Lima bean, Wheat germ, Chive, Peanut Lettuce, Apricot (dr.), Savoy cabbage, Peas (dr.) Raisins, Black currant, Dates, Snap beans, Chestnut Leek, Pumpkin seeds, Onion-green, Parsnip Cabbage, Peach (dr.), Macadamia nut, Wheat, Orange Celery, Turnip, Cashew nut, Rye grain, Carrot

CALCIUM

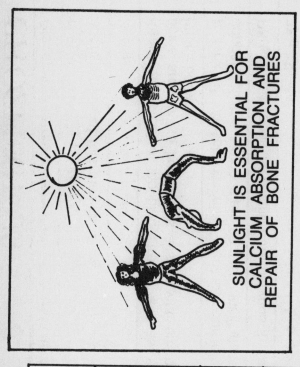

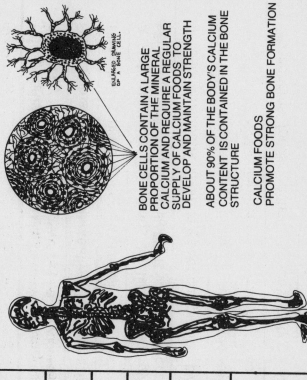

SUNLIGHT IS ESSENTIAL FOR CALCIUM ABSORPTION AND REPAIR OF BONE FRACTURES

ENLARGED DRAWING OF A BONE CELL.

BONE CELLS CONTAIN A LARGE PROPORTION OF THE MINERAL CALCIUM AND REQUIRE A REGULAR SUPPLY OF CALCIUM FOODS TO DEVELOP AND MAINTAIN STRENGTH

ABOUT 90% OF THE BODY'S CALCIUM CONTENT IS CONTAINED IN THE BONE STRUCTURE

CALCIUM FOODS PROMOTE STRONG BONE FORMATION

Calcium ascorbate, which is formed with the chemical combination of Vit D (sunlight) and the mineral calcium, assists in the proper healing of all bone fractures and breakages.

Only when calcium levels are low can a virus infection occur.

The balance of Calcium and Phosphorus is severely affected by the continual intake of all forms of refined sugars. This often results in tooth decay, bone deformation of children and cancer sores and cramps in the body of adults.

Alcohol and chocolate cause a severe loss of calcium from the body.

The use of inorganic salt (table salt) also drives calcium out of the body.

Any calcium intake must be suitably balanced with the minerals, potassium and sodium. In all natural foods that are rich in calcium, these two minerals are always found in combination. (Celery, Almonds, Lettuce, Sesame Seeds).

Cancer research has shown that, cancerous tissues are abnormally low in calcium. Due to a lack of calcium, these cancer cells will spread to other parts of the body. Calcium foods also prevent anemia.

Reduces fatigue and increases the body's general resistance to fight infections. Excess intake of fatty based foods, hinders Calcium absorption.

Calcium improves the vital acid—alkaline balance of the body.

Calcium plays a major role in providing firmness and elasticity for the skin and all the cells and tissues of the body. Calcium foods deter acne.

When the body is in an acid condition and is lacking the mineral sodium, the calcium reserves of the body are precipitated from the bone structure, such as in cases of arthritis. Natural Foods give you balanced Health.

A prolonged Calcium deficiency may lead to any of the following ailments. Lung disease, Asthma, Kidney disease, poor vision and sensitivity to light, poor appetite, varicose veins, poor growth of children, skin disorders, freckles, weak muscles, eczema, rheumatism, irregular heartbeat and arthritic complaints.

PHOSPHORUS

– P – *Acid mineral*

Phosphorus is part of every living cell and chemical reaction within the body.

The phosphorus content of the body is renewed over a period of 3 years. Approx. 90% of this mineral is found in the bone structure, teeth and nails.

Is essential for the maintenance and repair of the entire nervous system.

Keeps acids out of the bloodstream and assists the transportation of fatty acids around the body. This assists vital energy distribution throughout the entire body.

Phosphorus foods strengthen the nervous system. (Spinal Cord & Brain).

A lack of phosphorus may lead to poor memory and weak abilities of concentration. Almonds are an excellent Phosphorus Food.

The phosphorus compounds, termed Lecethins, are found in the body's tissues, the lymphatic system, the white matter of the brain and the grey matter of the nerves. Phosphorus foods contain Lecethin.

Phosphorus Foods are essential for the Health of the skin, hair, nails and Brain.

Phosphorus foods improve blood circulation and normalize blood pressure levels especially for those people who have a very low blood pressure count.

Phosphorus foods promote creative ability, assisting artistic people and writers.

Phosphorus plays an important role in the transfer of hereditary characteristics

A lack of phosphorus leads to lack of energy, exhaustion, shyness and sensitivity. Vitamin D (Sunlight) is vital for correct Phosphorus balance.

Phosphorus foods improve a poor complexion, by stimulating blood circulation.

Use of refined sugar products will lead to a Phosphorus deficiency.

Phosphorus foods improve the utilization of Fats, Proteins and Carbohydrates.

Phosphorus foods reduce the possibility of Cancerous tissue formation.

MAIN TYPES OF HUMAN CELLS

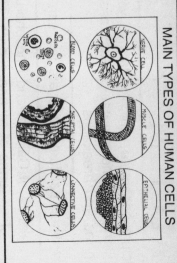

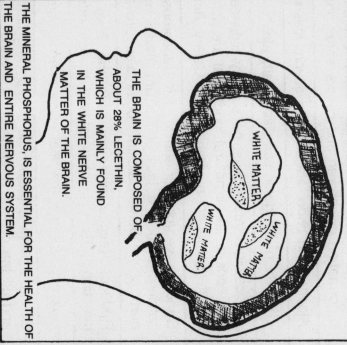

THE MINERAL PHOSPHORUS, IS ESSENTIAL FOR THE HEALTH OF THE BRAIN AND ENTIRE NERVOUS SYSTEM.

THE BRAIN IS COMPOSED OF ABOUT 28% LECETHIN, WHICH IS MAINLY FOUND IN THE WHITE NERVE MATTER OF THE BRAIN.

WHITE MATTER

WHITE MATTER

WHITE MATTER

Rice bran, Pumpkin seeds, Wheat bran, Wheat germ
Sunflower seeds, Brazil nut, Safflower seed
Sesame seed, Soya bean, Almonds, Peanut
Pistachio nut, Pinto beans, Cowpea, White bean
Red bean, Wheat, Broad bean, Lima bean, Walnut
Lentils, Rye, Cashew, Hickory nut, Mung bean, Millet
Hazel nut, Wild rice, Chick pea, Pigeon pea, Barley
Pecan nuts, Sorghum, Dulse, Kelp, Garlic, Rice
Chestnut, Macadamia nut, Mushroom, Peas

POTASSIUM

– K – Alkaline mineral

Potassium is the foundation mineral of all muscular tissues. It is essential for the repair and health condition of all the body's muscles.

Potassium combines with Iron to utilize oxygen in the body and is essential to keep the heart in a healthy condition. It also strengthens the heart muscles. Potasssium foods normalize heart action.

Potassium Foods assist in the elimination of blood impurities, via the kidneys.

Potassium in combination with Sodium prevents hardening of the arteries.

Cancer cells cannot live in a solution of potassium.

Potassium foods retard the ageing process, by improving blood circulation.

Excessive salt intake depletes the potassium reserve of the body.

A combination of potassium, sodium and calcium is recommended for lung diseases and chest infections. Also for the efficient functioning of the brain, nerves and heart. Olives are one of the best Potassium foods, eaten raw.

Potassium assists by balancing the acid alkaline levels of the body.

Assists repair of the liver and is essential for the formation of Glycogen from the liver. This substance is stored and converted in the liver, to Glucose which is a usuable energy source.

Potassium is the most effective healing mineral for the body.

Cooking and processing easily destroy the potassium content of foods.

Potasssium foods in combination with Phosphorus are vital for the transportation of Oxygen into the brain, which is essential for efficient mental functioning.

Alcohol & Coffee, taken in excess, will cause a severe Potassium deficiency. Potassium foods assist the body in the transfer of nerve impulses.

Other symptoms of a deficiency are, irritability, weariness, sleep walking and poor nerves. Diabetics are often Potassium deficient.

POTASSIUM IS THE 'MUSCLE MINERAL'

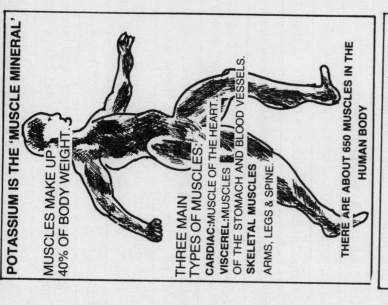

MUSCLES MAKE UP 40% OF BODY WEIGHT.

THREE MAIN TYPES OF MUSCLES:

CARDIAC: MUSCLE OF THE HEART.

VISCEREL: MUSCLES OF THE STOMACH AND BLOOD VESSELS.

SKELETAL MUSCLES ARMS, LEGS & SPINE.

THERE ARE ABOUT 650 MUSCLES IN THE HUMAN BODY

POTASSIUM IS THE MAIN HEALING MINERAL

COOKING DESTROYS THE POTASSIUM CONTENT OF FOODS

Kelp, Soya bean, Lima bean, Rice bran, White bean Wheat bran, Mung bean, Cowpea, Pea, Pinto bean Red bean, Pigeon pea, Pistachio nut, Chestnut Wheat germ, Chick pea, N.Z. Spinach, Lentils Almonds, Raisins, Parsley, Sesame seeds, Brazil nut Hazel nut, Peanut, Dates, Figs, Watercress, Avocado Pecan nut, Parsnip, Garlic, Rye, Cashew nut, Walnut Millet, Mushroom, Potato, Collard, Dandelion greens Fennel, Brussel sprouts, Broccoli, Kale, Banana Black currants, Wheat, Sorghum, Leek, Carrot Celery, Pumpkin, Beetroot, Radish, Peas, Barley

SULPHUR

— S — Acid mineral

Sulphur is contained in all the tissues of the body and as part of blood haemoglobin ,where it acts as an oxidyzing agent.

Sulphur foods are essential for optimal Protein absorption.

Has an antiseptic and cleansing effect on the digestive system. Also maintains the health of bile and pancreatic juices at a normal fluid level.

Is an excellent blood purifier, with antiseptic and cleansing effects for the digestive tract. Sulphur & Phosphorus must be balanced.

Sulphur Foods also assist by providing oxygen to the blood. Sulphur is also required in the formation of blood plasma. You can depend on Natural Foods.

Sulphur foods prevent the accumulation of waste body toxins.

Sulphur foods are essential for normal functioning of the heart muscles.

Assists growth in children and maintains healthy hair, teeth and skin.

Sulphur foods prevent the development of infections, such as Hepatitis.

Cooking destroys the sulphur content of foods.

Promotes a good complexion, by cleansing the body of any acid mucus poisons which are often the cause of such disorders as dandruff and acne.

SULPHUR FOODS PROMOTE A GOOD COMPLEXION
SULPHUR FOODS PREVENT DANDRUFF AND ACNE

The mineral Sulphur is part of the structure of Insulin, which is required for proper digestion and metabolism of Carbohydrates.

Sulphur is an ingredient of Keratin, a protein substance that improves skin and hair growth and condition.
Sulphur foods contain Keratin.

SULPHUR FOODS ALSO MAINTAIN HEALTHY HAIR, TEETH & SKIN.

SULPHUR FOODS ASSIST GROWTH OF CHILDREN.

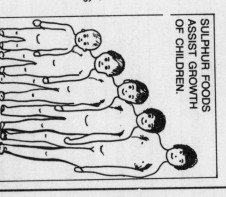

COOKING DESTROYS THE SULPHUR CONTENT OF ALL FOODS

SULPHUR FOODS KEEP YOUR BODY CLEAN.

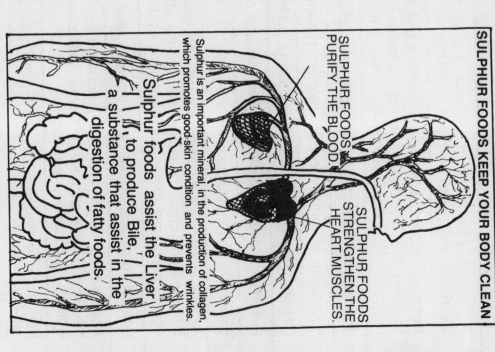

SULPHUR FOODS PURIFY THE BLOOD.

SULPHUR FOODS STRENGTHEN THE HEART MUSCLES.

Sulphur is an important mineral, in the production of collagen, which promotes good skin condition and prevents wrinkles.

Sulphur foods assist the Liver, to produce Bile, a substance that assist in the digestion of fatty foods.

Kale, Watercress, Cabbage, Brussel sprouts Snap beans, Turnips, Cauliflower, Kelp, Raspberry Spinach, Parsnip, Leek, Radish, Cucumber, Okra Lettuce, Chives, Peas (fr.), Celery, Red currant Avocado, Asparagus, Tomato, Hazel nut Black currants, Turnip greens, Carrots, Eggplant Pineapple, Brazil nuts, Sweet corn, Peach, Potato Dandelion greens, Fig, Onion, Soya beans, Artichoke Lima beans, Raisins, Mushrooms, Barley, Rhubarb Watermelon, Strawberry, Apple, Oranges, Limes

CHLORINE

— Cl – Acid mineral

Organic chlorine is essential for the production of vital gastric juices which aid digestion. Chlorine foods stimulate Hcl production.

Helps in regulating the heart action and normalizing blood pressure.

Helps eliminate poisons from the body and assists in purifying the blood.

Chlorine foods assist in the digestion of fats and especially Proteins.

Is helpful for those wishing to reduce weight, as it cleanses the body of excess fats. Chlorine foods assist the Liver.

In Japan, the high intake of salted fish has been traced to be the major cause of the high average incidence of high blood pressure. The higher the salt intake the more likely a person is to develop hypertension, the heart attack forerunner. *Chlorine foods assist in the rejuvenation of all the body's skin tissue.*

A deficiency may cause inability of human reproductivity, mumps which could lead to deafness, swollen glands and congestion.

Inorganic chlorine, which is not a naturally occurring substance, was used as a deadly war gas, and nowadays it is a common ingredient used in the bleaching of flour and as an ingredient in many modern day medicines such as pain killers and sleeping tablets. This causes contraction of the blood vessels and a paralyzing effect on the sensory nervous system.

Natural Chlorine foods prevent digestive disturbances. Chlorine foods help to regulate the Acid—Alkaline levels of the blood. Chlorine assists hormone distribution. Chlorine is usually associated with Sodium & Potassium.

Chlorine is avaible from fresh vegetables, in the form of Potassium Chloride and Sodium Chloride. Sodium Chloride is vital for the production of digestive juices.

An excess consumption of common table salt will lead to conditions of high blood-pressure, kidney failure and possibly arthritis. Most processed and refined foods have already a high salt level and the risk of excess Chlorine is very likely. With a high intake of table salt, the Potassium levels of the body are displaced. Without sufficient Potassium, the body cannot utilize Glucose,— the simplest form of Energy. The common result of excess table salt is likely to lead to obesity.

CHLORINE FOODS HELP YOU TO STAY SLIM

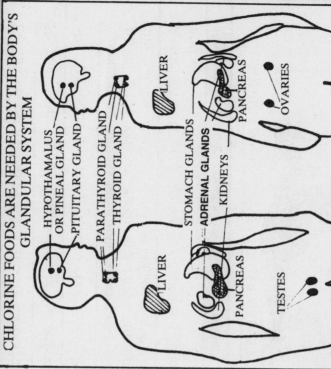

CHLORINE FOODS ARE NEEDED BY THE BODY'S GLANDULAR SYSTEM

HYPOTHAMALUS OR PINEAL GLAND
PITUITARY GLAND
PARATHYROID GLAND
THYROID GLAND
LIVER
STOMACH GLANDS
ADRENAL GLANDS
KIDNEYS
PANCREAS
OVARIES
LIVER
PANCREAS
LIVER
PANCREAS
TESTES

Tomato, Celery, Lettuce, Kelp, Cabbage, Parsnips Radish, Turnip, Watercress, Snap bean, Rhubarb Eggplant, Cucumber, Avocado, Sweet potato, Dates Dandelion greens, Cauliflower, Carrots, Leek Raspberry, Beetroot, Banana, Pineapple, Limes Chives, Raisins, Mango, Artichoke, Blackberry Guava, Potato, Lentils, Peas (fr.), Onion, Strawberry Watermelon, Sweet corn, Figs, Chick peas Sunflower seeds, Brazil nuts, Peaches, White beans Cherry, Hazel nuts, Cowpea, Soya bean, Grapes

SODIUM

— Na — Alkaline mineral

Sodium is essential for the production of saliva which is required for the proper digestion of all carbohydrate foods. (Bread, Grains & Legumes).

Prevents against conditions of Arthritis, as it keeps calcium in the body and expells waste inorganic elements from the system (Carbonic Acid).

Sodium foods are essential for the maintenance of normal blood pressure and prevents thickening of the blood. Sodium is required for Magnesium balance.

Sodium assist the proper elimination of Carbon dioxide waste from the lungs.

Sodium foods prevent hardening of the arteries and excess mucus levels.

Sodium foods provide a healthy condition to the skin tissues, hair and eyes.

Common household table salt is inorganic sodium (chloride) which causes harm to the kidneys, raises the blood pressure and promotes hardening of the arteries. Sodium is only valuable when it's Organic & balanced.

A sodium deficiency upsets the delicate balance of the minerals phosphorus and calcium.

Sodium is a main constituent of the Lymphatic system.

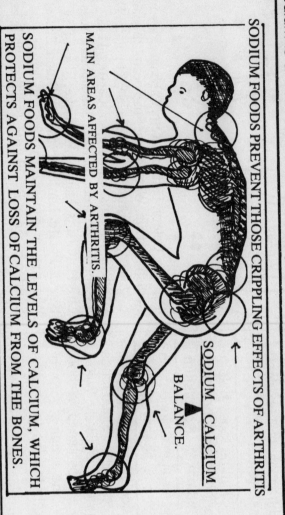

SODIUM FOODS PREVENT THOSE CRIPPLING EFFECTS OF ARTHRITIS

SODIUM CALCIUM BALANCE. ▶

MAIN AREAS AFFECTED BY ARTHRITIS.

SODIUM FOODS MAINTAIN THE LEVELS OF CALCIUM, WHICH PROTECTS AGAINST LOSS OF CALCIUM FROM THE BONES.

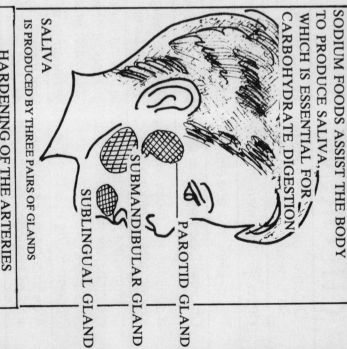

SODIUM FOODS ASSIST THE BODY TO PRODUCE SALIVA, WHICH IS ESSENTIAL FOR CARBOHYDRATE DIGESTION

PAROTID GLAND

SUBMANDIBULAR GLAND

SUBLINGUAL GLAND

SALIVA IS PRODUCED BY THREE PAIRS OF GLANDS

HARDENING OF THE ARTERIES

SATURATED FAT PARTICLES.

HARDENING IS OFTEN CAUSED BY ACCUMULATIONS OF SATURATED FAT PARTICLES. SODIUM FOODS PREVENT HARDENING AND HIGH BLOOD PRESSURE

NORMAL ARTERY SIZE

Kelp, Olives, Spinach, Celery, Dandelion, Kale Beetroot, Sesame seeds, Watercress, Turnip, Carrot Parsley, Artichoke, Collard, Cowpea, Lentil, Raisins Sunflower seed, Chick pea, Coconut, Cabbage, Garlic White bean, Radish, Cashew, Broccoli Brussel sprouts, Endive, Cauliflower, Parsnip Capsicum, Honeydew melon, Prunes, Pinto bean Onion, Red bean, Sweet potato, Lettuce, Rice Wheat bran, Kumquat, Mango, Wild rice, Pear Snap bean, Nectarine, Mung bean, Cucumber, Leek

FLUORINE

— F — *Acid mineral*

Fluorine is a trace mineral and found throughout every human bone.

Fluorine is an excellent beauty mineral and it also helps to preserve youth.

Organic fluorine helps to increase the number of blood cells in our bodies.

Gives sparkle to the eyes, and maintains delicate functions of the Iris of the eye. Fluorine foods improve the development of childrens teeth.

Inorganic Fluorine is highly toxic and dangerous to our bodies. It is contained in food preservatives, and also in some headache tablets,

Protects the tooth enamel and helps prevent curvature of the spine.

Fluorine is required in small amounts, compared to most other minerals.

About 90% of the body's Fluorine is contained in the bloodstream. Refined cereals and other Calcium deficient foods impair Fluorine absorption.

The Fluorine content of Natural foods is well balanced to ensure effective absorption and use by the body. The condition of soil is also a vital factor. Fluorine foods such as Garlic and Oats provide natural defence from disease.

Organic Fluorine contains both Sodium & Calcium Fluorine. Fluoridated water lacks the Calcium content to have long term beneficial effects for the teeth. Fluoridated water contains Sodium Fluoride. If Fluoridated water is taken excessively, it has a toxic effect on the body which can reduce the body's ability of Calcium absorption and therefore have subsequent deficiency effects.

A good intake of Fluorine foods improves the absorption and subsequent depositing of Calcium around the body's entire bone structure.

Fluorine foods reduce acidity of the mouth which therby deters tooth decay.

A Fluorine deficiency may lead to, retarded growth, decalcifying effect of the bones, impaired kidney, liver, heart and nervous and glandular system.

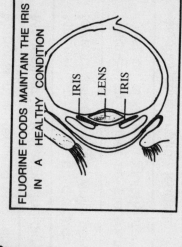

FLUORINE FOODS MAINTAIN THE IRIS IN A HEALTHY CONDITION

IRIS LENS IRIS

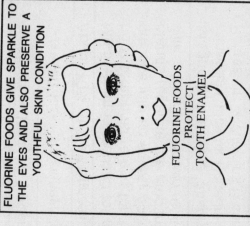

FLUORINE FOODS GIVE SPARKLE TO THE EYES AND ALSO PRESERVE A YOUTHFUL SKIN CONDITION

FLUORINE FOODS PROTECT TOOTH ENAMEL

FLUORINE FOODS PREVENT CURVATURE OF THE SPINE

Asparagus, Oats, Garlic, Rice, Cabbage, Goat milk Watercress, Rice bran, Beetroot, Endive, Corn Barley, millet, Wheat, Fresh vegetables, Fresh fruits

MAGNESIUM

— Mg – Alkaline mineral

Magnesium is essential for the formation of strong bones and teeth.

Magnesium foods promote steady nerves and reduce feelings of irritability.

Magnesium is required for the formation of lung tissues and all body tissues.

Magnesium is required in combination with calcium for proper digestion.

Magnesium foods assist the digestion of Protein and Carbohydrate foods.

Magnesium helps to build a good memory by activating all muscular activity and for nourishment of the white nerve fibre of the brain and spinal cord.

Magnesium cannot be stored in the body for long periods and therefore it must be obtained regularly from the diet.

Alcohol consumption leads to a magnesium deficiency, by an excessive loss from the kidneys. Magnesium foods protect against heart attacks.

A deficiency leads to hardening of the arteries and high blood pressure.

A severe lack of magnesium will lead to leukemia, arthritis and Neuritis.

About 70% of the Magnesium content is found in the bone structure.

Magnesium is required for regulating normal body temperature and for the conversion of glucose into an energy source. The Adrenal glands regulate the amount of Magnesium, with a hormone known as ALDOSTERONE.

Magnesium assists absorption of the minerals Calcium, Phosphorus, Sodium and Potassium & Vitamins B complex, C & E.

Magnesium is an alkaline mineral . An excess consumption of milk will lead to a Magnesium deficiency. Milk contains high amounts of Calciferol (Synthetic Vit D) which in excess has a tendancy to withdraw Magnesium from the bloodstream. Soy milk is an excellent substitute.

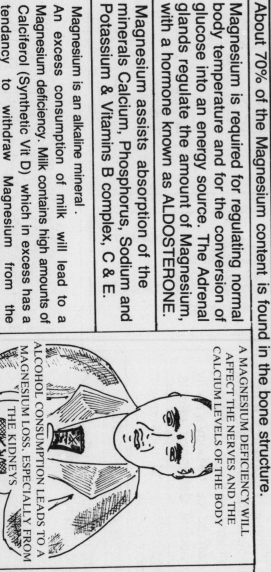

A MAGNESIUM DEFICIENCY WILL AFFECT THE NERVES AND THE CALCIUM LEVELS OF THE BODY

ALCOHOL CONSUMPTION LEADS TO A MAGNESIUM LOSS, ESPECIALLY FROM THE KIDNEYS

THE NERVOUS SYSTEM

MAGNESIUM FOODS IMPROVE THE MEMORY

THE PARATHYROID GLANDS PLAY AN IMPORTANT ROLE IN REGULATING THE DAILY INTAKE & ABSORPTION OF MAGNESIUM.

Magnesium foods regulate heart action

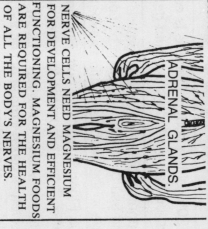

ADRENAL GLANDS.

NERVE CELLS NEED MAGNESIUM FOR DEVELOPMENT AND EFFICIENT FUNCTIONING. MAGNESIUM FOODS ARE REQUIRED FOR THE HEALTH OF ALL THE BODY'S NERVES.

Magnesium foods control the Cholesterol levels of the blood and are also effective in preventing kidney stone formation and hardened arteries.

Kelp, Wheat bran, Almonds, Wheat germ, Cashew Soya bean, Cowpea, Brazil nut, Dulse, Peanut Hazel nut, Lima bean, Sesame seeds, Walnuts, Millet White bean, Red bean, Wheat, Hickory nut Pistachio nut, Pecan nut, Wild rice, Rye, Pigeon pea Beetroot greens, Spinach, Rice, Lentils, Dates Turnip greens, Collard leaves, Sweet corn, Avocado Chestnut, Okra, Parsley, Coconut, Prune, Kale Barley, Dandelion greens, Garlic, Raisins, Peas Potato, Banana, Chives, Parsnip, Beans, Blackberry Brussel sprouts, Loganberry, Beetroot, Carrot

IRON

– Fe – Alkaline mineral

Iron is the nucleus of every cell in the body. It is essential in the formation of rich red blood cells. 90% of the Iron content in the body is contained in the blood. A combination of protein and iron are required for the formation of blood haemoglobin. Iron foods improve Protein metabolism.

Iron is stored in the body, in the bone marrow until required.

Fresh oxygen is required in combination with iron for oxygen transfer throughout the body. Iron foods improve Oxygen transfer.

Is required to burn up waste matter in the body and then to build new cells.

Women need extra amounts of Iron, especially during the menstruation period. An average loss of 30 mgs. per month is normal. This amount should be restored to the body by those foods that are natural and rich in iron content.

Laxatives cause a great loss of iron from the body.

Other effects of a deficiency are, dizziness, fainting, anaemia, fevers, muscle fatigue, difficulties in breathing and constipation.

The absorption of Iron from foods takes about 4 hours and only about 4% of the Iron content is absorbed into the bloodstream.

The continual drinking of Coffee and Tea retard the absorption of the mineral Iron.

Iron is required in the formation of MYOGLOBIN which is essential for oxygen distribution to all the body's muscular cells.

The minerals Calcium and Copper are required for effective Iron absorption. Natural foods are always balanced.

A regular supply of B group vitamins are most essential for secretion of Hcl:(Stomach) which is required to dissolve the Iron content of food.

FRESH STRAWBERRY JUICE IS A MOST DELICIOUS WAY TO GET NATURAL IRON.

BLOOD CELLS ARE COMPOSED OF
98% WHITE CELLS
1.8% RED CORPUSCLES
.2% PLATELETS

PLATELETS.
RED CELL.
WHITE CELL.
WHITE CELL.
RED CELLS.
RED CELL.
RED CELL.

A RED CELL OR CORPUSCLE IS A COMPLEX PROTEIN, CONSISTING OF A PROTEIN— GLOBIN AND AN **IRON** PIGMENT CALLED— HAEMATIN—HAEMOGLOBIN.

IRON FOODS ARE ESSENTIAL IN THE FORMATION OF RICH HEALTHY BLOOD.

WOMEN NEED EXTRA AMOUNTS OF IRON FOODS REGULARLY.

PROTEINS.
CARBOHYDRATES.
MINERALS. **IRON.**
VITAMINS.
FATS & OILS.
LYMPHATIC SYSTEM ABSORBS FATS AND SOME VITAMINS.

BLOOD STREAM.
LYMPHATIC SYSTEM.

BLOOD CELL. IRON.
IRON IS THE NUCLEUS OF EVERY BLOOD CELL.

Dulse, Kelp, Rice bran, Wheat bran, Pumpkin seeds Sesame seeds, Wheat germ, Soya bean, Pigeon pea White bean, Lima bean, Mung bean, Pistachio nut Sunflower seeds, Broad bean, Red bean, Chick pea Lentil, Millet, Pinto bean, Parsley, Cowpea, Almonds Sorghum, Wild rice, Prunes, Cashew, Rye, Raisins Wheat, Pilinut, Artichoke, Chestnut, Walnut Beetroot greens, Dandelion, Spinach, Dates, Figs Fennel, Kale leaves, Barley, Pecan, Hickory nut Peanut, Lettuce, Macadamia nut, Peas, Turnip

MANGANESE

— Mn — Alkaline mineral

Manganese is required for the healthy functioning of all the body's glands.

Manganese foods are essential for proper formation of red blood cells.

Assists the transportation of oxygen from the lungs to all the cells of the body. Manganese foods nourish the nerves and brain.

The majority of manganese in the body is contained in the liver, pancreas and the adrenal glands.

Manganese is essential for regulating menstrural periods.

Manganese foods are essential for expectant mothers and during lactation.

Manganese is a good memory builder.

Manganese is a trace mineral which is also required for various digestive and Enzyme reactions. Manganese foods, improve the absorption of the following, Vitamin B complex, Choline, Biotin, Thiamine and also Vitamin C.

Manganese foods are essential for effective Protein, Fat and Carbohydrate metabolism (Digestion, Absorption and Utilization), as a source of energy.

Manganese foods assist in hormone production. Both male and female, need Manganese foods, for healthy sex—hormone production.

MANGANESE FOODS ARE ESSENTIAL FOR EXPECTANT MOTHERS AND DURING LACTATION

A HEALTHY CHILD NEEDS A HEALTHY MOTHER

Manganese foods assist the maintenance of normal blood sugar levels.

Manganese foods improve the co—ordination of nerves and nerve impulses.

Manganese foods may also be beneficial in cases of Diabetes, Asthma, Muscular and Mental fatigue and Epilepsy.

Manganese in combination with the minerals: Iron & Copper, are essential in the formation of healthy red blood cells. Manganese in combination with B group vitamins, stimulates the transmission of impulses between nerves and muscles.

MANGANESE FOODS ARE REQUIRED FOR THE HEALTHY FUNCTIONING OF THE GLANDULAR SYSTEM

HYPOTHAMALUS
PINEAL GLAND
PITUITARY GLAND
PARATHYROID GLAND
THYROID GLAND
THYMUS GLAND
LIVER
GALL BLADDER
PANCREAS
ADRENALIN GLANDS
KIDNEYS
PROSTRATE—MALE
OVARIES—FEMALE

YOUR GLANDS CONTROL
— PHYSICAL HEALTH
— MENTAL HEALTH

THE MAJORITY OF MANGANESE IS CONTAINED IN THE LIVER, PANCREAS, ADRENAL GLANDS

Manganese foods assist in hormone production. Both male and female need Manganese for healthy hormone production.

Chestnuts, Brazil nuts, Hazel nut, Almonds, Peanuts Pecan nut, Coconut, Walnut, Buckwheat, Barley Kidney beans, Lima beans, Pineapple, Grapes Beetroot, Parsley, Lettuce, Watercress, Apricots Bananas, Cherries, Green beans, Kale, Artichoke Avocado, Blackberries, Dates, Carrots, Celery Cucumber, Dandelion, Figs, Lemons, Pears, Apples Melons, Parsnips, Chive

SILICON
— Si — Acid mineral

Silicon is one of the most abundant minerals in the soil. With fresh fruits and vegetables, Silicon is mainly concentrated in the outer skin layer.

Silicon foods are essential for healthy hair, skin and teeth. Silicon is a main beauty mineral, required for hair growth, proper eyesight and repair of damaged skin tissues. Silicon is vital for efficient cell growth.

Silicon is also a cleansing mineral. It promotes the formation of healthy red blood cells and is essential for proper blood circulation.

Silicon foods protect against mental fatigue, nervous exhaustion, baldness, infection and poor vision. The action of Silicon is dependant on the mineral fluorine.

A Silicon deficiency is often related to the formation of Arthritic conditions.

Silicon foods protect the body against the development of cancerous tissue.

Lettuce, Parsnip, Asparagus, Dandelion, Rice bran Spinach, Onions, Cucumber, Strawberry, Cabbage Leek, Sunflower seeds, Artichoke, Pumpkin, Celery Rhubarb, Cauliflower, Cherries, Apricot, Figs Beetroot, Tomato, Carrot, Watermelon, Sweet potato Millet, Apples, Turnips, Potato, Peas (fr.), Radish Gooseberry, Banana, Plums, Mushrooms, Wheat Grapes, Wheat bran, Blueberries, Rice, Pears Lemons, Guava, Rye, Soya beans, Oranges White bean, Avocado, Walnuts, Peanut, Almond

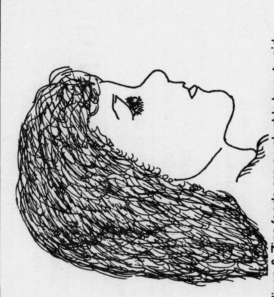

ZINC

Zinc foods are vital for development of children's bones and teeth and for repair of bone fractures. Zinc is one of the main healing minerals.

Zinc foods are essential for healthy hair and proper digestion of proteins and carbohydrates. Zinc is a component of numerous essential enzymes.

Refined Carbohydrates are often lacking in their original Zinc content. Zinc is essential for the proper action of insulin: sugar conversion.

Zinc is essential for the health of the prostrate gland and also for the manufacture of various male hormones and development of the genital organs.

Zinc is an essential mineral for growth: nearly all human tissues contain Zinc, especially the thyroid gland, pancreas and reproductive organs.

A prolonged deficiency of Zinc may lead to any of the following ailments: arteriosclerosis, diabetes, acne, dermatitis, retarded growth and ulcers.

Zinc is also an ingredient of the enzyme that is required to break down alcohol. Regular consumption of alcohol can lead to a Zinc deficiency.

Zinc is an active ingredient with numerous digestive enzymes and it is required for the action of vitamins, especially the B complex vitamins.

Other signs of a Zinc deficiency are — fatigue, decreased alertness, poor hair condition, susceptibility to infection and retarded sexual activity.

Silicon & Zinc foods are a valuable beauty aid and they promote the growth of hair.

Brazil nuts, Almonds, Cashew, Hazel nuts, Walnuts Rice Barley, Sunflower seeds, Rye, Sesame seeds Wheat, Olives, Pumpkin seeds, Wheat bran, Wheat germ, Brewers yeast, Millet, Garlic, Onions, oats, Soya beans, Asparagus, Lettuce Brussel sprouts, Blackberries, Avocado, Cauliflower Radish, Peas (fr.), Banana, Oranges, Peaches, Tomato Cucumber, Artichoke, Green beans, Spinach

COPPER

— Cu — Acid mineral

Most of the copper content of the body is stored in the muscles, liver and bones. Copper is a trace mineral and part of every body tissue.

The Copper content of Natural foods is absorbed into the bloodstream shortly after digestion and stored in the Liver, Kidneys, Heart, Brain, Bones and Muscles. 50% of the total copper content is found in the bone structure.

Copper is required in combination with manganese for the proper assimilation of iron.

Copper is an ingredient of many digestive enzymes. Copper foods improve the functions of the digestive system. (Liver, Small intestines and Pancreas.)

Copper foods assist tissue respiration and protect the lungs from infection.

Copper foods are required to convert the Amino acid Tryosine into the various respective colours of skin and hair pigment.

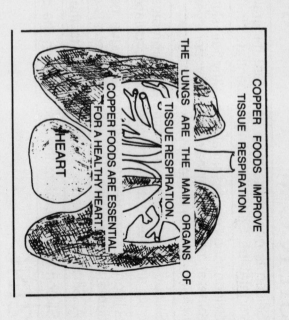

COPPER FOODS IMPROVE TISSUE RESPIRATION

THE LUNGS ARE THE MAIN ORGANS OF TISSUE RESPIRATION.

COPPER FOODS ARE ESSENTIAL FOR A HEALTHY HEART.

HEART

IODINE

— I — Acid mineral

Iodine is essential for regulating the thyroid gland. Iodine is stored in the thyroid gland and it's purpose is to control the metabolism of the entire body.

Iodine foods assist in regulating the body's metabolism and activity, therby affecting growth, development and the rate of digestion. Iodine foods assist the body to burn up excess fat.

Thyroxine is the hormone produced by the Thyroid gland. Thyroxine regulates Cholesterol levels. About 30% of iodine intake is required by the Thyroid gland for effective functioning.

A deficiency of Iodine. may show as the condition Goiter which is a Thyroid enlargement and leads to a slow rate of hormone secretion.

A deficiency of Iodine may also lead to irregular heart beat, hardening of the arteries, rapid pulse, nervousness, iritability, dry hair, obesity and poor mental abilities, such as concentration.

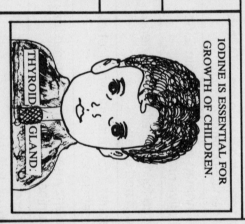

IODINE IS ESSENTIAL FOR GROWTH OF CHILDREN.

THYROID GLAND.

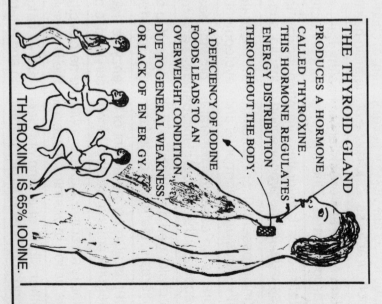

THE THYROID GLAND PRODUCES A HORMONE CALLED THYROXINE. THIS HORMONE REGULATES ENERGY DISTRIBUTION THROUGHOUT THE BODY.

A DEFICIENCY OF IODINE FOODS LEADS TO AN OVERWEIGHT CONDITION DUE TO GENERAL WEAKNESS OR LACK OF EN ER GY.

THYROXINE IS 65% IODINE.

GASSEOUS & MINERAL COMPOSITION OF THE BODY

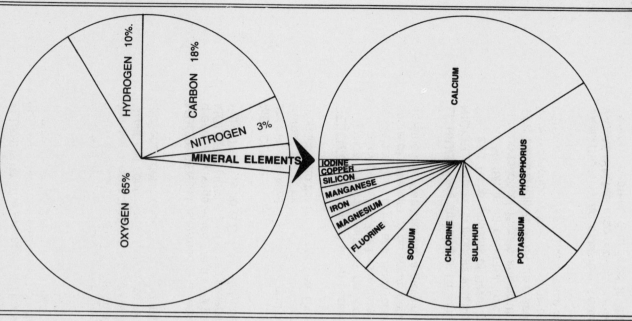

GASSEOUS ELEMENTS	BODY WEIGHT	MINERAL ELEMENTS	BODY WEIGHT
OXYGEN	65%	CHLORINE	0.25%
CARBON	18%	SODIUM	0.25%
HYDROGEN	10%	FLUORINE	0.20%
NITROGEN	3%	MAGNESIUM	0.05%
WATER H20	75%	IRON	0.008%
CALCIUM	2%	MANGANESE	0.003%
PHOSPHORUS	1%	SILICON	0.002%
POTASSIUM	0.4%	COPPER	0.002%
SULPHUR	0.25%	IODINE	0.00004%

TRACE MINERALS

ALUMINIUM; The average adult body contains between 50-150 milligramms of Aluminium. There is no recognized need for ALUMINIUM to be part of Human Nutrition. Excess consumption of Aluminium can be fatal. The average daily amount ingested from the diet has been estimated to range from 10-100 mg. Cooking with Aluminium cookwear, cutlery and use of Aluminium food wraps are the main sources of this Trace Mineral. Excess Aluminium in the blood will lead to poisoning.

COBALT; is often referred to as an essential Trace Mineral, as it is part of the Vitamin B12 structure. Cobalt is an important Trace Mineral for the maintainance and development of red blood cells and other body cells. Cobalt must be supplied from the diet. It cannot be synthesized by the body. Such foods as fish and all sea foods are reliable sources of Cobalt. Most soil contains no Cobalt, so land-foods are lacking in this essential trace mineral There is no R.D.A. for Cobalt. A Cobalt defi ciency may lead to impaired red blood cell production, anemia, nervous disorders and poor growth.

MOLYBDENUM; is termed as an essential Trace Mineral. It is obtainable from both plant and animal sources. Legumes and green leafy vegetables are a very good source of this essential Trace Mineral (depending on the soil condition). MOLYBDENUM is part of two essential enzymes – Xanthine and Aldehyde oxidase: Xanthine is required for the oxidation of Fats. There is no R.D.A. for Molybdenum. The nervous system and brain also require Molybdenum.

MERCURY; is not an essential Trace Mineral. Mercury is widely distributed in the outer atmosphere and is also part of some chemical fertilizers, pesticides and other by-products from some factories. Mercury is a threat to the enviroment and the Human body. Fish from inland waters are often contaminated with Mercury, as a result of factories which dump waste products into the rivers and sea. Excess Mercury will have adverse effects on the functioning of the entire Nervous system.

SELENIUM; is termed as an essential Trace Mineral. The function of Selenium is closely related with Vitamin E, as an antioxidant, which promotes the body's ability to utilize Oxygen and also delays the rate of oxidation of the poly unsaturated fatty acids, which is vital for the preservation and elasticity of all skin tissues. The Selenium content of food is directly related to the condition of the soil. Such foods as whole grains and vegetables are usually a good supply of Selenium. Tuna is a rich soure of selenium. A Selenium deficiency is related to premature aging. Selenium has also been succesfully used in the treatment of Kwashiorkor: a protein deficiency disease. Trace amounts are all that is required.

LITHIUM: trace amounts of Lithium are present in the Human body, however the function of Lithium is not known.
NICKEL: is used in industry and food processing, for the hydrogenation of Oils, which is why trace amounts are present.
SILVER: Trace amounts of Silver have been recorded to be present in the Human body. Silver has no known function.
CHROMIUM; is an essential Trace Mineral, used for the metabolism of Glucose into the form of Energy and for the transportation of Protein around the bloodstream. Brewers yeast is a very good source, Fruits and Vegetables also.
TIN; Trace amounts of Tin are present in the Human body, possibly due to the widespread use of canned foods. There is no known function of this trace mineral.
RUBIDIUM: is also found in trace amounts, however there is no known function of this Trace mineral.

VANADIUM is an essential Trace Mineral. The body uses Vanadium for the regulation of blood circulation. VANADIUM has also proved to inhibit the formation of Cholesterol in the blood vessels (brain) and also the Central nervous system. Sea food is the most reliable source of Natural Vanadium. Vegetables also supply varying amounts

ENZYMES

ENZYMES: This chart provides a summary of information, from pages 19–20, 85, 103 and 125. Enzymes assist the conversion of food; of starches into simple sugars, of complex proteins into individual amino acids and of fats into fatty acids. All fresh food contains life-enzymes. The human body also produces enzymes, for food digestion and metabolism. When food is cooked and heated above 48 C., or 118 F., all food-enzymes are destroyed. When food is cooked or frozen, the enzymes are restricted from their normal activity — "ripening of fruits" etc., thereby preserving the life of fresh foods. Enzymes are destroyed by processing, refinement and oxidation. Enzymes are the essential micro-nutrient, required for all digestive processes. A deficiency of enzyme-food is a common cause of illness. Fresh fruits and vegetables sprouted foods and fermented foods are the best enzyme-providing foods. Freshly prepared fruit or vegetable juices are the most delicious and rewarding enzyme-drinks, have some daily, for life.

The R.D.A. (recommended dietary allowances) chart below, is based on information from the National Research Council, Academy of Sciences, U.S. The amounts should be considered as a guide to the "average requirements". On page 198, the Vitamins R.D.A. chart is provided. For some minerals, there are no available R.D.A. figures. By maintaining a complete, well balanced natural food diet, a full range of all essential nutrients is obtainable (see pages 11, 13, 18, 43, 61, 97, 117 and 219–220 for details).

FOOD TYPE	ENZYME	SITE	DIGESTIVE FUNCTION
STARCH.	PTYALIN.	SALIVA.	Converts cooked STARCH into MALTOSE.
PROTEIN.	PEPSIN.	STOMACH.	Converts Proteins into PEPTONES in the presence of HYDROCHLORIC ACID.
MILK.	RENNIN.	STOMACH.	Converts CASEINOGEN (Milk) into CASEIN. (children only).
PROTEIN.	TRYPSIN.	PANCREAS.	Converts PEPTONES (Proteins) into AMINO ACIDS.
STARCH.	AMYLASE.	PANCREAS.	Converts all STARCH into MALTOSE.
FAT.	LIPASE.	PANCREAS.	Converts FATS into FATTY ACIDS.
SUGARS.	MALTASE.	SMALL INTESTINE.	Converts MALTOSE into GLUCOSE.
SUGARS.	INVERTASE.	SMALL INTESTINE.	Converts Cane sugar into GLUCOSE.
PROTEIN.	EREPSIN.	SMALL INTESTINE.	Converts PEPTONES into AMINO ACIDS.
	ENTEROKINASE.	SMALL INTESTINE.	Assists TRYPSININ in converting PEPTONES into AMINO ACIDS.

R.D.A. CHARTS

The R.D.A. Chart below; is based on figures supplied by the National Research Council-(National Academy of Science)

		CHILDREN.				GIRLS.				WOMEN.			BOYS.			MEN.	
		0-6 months	1-3	4-6	7–10	11-14	15-18	19-22	23-50	pregnant,	lactating.	51+	11-14	15-18	19-22	23-50	51+
CALCIUM	mg.	360	800	800	800	1,200	1,200	800	800	1,200	1,200	800	1,200	1,200	800	800	800
PHOSPHORUS	mg.	240	800	800	800	1,200	1,200	800	800	1,200	1,200	800	1,200	1,200	800	800	800
POTASSIUM	mg.	Average Daily Intake ——————————————— 1,950–5,850 ———————————														
SODIUM	mg.	Average Daily Intake ——————————————— 2,300–6,900mg. ———————————														
MAGNESIUM	mg.	60	150	200	250	300	300	300	300	450	450	300	350	400	350	350	350
IRON	mg.	10	15	10	10	18	18	18	18	18+	18	10	18	18	10	10	10
IODINE	mcg.	35	60	80	110	115	115	100	100	125	150	80	130	150	140	110	110

MINERALS FOOD CHARTS

	EXCELLENT SOURCE	GOOD SOURCE	FAIR SOURCE
CALCIUM ESSENTIAL ASSOCIATED NUTRIENTS FOR EFFECTIVE ABSORPTION: Iron, Magnesium and Phosphorus. Vitamins: A, C, D, F. Protein. NUTRIENT INHIBITING FACTORS: Lack of: Sunlight, Exercise, Magnesium and Phosphorus foods. Refined foods, chocolate and excess stress. (alkaline mineral)	Sesame seeds, Kelp Collard + Kale leaves Turnip greens, Almonds Soya beans, Hazel nuts Parsley, Dandelion greens Brazil nut, Watercress Chick pea, White bean Pinto bean, Pistachio nut Fig (dr.), Sunflower seed Beetroot greens, Wheat bran Mung bean, Olives, Broccoli Broad bean, English walnut Rhubarb, Spinach, Okra Prune (dr.), Swiss chard	Endive, Lentils, Rice bran Cowpea, Pecan nut, Lima bean Wheat germ, Chive, Peanut Lettuce, Apricot (dr.) Savoy cabbage, Peas (dr.) Raisins, Black currant, Dates Snap beans, Chestnut, Leek Pumpkin seeds, Onion-green Parsnip, Cabbage, Peach (dr.) Macadamia nut, Wheat, Orange Celery, Turnip, Cashew nut Rye grain, Carrot, Brussel sprouts Fig (fr.), Loganberry, Pear (dr.) Radish, Barley, Banana (dr.)	Blackberry, Red + White currant Sweet potato, Brown rice Apple (dr.), Black raspberry Garlic, Sorghum, Cauliflower Cucumber, Asparagus, Pumpkin Strawberry, Loquat, Papaya Coconut water, Millet, Yam Apricot, Pineapple, Grapefruit Grapes, Coconut milk, Beet Blueberry, Cantaloupe, Melon Tomato, Eggplant, Mango Peach, Capsicum, Pear, Apple Mushroom, Nectarine, Sweet corn
PHOSPHORUS ESSENTIAL ASSOCIATED NUTRIENTS FOR EFFECTIVE ABSORPTION: Calcium and Manganese. Vitamins: A, D, F. Protein. NUTRIENT INHIBITING FACTORS: Excess stress, fatty fried foods, antacids, sugar and refined foods. (acid mineral)	Rice bran, Pumpkin seeds Wheat bran, Wheat germ Sunflower seeds, Brazil nut Safflower seed, Sesame seed Soya bean, Almonds, Peanut Pistachio nut, Pinto beans Cowpea, White bean, Red bean Wheat, Broad bean, Lima bean Walnut, Lentils, Rye, Cashew Hickory nut, Mung bean, Millet Hazel nut, Wild rice, Chick pea Pigeon pea, Barley, Pecan nuts	Sorghum, Dulse, Kelp, Garlic Rice, Chestnut, Macadamia nut Mushroom, Peas, Sweet corn Raisins, Coconut, Kale leaves Artichoke, Collard leaves Brussel sprouts, Prunes, Figs Broccoli, Parsnip, Dandelion Kale leaves, Mung bean sprouts Soya bean sprouts, Parsley Dates, Asparagus, Cauliflower Cabbage, Endive, Watercress Potato, Spinach, Leek, Onions	Chives, Pumpkin, Snap beans Avocado, Guava, Beetroot greens Black currant, Loquat, Beetroot Radish, Turnips, Celery, Tomato Banana, Eggplant, Lettuce Apricot, Red + White currants Kumquat, Raspberry, Strawberry Grapes, Olives, Blackberry Cherries, Peaches, Rhubarb Cantaloupe, Melons, Papaya Blueberry, Mango, Pear, Apple Watermelon, Pineapple

MINERALS FOOD CHARTS

	EXCELLENT SOURCE	GOOD SOURCE	FAIR SOURCE
POTASSIUM ESSENTIAL ASSOCIATED NUTRIENTS FOR EFFECTIVE ABSORPTION: Sodium, Phosphorus, Sulphur and Chlorine. Vitamin B6. NUTRIENT INHIBITING FACTORS: Salt, Alcohol, Coffee, Sugar and excess stress. (alkaline mineral)	Kelp, Soya bean, Lima bean Rice bran, White bean Wheat bran, Mung bean Cowpea, Pea, Pinto bean Red bean, Pigeon pea Pistachio nut, Chestnut Wheat germ, Chick pea N.Z. Spinach, Lentils Almonds, Raisins, Parsley Sesame seeds, Brazil nut Hazel nut, Peanut, Dates Figs, Watercress, Avocado Pecan nut, Parsnip, Garlic	Rye, Cashew nut, Walnut Millet, Mushroom, Potato Collard, Dandelion greens Fennel, Brussel sprouts Broccoli, Kale, Banana Black currants, Wheat Sorghum, Leek, Carrot Celery, Pumpkin, Beetroot Radish, Peas, Barley Cauliflower, Nectarine Endive, Guava, Apricot Sweet corn, Asparagus Turnip, Macadamia nut	Lettuce, Coconut, Melon Cantaloupe, Rhubarb, Chive Okra, Tomato, Sweet potato Snap beans, Kumquat, Papaya Cabbage, Onions, Wild rice Mung bean spouts, Eggplant Rice, Capsicum, Peaches Oranges, Black raspberry Fresh figs, Cherry, Grapes Blackberry, Loganberry Lychees, Strawberry Cucumber, Gooseberry Pineapple, Lemons, Pear
SULPHUR ESSENTIAL ASSOCIATED NUTRIENTS FOR EFFECTIVE ABSORPTION: Vitamins: B group. NUTRIENT INHIBITING FACTORS: High temperatures. (acid mineral)	Kale, Watercress, Cabbage Brussel sprouts, Snap beans Turnips, Cauliflower, Kelp Raspberry, Spinach, Parsnip Leek, Radish, Cucumber, Okra Lettuce, Chives, Peas (fr.) Celery, Red currant, Avocado Asparagus, Tomato, Hazel nut	Black currants, Turnip greens Carrots, Eggplant, Pineapple Brazil nuts, Sweet corn, Peach Potato, Dandelion greens, Fig Onion, Soya beans, Artichoke Lima beans, Raisins, Mushrooms Barley, Rhubarb, Watermelon Strawberry, Apple, Oranges Limes, Cherries, Pumpkin	Gooseberry, Grapes, White bean Apricot, Pear, Blueberries Lemons, Banana, Dates, Lentils Chick pea, Guava, Sweet potato Plums, Grapefruit, Almond nut Blackberry, Sunflower seeds Prunes, Coconut, Beetroot, Walnuts, Rye, Sorghum, Rice Watercress, Rice bran, Wheat
CHLORINE ESSENTIAL ASSOCIATED NUTRIENTS FOR EFFECTIVE ABSORPTION: Sodium and Potassium. NUTRIENT INHIBITING FACTORS: Chlorine is easily lost with cooking. (acid mineral)	Tomato, Celery, Lettuce, Kelp Cabbage, Parsnips, Radish Turnip, Watercress, Snap bean Rhubarb, Eggplant, Cucumber Avocado, Sweet potato, Dates Dandelion greens, Cauliflower Carrots, Leek, Raspberry	Beetroot, Banana, Pineapple Limes, Chives, Raisins, Mango Artichoke, Blackberry, Guava Potato, Lentils, Peas (fr.) Onion, Strawberry, Watermelon Sweet corn, Figs, Chick peas Sunflower seeds, Brazil nuts	Peaches, White beans, Cherry Hazel nuts, Cowpea, Soya bean Grapes, Barley, Grapefruit Red + White currants, Pumpkin Oranges, Sorghum, Peanuts Apricots, Lemons, Almond nut Black currants, Wheat, Rice Lima beans, Chestnuts, Rye

MINERALS FOOD CHARTS

	EXCELLENT SOURCE	GOOD SOURCE	FAIR SOURCE
SODIUM ESSENTIAL ASSOCIATED NUTRIENTS FOR EFFECTIVE ABSORPTION: Chlorine and Potassium. Vitamin D. The adrenal glands regulate Sodium metabolism. NUTRIENT INHIBITING FACTORS: Excess salt. (alkaline mineral)	Kelp, Olives, Spinach, Celery, Dandelion, Kale Beetroot, Sesame seeds, Watercress, Turnip, Carrot Parsley, Artichoke, Collard Cowpea, Lentil, Raisins Sunflower seed, Chick pea Coconut, Cabbage, Garlic White bean, Radish, Cashew	Broccoli, Brussel sprouts Endive, Cauliflower, Parsnip Capsicum, Honeydew melon Prunes, Pinto bean, Onion Red bean, Sweet potato Lettuce, Rice, Wheat bran Kumquat, Mango, Wild rice Pear, Snap bean, Nectarine Mung bean, Cucumber, Leek	Peanut, Pigeon pea, Soya bean Avocado, Guava, Almond nut Lima bean, Potato, Tomato Black currant, Grapes, Papaya Walnut, Wheat, Wheat germ Cherries, Figs, Lemons Oranges, Pear, Hazel nut Asparagus, Eggplant, Apple Apricot, Banana, Blackberry
MAGNESIUM ESSENTIAL ASSOCIATED NUTRIENTS FOR EFFECTIVE ABSORPTION: Calcium and Phosphorus. Vitamins: B6, C, D. Protein. NUTRIENT INHIBITING FACTORS: Coffee, Tobacco and Alcohol. (alkaline mineral)	Kelp, Wheat bran, Almonds Wheat germ, Cashew, Soya bean Cowpea, Brazil nut, Dulse Peanut, Hazel nut, Lima bean Sesame seeds, Walnuts, Millet White bean, Red bean, Wheat Hickory nut, Pistachio nut Pecan nut, Wild rice, Rye Pigeon pea, Beetroot greens Spinach, Rice, Lentils, Dates	Turnip greens, Collard leaves Sweet corn, Avocado, Chestnut Okra, Parsley, Coconut, Prune Kale, Barley, Dandelion greens Garlic, Raisins, Peas, Potato Banana, Chives, Parsnip, Beans Blackberry, Brussel sprouts Loganberry, Beetroot, Carrot Broccoli, Cauliflower, Leek Olives, Celery, Asparagus	Turnip, Watercress, Mango Capsicum, Cantaloupe, Eggplant Rhubarb, Black currant, Radish Tomato, Grapes, Guava, Nectarine Pineapple, Cabbage, Mushroom Apricot, Grapefruit, Onions Strawberry, Pumpkin, Oranges Artichoke, Lettuce, Peaches Endive, Goodseberry, Plums Apple, Lemon, Watermelon, Pear
IRON ESSENTIAL ASSOCIATED NUTRIENTS FOR EFFECTIVE ABSORPTION: Vitamins: B12, C, E and Folic acid. NUTRIENT INHIBITING FACTORS: Coffee and Tea. During conditions of fever, extra Iron is required. (alkaline mineral)	Dulse, Kelp, Rice bran Wheat bran, Pumpkin seeds Sesame seeds, Wheat germ Soya bean, Pigeon pea White bean, Lima bean Mung bean, Pistachio nut Sunflower seeds, Broad bean Red bean, Chick pea, Lentil Millet, Pinto bean, Parsley Cowpea, Almonds, Sorghum Wild rice, Prunes, Cashew Rye, Raisins, Wheat, Pilinut	Artichoke, Chestnut, Walnut Beetroot greens, Dandelion Spinach, Dates, Figs, Fennel Kale leaves, Barley, Pecan Hickory nut, Peanut, Lettuce Macadamia nut, Peas, Turnip Olives, Coconut, Watercress Endive, Rice, Collard leaves Brussel sprouts, Garlic Mung bean sprouts, Loganberry Black currant, Cauliflower Broccoli, Cucumber, Leek Strawberry, Asparagus, Onion	Radish, Soya bean sprouts Blackberry, Guava, Raspberry Cabbage, Mushroom, Pumpkin Rhubarb, Snap beans, Banana Guava, Beetroot, Carrot Sweet corn, Eggplant, Parsnip Capsicum, Avocado, Potato Apricot, Nectarine, Peaches Pineapple, Plums, Watermelon Tomato, Turnip, Cherry, Grape Kumquat, Loquat, Cantaloupe Melons, Oranges, Pear, Apple Papaya, Celery, Lemons, Lime

MINERALS FOOD CHARTS

	EXCELLENT SOURCE	GOOD SOURCE	FAIR SOURCE
FLUORINE Fluoridated water lacks a balance of Calcium Fluoride (acid mineral)	Asparagus, Oats, Garlic, Rice Cabbage, Goat milk, Watercress	Rice bran, Beetroot, Endive Corn, Barley, millet, Wheat	Fresh vegetables, Fresh fruits
MANGANESE ESSENTIAL ASSOCIATED NUTRIENTS FOR EFFECTIVE ABSORPTION: Calcium and Phosphorus. Vitamins: B1 and E. (alkaline mineral)	Chestnuts, Brazil nuts, Hazel nut Almonds, Peanuts, Pecan nut Coconut, Walnut, Buckwheat Barley, Kidney beans, Lima beans	Pineapple, Grapes, Beetroot Parsley, Lettuce, Watercress Apricots, Bananas, Cherries Green beans, Kale, Artichoke	Avocado, Blackberries, Dates Carrots, Celery, Cucumber Dandelion, Figs, Lemons, Pears Apples, Melons, Parsnips, Chive
SILICON (acid mineral)	Lettuce, Parsnip, Asparagus Dandelion, Rice bran, Spinach Onions, Cucumber, Strawberry Cabbage, Leek, Sunflower seeds Artichoke, Pumpkin, Celery	Rhubarb, Cauliflower, Cherries Apricot, Figs, Beetroot, Tomato Carrot, Watermelon, Sweet potato Millet, Apples, Turnips, Potato Peas (fr.), Radish, Gooseberry	Banana, Plums, Mushrooms, Wheat Grapes, Wheat bran, Blueberries Rice, Pears, Lemons, Guava, Rye Soya beans, Oranges, White bean Avocado, Walnuts, Peanut, Almond
COPPER ESSENTIAL ASSOCIATED NUTRIENTS FOR EFFECTIVE ABSORPTION: Cobalt, Iron and Zinc. (acid mineral)	Sunflower seeds, Sesame seeds Brazil nuts, Hickory nuts Hazel nuts, Pecan nuts, Walnuts Pistachio nuts, Almond nuts Chestnut, Coconut, Peanuts	Wheat, Buckwheat, Rye, Soya bean Rice, Wheat germ, Parsley, Spinach, Olives, Dates, Apple Apricots, Beetroot, Broccoli Pears, Bananas, Green beans	Carrots, Berries, Garlic, Oats Celery, Prunes, Lettuce, Onion Peas, Lemons, Tomato, Peaches Capsicum, Pumpkin, Radish Black currants, Cabbage, Leek
IODINE (acid mineral)	Kelp, Dulse, Turnip greens Watermelon, Cucumber, Spinach Asparagus, Kale, Turnip, Okra Blueberry, Peanut, Strawberry	Capsicum, Collard, Artichoke Eggplant, Loganberry, Peaches Snap beans, Onions, Lettuce Banana, Carrot, Potato, Apple Tomato, Beetroot, Cabbage	Celery, Sweet corn, Figs, Plum Walnuts, Broccoli, Pineapple Papaya, Almond nut, Chestnut Hazel nuts, Rice, Grapefruit Rye, Wheat, Dates, Lemons
ZINC ESSENTIAL ASSOCIATED NUTRIENTS FOR EFFECTIVE ABSORPTION: Calcium, Phosphorus and Copper. Vitamins: A and B group.	Brazil nuts, Almonds, Cashew Hazel nuts, Walnuts, Rice Barley, Sunflower seeds, Rye Sesame seeds, Wheat, Olives	Pumpkin seeds, Wheat bran Wheat germ, Brewers yeast Millet, Garlic, Onions, oats Soya beans, Asparagus, Lettuce	Brussel sprouts, Blackberries Avocado, Cauliflower, Radish Peas (fr.), Banana, Oranges Peaches, Tomato, Cucumber Artichoke, Green beans, Spinach

MINERALS — DIGESTION

MINERALS--ORGANIC SALTS AND VITAL ELECTRICITY.

MINERALS are the conveyors of vital electricity and magnetic forces, which are constantly required to furnace the 'Human Generator' into all the various activities of Life. As soon as food is eaten the Digestive system begins to seperate food into minute particles and compounds, which are then capable of passing through the walls (Epithelium Cells) of the small Intestine and then into the bloodstream. The movement of minute food particles, from one side of the intestinal wall to the outer side is known as (Osmosis). This continuous movement of nutrient, can only take place when there are various Mineral Elements available from a food source. A lack of Mineral Elements, due to (Refinement, Processing etc.) results in food wastage, impurities entering the bloodstream, general decline in health, constant need for food, excess eating, expensive food bills and a deteoration of mental and physical abilities, to mention a few. Every (Epithelium cell) of the small Intestine is a Living part of the body and requires nutrition in the form of "ORGANIC SALTS" to perform the process of OSMOSIS. The availability of Mineral Elements from a meal is essential to assist the transfer of all nutrients, from the small Intestine into the bloodstream and Lymphatic system. When Minerals (Organic Salts) are seperated (by the process of Digestion), the pressure exerted by molecules on the Intestinal wall, varies with each individual Mineral Element. The minute cells (Epithelium) are constantly maintaining the balance; passing nutrients through and receiving others in return, (usually waste products). The 'Osmotic Pressure' between these Living cells is constantly reliant on good quality Natural Whole foods, in their Natural state. A lack of Minerals in the food, leads to an imbalance, which will lead to a loss of other Minerals from the body and a rapid decline in Health.   Natural foods give you Life.

MINERALS are converted into Organic Salts and when these Organic Salts are dissolved in the body fluids (Water & Blood), they break-up into the form of 'IONS', which can be either Positively or Negatively charged, depending on their Original Mineral Element source. When these IONS are dissolved in the body fluids, the solution will conduct 'Electrical Energy'. Similiar Electrical particles will repel and opposite charged IONS will attract one another. The Minerals Sodium & Potassium for example are both Positively charged, while the Minerals Fluorine & Chlorine are Negatively charged. The functions of a Mineral is very complex when we realize the ways of Energy transfer throughout the body. Both functions (Repel & Attract) are essential for a multitude of body movements, such as relaxation & contraction of muscles and also the transmission of Nerve impulses, from the Spinal cord & Brain to all parts of the body.

MINERALS play an important role in regulating the Acid—Alkaline levels of the body. A normal diet should consist of : **75% ALKALINE FORMING FOODS: 25% ACID FORMING FOODS.**

MAIN ALKALINE FORMING FOOD GROUPS:
Fresh Fruits, Vegetables, Almonds, Soy Beans, Millet & Rice.

MAIN ACID FORMING FOOD GROUPS:
Whole Grains, Nuts, Legumes, Seeds, Meat, Poultry, Fish, Eggs, Refined Bread, Processed foods, Coffee, Alcohol, Sugar, Preservatives, Cooked Food. The Blood must remain at an Alkaline level for the body to be capable of Natural Self Defense against all forms of illness and Disease. A mainly Acid Food diet is the common cause of most sickness.

ACID—ALKALINE – MINERALS – FOOD CHARTS

ACID MINERALS: PHOSPHORUS SULPHUR SILICON CHLORINE FLUORINE IODINE

ALKALINE MINERALS: POTASSIUM SODIUM CALCIUM MAGNESIUM IRON MANGANESE

ALKALINE FORMING FOODS		ALKALINE FORMING FOODS		ACID FORMING FOODS		
APPLES	.8 — 3.7.	BEETROOT	8.9 — 11.4.	ASPARAGUS	neutral	
ALMONDS	12 — 18.3.	BROCOLLI	3.6 — 4.9.	CAPSICUM	neutral	
APRICOTS	4.8 — 8.4.	CABBAGE	1.4 — 8.2.	HUMAN MILK	neutra.	
BANANAS	4.4 — 7.9.	CARROTS	4.4 — 10.8.	HONEY	.4 — 4.6.	1.1.
CANTALOUPE	7.5.	CAULIFLOWER	1.4 — 5.3.	LENTILS	0.4 — 2.0.	5.2 — 17.8.
CHERRIES	1.7 — 7.3.	CELERY	2.5 — 11.1.	OATS		1.5 — 13.2.
COCONUT	4.1 — 7.0.	CUCUMBERS	3.2 — 31.5.	PEANUTS		3.9 — 16.4.
CURRANTS	.7 — 8.8.	EGGPLANT	4.5.	BARLEY		6.0 — 17.5.
SWEET CORN	1.8.	GARLIC	neutral.	RYE		11.3.
DATES	5.5 — 12.4.	KALE	4.0 — 17.	WHEAT		11
FIGS	neutral	LEEKS	5.5 — 11.3.	BREAD WHITE		1.5 — 7.1.
FIGS DRIED	10 — 100.	LETTUCE	3.8 — 14.1.	BUTTER		.4 — 4.3.
GRAPEFRUIT	6.4.	ONIONS	.2 — 8.4.	CHEESE HARD	3.6 — 5.1.	0.3 — 11.8.
GRAPES	2.7 — 7.2.	POTATOES	7 — 12.8.	CRABS		39.5.
LEMONS	5.5 — 9.9.	PUMPKIN	.3 — 7.8.	EGGS		11.1 — 24.5.
ORANGES	5.6 — 9.6.	RADISH	2.9 — 7.2.	EGG YOLK		25.3 — 51.8.
PEACHES	3.8 — 6.1.	SPINACH	5.1 — 39.6.	BEEF		
PEARS	3.6.	TURNIPS	2.7 — 10.2.	FISH		8.5 — 19.7.
PINEAPPLE	2.2 — 7.	WATERCRESS	8.1.	LIVER		9.4 — 49.5.
PRUNES DRIED	7.8 — 20.	WATERMELON	2.2.	LOBSTER		38.4.
RAISINS	23 — 27.	LIMA BEANS	14.	MUTTON		4.5 — 22.5.
RASPBERRIES	4 — 6.	BROWN RICE	neutral	PORK	neutral	7.7 — 28.6.
STRAWBERRIES	2.7.	SOYA BEANS	neutral	TURKEY	neutral	10.4 — 19.5.

Every food has both Acid and Alkaline elements as part of the Original composition. A food type is termed Acid or Alkaline, according to the reaction on the body and the end product after Digestion, when all particles have been converted into Acid or Alkaline Ash. The Ash will be left after the body has used the food as Energy. A normal Diet should consist of 75% Alkaline Forming Foods and 25% Acid Forming Foods.

Minerals are the main controllers of the Acid-Alkaline.

The Pituitary Gland is the main controller of the Acid-Alkaline levels of the human body. Alkalinity is essential for the reproduction of Life. Seeds cannot germinate unless they are Alkalinized by water. Life is dependant on Alkaline Elements.

75% ALKALINE FORMING FOODS.

25% ACID FORMING FOODS.

The chart above shows the variation between the acid – alkaline content of food. The two groups of food on the left side: Fruits, Vegetables, some Grains and Legumes, all have an alkaline reaction, after the process of digestion. Those foods listed on the right hand side column are all acid forming foods, except for the first three mentioned. Some of the foods listed have one amount only, others show a variation of alkalinity, acidity or both. To obtain an average value for those foods having a variable amount, halve the numerical difference and add that to the lowest amount, for example: apples .8-3.7, the numerical difference is 2.9, half of that is 1.4, added to .8 = 2.2. The most important point to realise is that, such foods, as: meat, eggs, poultry, crabs, lobster and seafood all have a high concentration of acid forming elements, they should be restricted and when having such meals, balance other meals of the day with alkaline forming foods, especially fruits.

BLOOD

Blood is the carrier of nutrients and nourishment,

Blood is the carrier of all nutrients and nourishment that the human body requires. These nutrients are in the form of GLUCOSE, AMINO ACIDS, VITAMINS and MINERALS.

Blood is our Lifeline, once it is loaded with impurities, the body will be strained and have difficulties in obtaining those essential elements of nutrition. Every time we give our body's food, that is unnatural, we are starving the bloodstream and accumulating a poor quality blood supply, which will lead to easy access for sickness and disease to follow. Once the trend of eating processed, refined and unnatural foods has been adopted, it will only be a matter of time for deteoration to become evident and eventually affect the entire body, unless the quality of the blood is improved to overcome such deteoration. It is possible for anyone to improve the quality of their blood over a short period of time, by utilizing those natural foods that only nature can provide.

Blood conveys Oxygen to all the body's tissues

Blood conveys OXYGEN to all the body's tissues in the form of red blood cells, (HAEMOGLOBIN). This substance is a Protein, which requires the mineral IRON for its healthy development.

Blood removes waste tissues from the body and is essential for the formation of new body cells and tissues. Blood removes this waste through the following organs of the body;

a) LUNGS remove Carbon Dioxide.

b) LIVER removes Urea.

c) KIDNEY'S, LUNGS and SKIN remove excess water.

Blood transfers chemical messages in the form of HORMONES.

Blood supplies anti-bodies to areas of infection and disease.

The average person's bloodstream is composed of 25 billion cells, that is a person in good health. These blood cells travel around the body every 20 seconds, passing through the heart, where they are replinished with fresh Oxygen and dispose of the waste which is in the form of oxygen exausted, Carbonic Acid Gas, which is expelled through the lungs by the movements of breathing out (Exhalation).

When blood is pure of toxic waste, it's efficiency and activity is greatly improved and this promotes an active mind and body.

Blood is our Lifeline

WHITE CELLS: Polymorpho-nucleur Leucocyte-75%. Lymphocytes 25%

POLYMORPHO. These cells are slightly larger than the red cells and also fewer in number. (500–1)

The two important functions of the WHITE Cells are:

1) To protect the body against harmfull Bacteria. To remove injured or dead cells from the body. When bacteria is powerfull enough, these white cells are destroyed, (remaining in the form of Pus). When these cells are healthy, they will remove the bacteria via the organs of excretion.

LYMPHOCYTES

These act as the defence force against possible infection. They are formed in the Lymphatic Glands, Spleen and Thymus. When an infection occurs, their number increases until the condition is relieved. Radiation can seriously affect the number of these cells and inhibit the body's ability to fight an infection.

BLOOD PLATELETS

The main function of the blood Platelets, is for the clotting of the blood. The essential change during the process of blood clotting is the conversion, of a protein substance called FIBRINOGEN, into FIBRIN. This forms a thread, which entangles the blood cells causing them to contract into a firm mass, which prevents further loss of blood. This process of blood clotting, relies on an adequate supply of Calcium Salts and Vitamin K, both of which are found abundantly in green leafy vegetables, especially Spinach and the outer green leaves of lettuce.

BLOOD PLASMA

Blood Plasma is a liquid substance, in which blood cells float. This is composed of three types of Protein. ALBUMIN, GLOBULIN, FIBRINOGEN.

RED CORPUSCLES (ERTHYROCYTES)

These Red Corpuscles, contain a substance called **HAEMOGLOBIN.** These red corpuscles have no nucleus and are therefore not cells, but flat circular discs, which contain a membrane with a concave surface. Their function is to carry Oxygen around the body. Haemoglobin, consists of a complex protein called, GLOBIN and a pigment containing IRON, termed HAEMATIN. Organic Iron is essential in the diet for the formation of this Haemoglobin. When the diet lacks Iron, the percentage of Red Corpuscles is reduced and the body's ability to transport Oxygen will be impaired. Anemic conditions and lack of resistance to fight infection will follow. Oxygen absorption occurs primarily in the Lungs, where blood from the Veins (blue coloured) is replinished with Oxygen and then passes into the Arteries (red coloured). Red blood cells are formed in the bone marrow where they are seperated into smaller cells, which are the red coloured nucleus.

ESSENTIAL NUTRIENTS OF RED CORPUSCLES.

1) Organic Iron.

2) A diet of protein, vit B, vit C, and the elements Cobalt and Copper.

3) B 12, is required for the formation of the large red cells into smaller cells in the process of HAEMOGLOBIN formation.

4) A diet of the essential minerals, vitamins and other nutrients to assist in he utilization of the above essential ingredients.

BLOOD

EPITHELIAL CELLS · CONNECTIVE CELLS · MUSCLE CELLS · SKELETAL CELLS · NERVE CELL · BLOOD CELLS (Red Cells, White cells)

PLASMA MAKES UP 55% OF TOTAL BLOOD. CELLS ARE 45% OF TOTAL BLOOD. TOTAL BLOOD.

SOLIDS. WATER. BLOOD PLASMA. WATER MAKES UP 90% BLOOD PLASMA. 10% SOLIDS—PROTEINS. MINER.

WHITE CELLS. PLATELETS. RED CELLS. BLOOD CELLS. RED CELLS ARE 95% BLOOD CELLS. PLATELETS 3%. WHITE CELLS 1.5%.

DIAGRAM SHOWING COMPONENTS OF WHOLE BLOOD.

Blood is what makes Life count': you may rarely see your blood or the inside of your precious body, but it does not disguise the fact that all the internal organs are constantly relying on healthy food and good quality blood for their life.

Blood feeds the Body: When human tissue is examined under a microscope, the cells that make up the tissues can be seen as an organized arrangement which combine to make up the different organs of the body. A body cell grows with the addition of blood and depends entirely on the quality of the blood to form new healthy cells. In a period of two months, the entire body's blood-cells are renewed, either to a healthy state or to a sick state.

Blood contains 16 mineral elements, which can only be renewed with the right mineral ingredients, natural minerals. It is impossible to obtain all the necessary elements of the blood, from any unnatural source. The human body is as much a part of nature as the plants, trees and animals, which all rely on nature for life.

TOTAL VOLUME OF BLOOD(average person). 6 litres; 10 pints. One twentieth of the body weight.

NORMAL BLOOD CONTAINS:
Red corpuscles: 5,000,000, cu milimetre.
White cells: 8,000 cu. milimetre.
Platelets: 250,000, cu milimetre.

	SODIUM.	POTASSIUM.	CALCIUM.	MAGNESIUM.	CHLORINE.	IODINE.	IRON.
PLASMA	340.	20.	10.	2.7.	370.	0.001.	0.1.
CELLS Red & White.	0	420.	0.	6.0	190.	—	100.
WHOLE BLOOD	160.	200.	5.	4.0	250.	—	50

Plasma. Red cells and Whole blood. Average amounts in milligrams per 100 cc.

ALCOHOL

Alcohol is defined as a colourless, volatile, intoxicating, inflammable liquid. The chemical composition is C_2H_5OH, commonly known as ethyl alcohol.

Alcohol consumption has numerous and varied effects on the body and mind. Initially, after alcohol enters the digestive system, a portion of the ethyl alcohol will be absorbed through the linings of the stomach. It will then enter the bloodstream and quickly travel to all parts of the body and mind. Most of the alcohol will pass into the lower digestive system, and because it requires no digestion, alcohol will be absorbed directly from the small intestine and be conveyed into the blood, travelling quickly to all cells within the body and eventually, the liver will collect some of the alcohol and prepare to convert it into a usable energy form. A special enzyme, alcohol dehydrogenase, is present within the liver, specifically to convert ethyl alcohol, however it is a slow process. It takes approx. one hour for the liver to convert the alcohol of one standard drink — i.e. a glass of wine, or 285 ml. glass of beer, or a glass of sherry or one ounce of a standard spirit, all equal to approx. one tablespoon of ethyl alcohol. Once the enzyme has performed, the ethyl alcohol is converted into another fairly harmful substance called aldehyde, that is defined as colourless, volatile fluid of suffocating smell, obtained by oxidation of alcohol. Another enzyme within the body will convert the aldehyde into a form of vinegar and once that is oxidised, the final product is carbon dioxide, a colourless heavy gas. During these various processes of alcohol conversion, energy is produced and depending on the type of activity, the 7 calories per gram of alcohol may be used directly or otherwise, converted into body fat. For some people, the alcohol intake is limited directly because it can easily lead to obesity. Alcoholic drinks are very likely to cause obesity because once the mind becomes relaxed from the effects of the alcohol, there may be less chance to take part in some activity or dance. If the alcohol within the system is used directly for activity, the after-effects of the drinks are greatly reduced, thereby protecting against "hangovers".

For some people many hours of the day or night are spent drinking and apart from some social entertainment, very little other 'attainment' is developed from hours of steady drinking, except for the continuous destruction of body cells and a definite decline in physical and mental health. Once alcohol starts to take the place of food, the effects of the alcohol will eventually poison the entire body and mind. Natural foods are capable of providing great protection against the effects of alcohol and more specifically, fructose, or fruit sugar is the most effective substance available to assist and promote the conversion of alcohol. Even though large quantities of fructose or fresh fruit drinks would be required to change a person from the state of temporary drunkenness into sobriety, a regular intake of fresh fruit drinks is the best cure for the alcohol headaches and other physical side effects. By having one glass of a freshly prepared fruit juice — apple, orange, pineapple, grape or tomato, per standard glass of alcohol, there would be numerous benefits obtained and the body could make better use of the alcohol. The party may become more lively and nobody would complain the next day. Alcohol is not the only party drink, there are so many wonderful fresh fruit cocktails to be made and by serving them at parties or with any occasion, you can be sure about maintaining good health and a genuine friendly atmosphere.

The illustration on the right displays five different groups of social alcohol levels and depending on the duration with a particular group, there may be an increased risk of health problems. The two groups presented on top: periodic drinker and the environmental drinker both have a fairly good chance to maintain their health if their diet is based on natural foods and fresh juices. The development of drinking habits will generally tend to rely on an increased intake of alcohol drinks in order to obtain the same as the original stimulation. With some control, a person can obtain their favourite wine or drink every evening without making a meal of it, and be at the same time "extra pleased" to know that their body can cope with the otherwise, detrimental effects of alcohol. With such wisdom, alcohol could be considered a special drink rather than the common life-destroying effects that occur to the compulsive drinker, the symptomatic drinker or finally, the patient. 'A natural wine could help the evening start to shine' and with natural foods, every day can be the start to a new life, of health and happiness.

"SOCIAL ALCOHOL LEVELS"

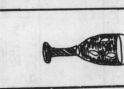

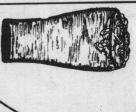

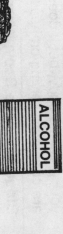

ALCOHOL

PERIODIC DRINKER;
The party drinker and the 'once in a while'

ENVIROMENTAL DRINKER;
The person who drinks to be sociable

COMPULSIVE DRINKER;
The person who is "forced" to drink, due to emotional instability and other forms of social problems.

SYMPTOMATIC DRINKER;
The person who drinks excessively, with the result of temporary and permanent physical and mental illness

THE PATIENT;
The person who has indulged excessively, either as a Symptomatic, Compulsive or Enviromental drinker, with the result of numerous damaged organs, mental deteoration and a drastic decline in physical and mental abilities.

ALCOHOL

	Grapes	BARLEY	Apples	WINES	MARTINI	RUM. WHISKY. GIN. VODKA.	BEER
CALORIES.	70	348	32	150	140	245	46
CARBOHYDRATES.	18	77	13	8	.3	.01	4
CALCIUM.	12	34	6.6	7	5	0	5
PHOSPHORUS.	21	290	9.3	0	1	0	30
POTASSIUM.	152	296	99	80	0	3.5	25
IRON.	.4	2.7	.27	4	.1	0	trace
SODIUM.	3.2	3	1.1	4	0	.01	7
MAGNESIUM.	6.4	35	7.9	10	0	0	0
COPPER.	.10		.8	0	0	0	0
MANGANESE.	.84	1.6	.069	30	0	0	0
ZINC.			.04	0	0	0	.02
A.	106		82	0	4	0	0
C.			3.8	0	trace	0	0
E.			.71	0	0	0	0
B1.	.05	.21	.02	.01	trace	0	.005
B2.	.03	.07	.018	.02	trace	0	.03
B3.	.35	3.7	.1	.21	trace	0	.60
B5.	.8	.5	.10	.03	0	0	.03
B6.	.79	.22	.027	.05	0	0	.08
BIOTIN.	2.1	0	.97	0	0	0	trace
FOLIC ACID.	.07	0	.017	0	0	0	0

CEREBRAL CORTEX: The Centre of thought and self consciousness and realization.

THALAMUS: 5
The co-ordinator of messages from the brain stem, to the Cerebral Cortex.

CEREBRAL CORTEX: 4
Is the first area of the brain affected by the intake or Alcohol, resulting in a relaxation of mental activity, slurred speach, slow reactions and eventual mental confusion.

The Pineal Gland is composed of mainly the Minerals- Magnesium & Phosphorus, both of which are eliminated by excess and regular alcohol consumption. The result is a deteoration of abilities to reconize the spiritual aspects of Life. **6**
The PINEAL GLAND is one of the main psychic sense organs, which has the ability to transfer spiritual knowledge to the Mental & Physical receptive parts of the body.

7 HYPOTHALAMUS: Controls the Pituitary Gland and regulates blood pressure and body temperature.

8 PITUITARY GLAND: Master Gland of the body, which controls the activity of all other glands. Also produces various Hormones, one such controls the functioning of the Adrenal, Thyroid and Sex Glands.

CEREBELLUM: Co-ordinator of all muscles and the sense of balance. **9**
The CEREBELLUM is poisoned by the intake of Alcohol, which leads to death of brain cells and temporary and permanent lack of co-ordination.

10 RETICULAR ACTIVATING SYSTEM: Passes messages from the brain stem, to the higher centres of the brain. Alcohol depresses the transfer of messages from the brain stem-Spinal Cord, to the higher centres if the brain which leads to drowsiness and eventual unconsciousness.

11 BRAIN STEM: The conecting point from the Spinal Cord to the brain.

CIRRHOSIS of the LIVER.
Excess and regular consumption of Alcohol, will result in a decreased tolerance to Alcohol as the Liver will form Fatty scar tissues, due to the effects of the Alcohol and lack of essential daily nutrients, which are required to build and replace worn out and damaged cells.

Depending on the alcohol drink, the concentration of ethyl alcohol will vary. On average, beer will supply 5% ethyl alcohol, wines will vary from 7-15%, sherry and port frange from 16-18% and the spirits and liqueurs will supply from 40-60% ethyl alcohol content. A drink with a 50% ethyl alcohol content is also termed as 100 proof. The level of alcohol intoxication is given as 100mg per 100ml or 10% blood-alcohol level.

FIGURES ARE CALCULATED TO APROXIMATE 100 GRAMMS.

ALCOHOL – EFFECT ON MINERALS – VITAMINS – HEALTH

Natural foods and drinks will provide positive protection from the effects of alcohol and by ensuring a well balanced diet, the desire for alcohol will be naturally limited as the body will obtain positive stimulation from the natural diet, thereby providing a proper substitute for the temporary stimulation of the alcohol.

The initial effect of alcohol may provide a soothing, relaxing feeling, as alcohol will slow down physical and mental activity, by impairing the efficiency of the nervous system and brain. After a person obtains approx. two standard drinks in the hour, the body will struggle to convert the alcohol and a saturation within the entire body will result. At this stage the alcohol will act as a poison and continue to cause health problems until such time that the alcohol is converted into a harmless form. The main initial health problems are associated with numerous nutrient deficiencies, caused by the empty calorie content of the alcohol drinks and unless the diet is providing a suitable replacement of nutrients, the risk of impaired health is definite, even though a person may appear to be all right, the damage to cells within may eventually spread outwards to make it quite obvious. The human body can maintain a remarkable resistance to alcohol, providing that the input of nutrients, natural foods and drinks is obtained regularly, daily. As alcohol provides 7 calories per gram, the concentration of energy per drink should promote greater activity, however, as there are no active nutrients supplied, those 7 calories could be wasted, or stored as body fat. When a well balanced natural diet is obtained, the body will have a better chance to make use of the energy and thereby protect against obesity and the numerous health problems.

VITAMIN B1 FOODS: Wheat germ, Soya beans, Sunflower seeds, Peanut Sesame seeds, Brazil nuts (see page 195)

Vitamin B1 is termed the 'morale vitamin'. It is essential for a healthy nervous system. Alcohol consumption reduces the body's store of this 'everyday vitamin.' A deficiency may lead to impaired learning and mental abilities and possible cardiac damage; weak heart muscles and irregular heartbeat.

VITAMIN B2 FOODS: Almonds, Wheat germ, Millet, Parsley, Cashew nut, Sesame seeds, Broccoli. (see page 198).

Vitamin B2 must be obtained regularly from the diet. Alcohol will quickly deplete the body's store of B2 and a prolonged deficiency may lead to cracks and sores of the mouth, baldness, general weakness, various nervous disorders, ulcers, arthritis, poor skin condition, and weak eyesight.

VITAMIN B3 FOODS: Peanut, Sesame seeds, Sunflower seeds, Rice, Whole wheat, Almonds. (see page 199).

Vitamin B3 is possibly the most affected vitamin, due to a prolonged or regular consumption of alcohol. B3 is essential for healthy nerves and proper mental abilities. A prolonged deficiency of B3 may lead to: poor skin condition, acne, headaches, depression, fatigue, indigestion and numerous types of nervous disorders.

VITAMIN B COMPLEX FOODS: (see pages 195-196).

As the B complex vitamins work as a team, a deficiency of B1, B2 and B3 will greatly affect the ability of other B complex vitamins (see pages 197-208).

VITAMIN C FOODS: Red & Green Capsicum, Parsley, Black currants, (see pages 186-187).

Alcohol consumption causes numerous types of body stress. Vitamin C is most effective for prevention of stress. A prolonged deficiency of Vitamin C can lead to numerous disorders (see page 186-187).

MAGNESIUM FOODS: Almonds, Cashew nuts, Soya beans, Walnuts, Green vegetables (see pages 160 & 170)

Excess and prolonged intake of alcohol will lead to an increased loss of Magnesium, via the kidneys. A Magnesium deficiency may lead to: diarrhea, weak bone development, arthritis, nervousness, blood clots and mental illness. Magnesium is termed 'the nerve mineral.'

ZINC FOODS: Brazil nuts, Almonds, Cashews, Hazel nuts, Walnuts, Whole Grains. (see pages 163 & 171)

Zinc is an essential trace mineral. It is a vital ingredient of the enzyme that is used to break down alcohol. A prolonged deficiency of Zinc may lead to poor healing of wounds, fatigue, sterility and prostate gland disorders. Zinc is often termed a 'healing mineral.'

CIGARETTES – SMOKING

Cigarette smoking and alcohol drinking often go hand-in-hand as an established social custom. The most active ingredient of cigarettes is nicotine: $C_{10}H_{14}N_2$, defined as a very poisonous volatile alkaloid. The name nicotine was given after a French diplomat, Jacques Nicot, introduced tobacco in France during the 16th century. Tobacco is obtained from the Nicotiana family of plants, Solanaceae, a native to tropical America. Nicotine is an addictive drug and therefore it becomes very difficult to resist another cigarette-dose once a person has acquired the habit. Similar to alcohol, the urge to have another cigarette is developed from a physical and mental addiction, over a period of a few years. The social acceptance of cigarettes has provided reason for an increased number of people to start or continue with the smoking habit. There are numerous reasons as to the popularity of cigarette smoking, apart from the social side of life, and they are mainly based on the stimulation that occurs after inhalation of the cigarette smoke. Depending on the amount of inhalation, the nicotine can be a powerful activator of the involuntary nervous system. After entering the lungs, the nicotine-smoke is quickly absorbed and travels throughout the body via the bloodstream. When reaching the adrenal glands, the nicotine stimulates the secretion of adrenaline which is also produced by the glands, naturally, in times of stress, danger, excitement, anger and various other states of emotion. The presence of adrenaline within the bloodstream also causes numerous changes of metabolism, thereby providing the 'cigarette stimulation'. The adrenaline in the bloodstream will cause constriction of the arteries which then leads to an increased heartbeat, or an increased 'temporary state of activity'. Adrenaline also stimulates the liver, resulting in an increased conversion of glycogen (stored glucose) into the active form of glucose which then enters the bloodstream and provides energy, so as to assist with the 'emergency condition'.

As a result of the stimulating effects that are initiated by the nicotine on the adrenal glands, it becomes clear as to the reason for the dependence that people may have with the cigarette and once addicted to the stimulation, a person may have great difficulty to feel content, initially, without a cigarette.

The increased supply of adrenaline, caused by the nicotine, will lead to a relaxing of the involuntary muscles of the bronchi, the main inlet for each lung, and that results in a reduction of oxygen intake and temporarily relaxes the lungs. Over a prolonged period of smoking, the lungs become considerably less active and that promotes the development of numerous possible respiratory disorders. The smoke also damages lung tissues and cells and eventually the lungs may become so weak that it becomes difficult for the smoker to even take a few deep breaths of fresh air.

One of the main reasons for the very addictive effect of the nicotine is due to the saturation of nicotine residue, within cells throughout the body, all of which contribute a 'reminder' of the cigarette, thereby providing part of the initial urge to have another cigarette. To successfully quit the smoking habit, it is essential to maintain a very cleansing diet and obtain regular exercise, so as to eliminate all traces of the nicotine and cigarette toxins. An attempt to quit smoking without such a cleansing diet would be more difficult and take considerably more time. The powerful nicotine-urge must be overcome with a powerful mental and physical substitute, otherwise the 'impulse' to smoke will be preferred. The mental decision to have another cigarette may only take a few moments and possibly occur regularly during the first few days of the withdrawal, and at these moments it is vital to be prepared with a substitute. Place something in the hand, take a few deep breaths, have a piece of fruit or some almonds and think about the real benefits that will be obtained once the mental and physical addiction have been eliminated, or think about the number of years that you survived without a cigarette.

Cigarette smoking has become a convenient social way to 'have a break' at work, or whenever it seems time to change the pace of events or thoughts with a type of euphoric relaxing temporary feeling as a result; after which the body will attempt to repair the damage and try to maintain natural functioning, however, if the diet is poor, the physical stress alone may be sufficient encouragement for the thought of another cigarette, resulting in a continuous cycle of smoking and the depletion of nutrients and the destruction of cells.

EFFECTS OF CIGARETTE SMOKING

Many factors are involved when considering the effects of smoking in regards to health. In all cases, it is definitely not advisable to smoke or to consider smoking as a relaxing habit. Apart from the nicotine content, tobacco smoke may contain nearly 300 chemical compounds and at least a dozen of those compounds have been proven to cause cancer in research testing with animals. Such substances as carbon monoxide, cyanide, saltpetre (potassium nitrate) and other irritants are most common with the average cigarette and over a prolonged period the accumulation of those toxins within the human system, plus the added toxins from the environment, refined foods and chemical additives will all contribute towards poor health and a limited lifespan. In Australia, it has been estimated that 15,000 people die annually as a direct result of cigarette smoking. Thousands of other people are in poor health, due to dietary deficiencies and their smoking habits.

There are numerous natural foods that provide special benefits for protection from the effects of cigarettes-nicotine and toxins. The following is a summarised list of the main foods and their benefits: smoking destroys body cells, damages lung tissues and causes diseased arteries. Vitamin E foods will protect against scar tissue formation. They also promote regeneration of skin tissues and they protect against wrinkly skin, a most obvious sign of cigarette damage. Vitamin E foods will protect the heart muscles and promote efficient heart action and blood circulation. Almonds, apples, fresh apple juice, sesame seeds-tahini, wheat germ oil, hazel nuts are all excellent vitamin E foods, have them regularly and protect your wonderful body. Cigarette smoking will quickly deplete the body-store of vitamin C. One cigarette may destroy the equivalent vitamin C content of a fresh, delicious orange. Vitamin C is essential for the health of the adrenal glands and as they are most affected by the nicotine, special nutrition is required to prevent adrenal exhaustion; a condition which can show as aches and back pains, headaches and prolonged fatigue. Vitamin C is vital for healthy skin and for protection from toxins. Depending on the number of cigarettes and the amount of inhalation, an increased intake of vitamin C foods is highly recommended (see pages 176–177 for details).

Cigarette smoking is most damaging to the nervous system and only with an increased regular intake of vitamin B complex foods can the smoker protect against the multitude of nervous disorders and other ailments associated with a B vitamin deficiency (see pages 187–197 for details). Such foods as sunflower seeds, almonds, sesame seeds, walnuts, peanuts, fresh vegetables and whole grains are vital for complete protection from a vitamin B deficiency and in combination with some additional B vitamin supplementation, such as brewers yeast or B complex yeast tablets, the smoker could be well protected. Some of the B complex vitamins are required daily, and for the smoker, the possibility of a deficiency is likely to occur, thereby leading the way to a destruction of the nervous system and on a daily basis, the smoker may feel extra fatigued, miserable, anxious and other types of negative emotion, once the B complex vitamins are neglected, or, dispersed by the effects of smoking. A cigarette is not at all relaxing for the nerves.

Other essential nutrients for protection from the effects of smoking are: vitamin A & D and the minerals magnesium, phosphorus, calcium, potassium, sulphur, chlorine, sodium and zinc. The best way to ensure a complete supply of these nutrients is to maintain a complete natural diet, including fresh juices and a regular intake of seeds, nuts, whole grains, fresh fruits and vegetables (see pp. 158–161 and 182–186 for details on nutrient-food sources).

An interesting concept about cigarette smoking, related to its popularity, may be viewed as being a substitute for the fire and smoke that were once upon a time relied on for the preparation of cooked meals. A type of instinctive transition takes place when a cigarette is burning, a memory of the days when Man was dependant on the fire for warmth, food preparation and the sharing of relaxing moments. In summary of the information mentioned, it may now be evident that the smoking habit is based on numerous types of physical and mental dependance, all of which contribute to the powerful addiction that develops from the inhalation of cigarette smoke.

CHAPTER SIX

VITAMINS

VITAMINS

INTRODUCTION

Vitamins were first discovered to be an essential food-element over a century ago, however, at that time the word vitamin had not even been thought of, all that was known about vitamins was that some 'other substances' in food, apart from carbohydrates, proteins, lipids and minerals, were 'vital'. Vitamin is derived from Latin — for life = vita, plus 'amines' being derived from the word amine, a nitrogen — containing compound (see protein introduction). The name vitamines was first thought of by a Polish chemist, Casimir Funk, who also recognized the existence of 'other food substances', during the mid 1930's. Within the last half-century, chemists and scientists alike have gathered up remarkable information about the functions and requirements of specific vitamins and this information is now made available to an increasing number of people; the vitamin-boom has started a health-revival awareness and some food-factories continue to make 'vitamin-enriched' foods, others produce 'vitamin deficient foods' and for the chemical industry, they thrive on making vitamin tablets, all of which are not necessary.

The original discovery of the individual vitamins was made possible by their availability from a wide variety of natural foods, not from their presence in 'vitamin-enriched foods' or tablets. Vitamins are the most intricate food-substances, they are present in such small quantities in comparison to minerals or the three main food groups but they are always present and they must continue to remain with their associated food in order to assist digestion, metabolism and maximum health potential. Once a vitamin is isolated from a food, such as with vitamin tablets, it's efficiency is greatly retarded as the other associated nutrients with the food also provide essential elements, some of which cannot be utilized without vitamins, some others promote the function of vitamins. It has been estimated that over 80% of the people who take vitamin tablets are not absorbing them properly, as the small intestine may create a barrier against such chemically isolated elements, the value of a vitamin tablet may not be worth the expense! Only naturally produced vitamin supplements provide maximum tablet-potential, and only natural whole foods can provide the complete answer to vitamin requirements.

Numerous other 'socially accepted substances': foods, drinks and additives also have a deteriorating effect upon the store of vitamins within the body. Alcohol is a prime example, and even though the body may adjust to a regular intake of alcohol, cell deterioration does occur and gradually the entire body cells and organs degenerate. It is possible to overcome a majority of vitamin 'deficiency effects', even when taking alcoholic drinks regularly, that relies upon the assistance of freshly made fruit or vegetable juices, natural whole foods and regular exercise. It may be hard to avoid the alcohol parties as so many people partake in the excitement, however, you can repair most of the damage caused by alcohol (see pages 166–168 for details), by obtaining the best nutrition: natural whole foods in their natural state and freshly made juices, sprouted foods and, of course, a well balanced diet with natural foods. Throughout this chapter on Vitamins, there are numerous important summarized facts about the effects of alcohol upon Vitamin storage and effectiveness and also the effects of other substances: caffeine, tannin, tablets and processed foods with the body — store of vitamins. For those people who avoid alcohol, nicotine, caffeine, processed foods and drinks, they are capable of maintaining excellent health with a minimum vitamin intake: natural foods, but as soon as one or more of those vitamin-depleting substances enters the body, an increased intake of vitamins will be required to maintain good health.

VITAMINS

INTRODUCTION

Throughout this chapter on Vitamins, there are numerous facts about the functions, requirements, benefits and availability of vitamins from natural whole foods and it is interesting to discover the varied vitamin-potential of natural foods, some are an excellent source of a specific vitamin and other foods may supply none of that vitamin and an excellent source of some other vitamins. To ensure that your diet supplies a full range of Vitamins, it is advisable to check through the Vitamin food charts and the recommended dietary allowance chart – R.D.A., to see if the foods you obtain regularly are mentioned as a source of one or a few vitamins, if your diet is based on a wide range of natural foods, you can be sure of obtaining a good supply of the essential vitamins, if your diet is based on factory-foods, you may obtain positive health benefits by ensuring that, at least, the natural foods that you eat, are an excellent source of vitamins, refer to the food charts pages 194-196 for details. It is not essential to obtain a wide variety of natural foods in order to get the essential vitamins, you could live quite healthfully on a diet of less than a dozen natural foods, depending on your individual nutrient requirements, all of which differ from person to person. Apart from obtaining vitamins from food, many vitamins are easily used-up by the body, especially in cases of stress, mental and physical, and also for the conversion of food into energy; certain vitamins are required to assist energy production and if those vitamins are absent from the food, as with many processed and refined foods and drinks, a person may slowly or quickly notice the effects of a deficiency. As the human body has adapted to millions of evolutionary changes, it may also be possible for the human to eventually exist on a very limited amount of vitamins, however, at this present time, vitamins are essential for human life. Some vitamins are required daily, others may be obtained weekly, all are obtainable from natural whole foods. A persons diet may supply only a limited amount of a particular vitamin, that may retard the function and activity of other associated vitamins as well as minerals, glucose, amino acids and lipids, and over a prolonged period of such a vitamin deficiency, their body may show signs of sickness, even though their diet provided small quantities of that vitamin, in comparison to their food intake and emotional state, they should have obtained a better supply of that vitamin and avoided the intake of processed and refined foods and drinks, as each portion of food requires the assistance of vitamins to transport, digest, metabolize and promote cell life, a food without the right vitamins can lead to a life without the right vitality.

Environmental pollutants are prevalent in city air, they also have a deteriorating effect upon the store of vitamins, if you cannot avoid the city air, make sure that you obtain a regular supply of natural foods-drinks-vitamins. When one vitamin is missing, your body-mind will have more difficulty in feeling content, the only way to be sure of obtaining the right combinations of vitamins is to always use natural foods and drinks.

LIST OF COMMON FOOD ADDITIVES: PACKAGED FOODS and DRINKS, CANNED and BOTTLED
Acidifiers, Acidulants, Aerating agents, Alkalies, Antibiotics, Antibrowning agents, Anticaking agents, Antifirming agents, Antifoaming agents, Antimould agents, Antimycotic agents, Antioxidants, Antirope agents, Antistaling agents, Antisticking agents, Artificial colours, Artificial sweeteners, Bleaching agents, Bodying agents, Bread improvers, Buffering agents, Buffers, Carriers, Chelating agents, Clarifiers, Coating agents, Crisping agents, Crystalline inhibitors, Crystallization modifiers, Crumb-firming agents, Curing agents, Defoaming agents, Dough conditioners, Dusting agents, Emulsifiers, Extenders, Fillers, Fining agents, Firming agents, Fixatives, Flavour enhancers, Foaming agents, Food colours, Food dyes, Freshness preservers, Fumigides, Fungicides, Glazing agents, Humectants, Hydroscopic agents, Leavening agents, Lubricating agents, Maturing agents, Moisture-retaining agents, Mould inhibitors, Neutralizers, Nonnutritive sweeteners, Oleoresins, Preservatives, Propellants, Release agents, Sequestrants, Softeners, Solvents, Stabilizers, Washing agents.

VITAMIN A

— Retinol — fat soluble

Vitamin A is a Fat–soluble vitamin that can be stored by the body for a few days, depending on conditions of stress and other illnesses.

Vitamin A occurs naturally from two types of sources :

Preformed vitamin A.

Preformed Vitamin A is formed by tissues of animals and fish. Fish oils are an excellent source of Pre–formed Vitamin A.

Pro vitamin A.

Pro–vitamin A, commonly known as Carotene, is the other form of naturally occuring Vitamin A ingredients. Carotene is most abundant in Carrots, from where it's name was derived. Green leafy vegetables and fruits are also abundant sources.

Carotene is the finest source of nutrient that can be converted by the body, into the form of usuable Vitamin A. It takes about 6–7 hours for the absorption and conversion of Carotene to take place. Carrot juice is the best way to get Vit A.

Vitamin A is essential for the health of the Optic system. Carrots are often known to be good for the eyes. Vitamin A allows any person to have good night vision especially. Fresh vegetable juices are an excellent source of Vit.A.

Vitamin A is essential in the formation of Visual purple, which illuminates objects seen at night or in dim lighting. This illumination occurs within the eyes, only when sufficient amounts of Vitamin A are available. Vitamin A is also essential for correct colour vision abilities and for perepheral vision (Side vision).

Protects the body against possible infection, and provides a greater immunity to overcome diseases and illness. Vit.A assists the growth of children.

Is essential for the correct utilization of all vitamins and minerals especially Calcium and Phosphorus.

A deficiency may affect the respiratory tract, which looses its ability to resist infection and the common symptoms of colds and flu last longer when Vit A is undersupplied. Carotene in any quantity is not toxic. Carrot juice is excellent.

Vitamin A promotes the secretion of Gastric juices, which are essential for all types of Protein digestion especially. Hydrochloric acid and the Enzyme Pepsin.

It has recently been discovered that Vit.A is related to the synthesis of R.N.A. a nucleic acid, that assists in the transmission of chemical messages, instructions for the maintenance of good health and prolonged lifespan.

VITAMIN A IS ESSENTIAL FOR HEALTHY EYES

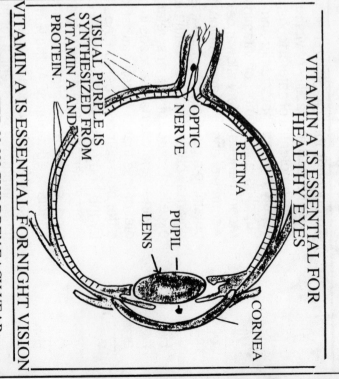

VISUAL PURPLE IS SYNTHESIZED FROM VITAMIN A AND PROTEIN.

OPTIC NERVE

RETINA

PUPIL

LENS

CORNEA

AN ESTIMATED 80,000 CHILDREN EACH YEAR, AROUND THE WORLD, BECOME PERMANENTLY BLIND, BECEAUSE OF A PROLONGED DEFICIENCY OF VITAMIN A.

VITAMIN A IS ESSENTIAL FOR NIGHT VISION

Dandelion greens, Carrot juice, Carrots Apricots (dr.), Kale, Collard, Sweet potato, Parsley Spinach, Turnip greens, Chives, Watercress, Mango Peach (dr.), Cantaloupe, Endive, Apricot, Broccoli Lettuce, Papaya, Prune, Pumpkin, Peach, Asparagus Tomato, Dried banana, Peas (fr.), Loquat Watermelon, Green beans, Okra, Brussel sprouts Tangerine, Capsicum, Sweet corn, Soya bean Black walnut, Avocado, Lima bean, Guava Cucumber, Black currant, Celery, Pistachio nuts Broad bean, Artichoke, Cabbage, Pigeon pea Raspberry, Pecan nut, Currants, Blueberry, Fig Cashew nuts, Rhubarb, Apple, Strawberry, Grapes Grapefruit, Mung bean, Olives, Pear (dr.), Pineapple Lentils, Pumpkin + Sunflower seeds, Dates

VITAMIN A

– Carotene – fat soluble

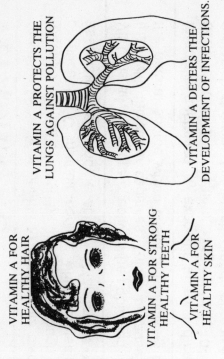

VITAMIN A FOR HEALTHY HAIR

VITAMIN A FOR STRONG HEALTHY TEETH

VITAMIN A FOR HEALTHY SKIN

VITAMIN A PROTECTS THE LUNGS AGAINST POLLUTION

VITAMIN A DETERS THE DEVELOPMENT OF INFECTIONS.

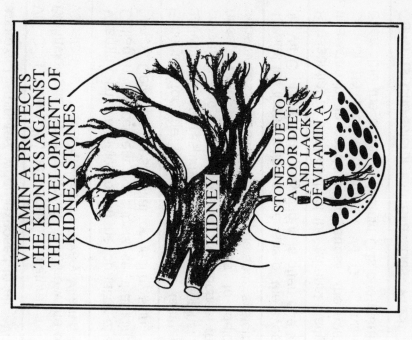

VITAMIN A PROTECTS THE KIDNEYS AGAINST THE DEVELOPMENT OF KIDNEY STONES

KIDNEY

STONES DUE TO A POOR DIET AND LACK OF VITAMIN A

Vitamin A is most important in fighting infections, as it provides strength to the cell walls which protect the minute mucous membranes of the cell against any infection or bacteria. Vitamin A will also retard the spreading of a infection.

Vitamin A helps to maintain healthy skin, by benefiting all cellular growth.

Vitamin A helps the body to stay and look young, preventing drying of the skin tissues and by promoting normal glandular activity, for the health of the body.

Helpful in cases of acne skin, as it nourishes the internal linings of the skin tissue. Also provides health and vitality to the hair, and promotes good teeth and bones. Aprox 90% of the Body's store of Vit.A is contained in the Liver.

With diets low in protein, Vit A absorption is limited.

A continued lack of Vit A can lead to falling hair and baldness.

Prevents the formation of cells that could develop into cancerous cells and slows the rate of already forming cells. Assists the reproduction of new cells which are capable of overcoming the rapid production of new cancerous cells, only when excellent sources of Vit A plus associated vitamins are given in a concentrated form. Diabetics cannot convert Carotene into Vit.A.

A deficiency can lead to the formation of stones in the gallbladder and kidneys. When Vit A is added in good amounts the stones will be assisted to dissolve naturally. Cigarettes and pollution retard Vit.A absorption.

Contraceptives deplete the reserves of Vit A which can have a serious effect on the health of the liver and other internal organs.

Protects the body against the harmful effects of radiation contamination, and for those people who have used the drug Cortisone.

Essential for mothers in pregnancy and lactation periods.

Protects the lungs against possible harm from the many pollutants in the air and in those places where car exhausts are prevelant. Ozone and Nitrogen dioxide are both common harmful pollutants in the air which can deteriorate the linings of the lungs.

VITAMIN C

— Ascorbic acid — water soluble

The human body is unable to produce its own supply of Vit C and so the required amounts must be obtained through the diet. Many animals can produce Vit C in their bodies which protects them against many of the associated deficiency effects.   Man is one of the exceptions.

Vit C is always more effective when obtained through a natural source rather than with tablets or capsules. This is because of the associated nutrients of the natural source which assist the functions of Vit C.

Is quickly destroyed by exposure to air and heat. This vitamin remains in the body for only a short time, ranging from 10—20 hours, and so it must be replenished every day. Freshly made orange juice looses its Vit C content in approx. 15 minutes when exposed to air. Vitamin C is water soluble.

Vit C is never formed alone in nature, it is always in combination with Bioflavionoids which are present in the white pulp of the associated fruits and vegetables.   Nature provides every Vitamin beautifully .

Vitamin C has a major role in the formation of a Protein substance — Collagen. Collagen is a cement like substance, that joins all skin tissues, ligaments and bones. Collagen is essential for healthy skin.

Essential for the formation of good teeth, growth of children, glandular activity, tissue respiration, protects against bacterial toxins, deteriorating vision, gastric ulcers, anaemia, headaches, rheumatic pains, bleeding of the nose, varicose veins and helps to detoxify harmful cancer causing substances, by reinforcing the defence system the body naturally possesses.

Is vital for the nutrition of the lens of the eyes. A healthy lens is always rich in Vit C. Deteorating eyesight is often due to a Vitamin C deficiency.

Is essential to the health of the adrenal glands which are the storehouse of this vitamin. In conditions of stress, the hormones released by the glands cannot be produced unless Vit C is available in sufficient amounts to overcome the stress. Vitamin C is often termed the stress Vitamin.

Converts Cholesterol into Bile acids, which is important for good digestion and prevention of gallstones and kidney stones. Vitamin C cleans the blood.

VITAMIN C IS ESSENTIAL FOR PRODUCTION OF A SUBSTANCE– COLLAGEN, WHICH JOINS ALL SKIN TISSUE TOGETHER AND PREVENTS PREMATURE AGING SKIN CONDITIONS.

VITAMIN C PREVENTS THE FORMATION OF PEPTIC ULCERS.

ULCER.

ACUTE ULCER.

PERFORATED ULCER.

VITAMIN C IS ESSENTIAL FOR GOOD EYESIGHT.

A HEALTHY LENS IS ALWAYS RICH IN VITAMIN C.

VITAMIN C FOODS PREVENT THE DEVELOPMENT OF ARTHRITIS. VITAMIN C ELIMINATES HARMFUL ACID POISONS FROM THE BODY.

VITAMIN C GIVES RELIEF FROM THE PAIN OF ARTHRITIS.

VITAMIN C

– Cevetamic acid – water soluble

Vit C is often called the youth vitamin, and as we grow older we require additional amounts. Vitamin C is required for the health of the nervous system.

Controls rapid oxidation in tissue cells and promotes a constant flow of many enzyme reactions which is essential and beneficial for the Pituitary, Adrenals, Ovaries, Heart, Brain and Eyes. Vitamin C keeps you young at heart.

Protects the body against invading infections, by increasing the number and speeding up the activity of the white blood cells which destroy all viruses and bacteria. **Vitamin C has to be replenished daily, for optimum health.**

Strengthens the blood capilaries and the bones and teeth.

Protects against excessive acidity of the body.

Enables the body to store Folic acid, which is necessary for normal blood and prevention of anaemia. Also important for the absorption of Iron from the digestive tract and subsequent storage in the bone marrow.

If you smoke, drink alcohol, inhale polluted air or are under conditions of stress, it is essential that you obtain extra amounts of this vitamin.

The pill upsets the delicate balance of glands in the body, and constitutes a chemical stress on the body and a subsequent loss of precious Vitamin C.

Lack of, may lead to hardening of the arteries and easy bruising.

During periods of menstruation, the Vit C level is drained.

When Vit C is lacking, the effects of vaccinations are harmful.

The ability of the body to absorb Vitamin C is greatly reduced by conditions of stress, cigarette smoking, fevers, anti–biotics, aspirin, alcohol and other forms of pain killers. Baking soda also reduces the levels of Vitamin C.

Vitamin C may provide sufficient relief from conditions of Arthritis, by allowing better movement and lubrication of bone joints.

Headaches are often a result of stressful conditions. Vitamin C or Ascorbic acid are far better to use than any tablet. Vitamin C powder is the ultimate headache tablet, obtainable from any of the good health food shops. Try it with orange.

If their were ever a vitamin that was deficient, it would be VITAMIN C.

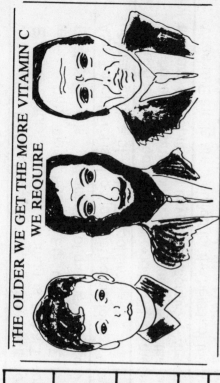

THE OLDER WE GET THE MORE VITAMIN C WE REQUIRE

No need to take an anti–acid tablet.

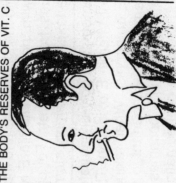

CIGARRETE SMOKING & ALCOHOL QUICKLY DEPLETE THE BODY'S RESERVES OF VIT. C

Acerola cherry, Guava, Capsicum, Black currants Kale leaves, Parsley, Collard leaves, Kale, Orange peel Turnip greens, Dock, Broccoli, Brussel sprouts Mustard greens, Watercress, Cauliflower, Jujube Strawberry, Lemon, Orange, Spinach, Lychee Currants, Pigeon pea (fr.), Lime, Grapefruit Kumquat, Turnip, Cantaloupe, Asparagus, Radish Tangerine, Fennel, Granadilla, Okra, Fresh beans Peas, Melon, Loganberry, Tomato, Blackberry Sweet potato, Mung bean sprouts, Lettuce, Pineapple Leek, Parsnip, Quince, Garlic, Avocado, Jujube

VITAMIN E

— Tocopherol — fat soluble

Vitamin E is found in unsaturated oils from plant foods. Seven types of vitamin E are available, the most common is Alpha Tocopherol, the other types are termed: Beta, Delta, Epsilon, Eta, Gamma & Zeta, they are all classed as Vit. E- Tocopherols. Tocopherol means ability to bear young.

Alpa Tocopherol is also the most potent form of Vitamin E. Wheat germ oil is the ultimate source of Alpha Tocopherol.

Vitamin E is termed as an anti-oxidant, which means it retards the oxidation and subsequent destruction of other nutrients in the body, especially the nutrients that are susceptible to oxygen deteoration.:-Vitamin C being the main one.

Vitamin E foods are required for the health of the Adrenal & Pituitary glands and their associated hormone production. Vitamin E protects these hormones from oxidation. Vitamin E is also essential for effective use of Linoleic acid (Fats).

Vitamin E creams which are applied locally to the skin surface, are absorbed directly into the skin tissues and mucous membranes. Vitamin E creams in combination with ingested Vitamin E (wheat germ oil), are excellent for healing of scar tissues, from burns etc. For optimum Vitamin E efficiency, wheat germ oil should be taken on an empty stomach.

Excess amounts of poly-unsaturated fats & margarines in the diet, will increase the rate of Vitamin E oxidation. The synthetic female hormone -Estrogen is a Vitamin E antagonist. When taking Vitamin E for the first time, such as pure Wheat germ oil, it is important to note that, a temporary rise in blood pressure will occur, until the body becomes accustomed to larger doses. Patients with a high blood pressure or rheumatic heart disease should be careful with taking Vitamin E in large doses especially. A healthy body can easily adjust to a tsp. of Vitamin E on a daily basis, with improved blood circulation as one of the benefits.

Vitamin E is one of the few vitamins that is affected by freezing. Processed and refined foods, such as many breakfast cereals, white rice, white bread & sweets are often very deficient in Vitamin E. Whole grains are an excellent source of Vitamin E. Proper storage of wheat germ oil is also important. About 90% of the Vitamin E content of whole grains is lost in the processes of refinement.

A deficiency of vitamin E may lead to Anemia, Angina Pectoris, Easy Bruising, Arteriosclerosis, Hypertension, Varicose Veins, Colitis, Epelipsy, Gallstones, Loss of hair, Dandruff, Headaches, Sinusitis, Arthritis, Constipation, Muscular Cramps, Common Cold, Emphysema, Mental Illness and Rheumatism.

VITAMIN E FOODS ARE REQUIRED FOR THE HEALTH OF THE PITUITARY, ADRENAL & KIDNEYS.

The PITUITARY Gland stimulates the THYROID Gland to produce THYROXIN, which regulates the speed of chemical reactions within the body.

THYROID.
The PITUITARY Gland produces a hormone (Vaso Pressin), which acts on the KIDNEYS, to regulate the balance of Water & Salts in the body.

The PITUITARY Gland stimulates the production of sex-hormones and for the production of Mother's milk, during lactation. The PITUITARY Gland is also responsible for the production of MELANIN, the substance which provides varying pigments, for peoples skin & hair.

Adrenal glands and contols childrens growth.

PITUITARY GLAND produces a Growth-Hormone (A.C.T.H.) which stimulates the

HYPOTHALAMUS

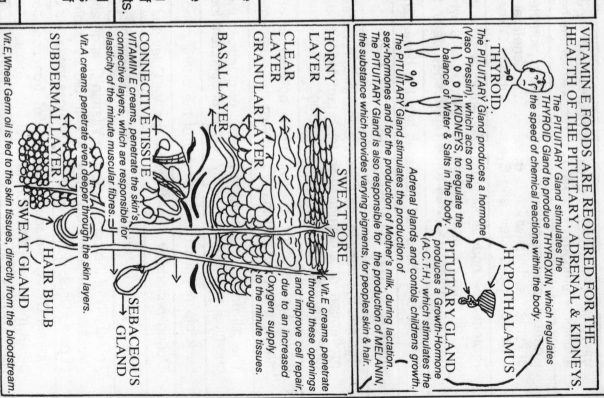

HORNY LAYER

CLEAR LAYER

GRANULAR LAYER

BASAL LAYER

Vit.E creams penetrate through these openings and improve cell repair, due to an increased Oxygen supply to the minute tissues.

SWEAT PORE

CONNECTIVE TISSUE
VITAMIN E creams, penetrate the skin's connective layers, which are responsible for elasticity of the minute muscular fibres.

Vit.A creams penetrate even deeper through the skin layers.

SUBDERMAL LAYER

Vit.E,Wheat Germ oil is fed to the skin tissues, directly from the bloodstream.

SWEAT GLAND

HAIR BULB

SEBACEOUS GLAND

Vitamin E is also essential for the synthesis and use of various Amino Acids.

VITAMIN E — *Alpha, Beta, Gamma and Delta Tocopherol*

Every cell in the body lives by burning up oxygen to produce warmth and energy. Vit E regulates this action and prevents cells from burning out too quickly. The normal life of a red blood cell is 120 days. A deficiency of Vit E reduces cell life to about 70 days.

Vitamin E assists the functioning of the entire nervous system (Spine & Brain).

Increases the power and activity of muscles, especially the heart muscles.

Vitamin E improves blood circulation by enlarging even the smallest blood vessels and arteries which provides Oxygen and nourisment to all body cells. Vitamin E retards ageing because of improved blood circulation.

Vitamin E also protects the B group vitamins from rapid oxidation.

Vitamin E regulates the body's use of Protein's and Fats from the daily diet.

Preserves the walls of the red blood cells and prevents their destruction.

Vitamin E increases and sets free blood platelets to those places where they are required, especially in cases of burns, scarring, wounds and intestinal ulcers.

Vitamin E improves the number, activity and potency of the male sperm cell.

Normalizes the activity of the ovaries in women, improving the periods regularity and preventing excessive bleeding, dryness and irritation of the genital passages. Vitamin E, improves male and female fertility.

Maintains the health and normal blood supply to the unborn baby in the early weeks and later stages in the mother's womb, often preventing miscarriages.

Vitamin E helps to detoxify such harmful substances as residue from pesticides, chemical fertilizers, industrial pollutants, car-exaust fumes and preservatives.

Vitamin C is required for improving the effectiveness of Vit A & C, Mineral Iron.

Vitamin E prevents unnecessary clotting in blood vessels. (Thrombosis).

The more Saturated Fats and Oils consumed, the greater the need for Vitamin E. Vitamin E was first discovered in 1922, from Wheat germ oil, the best source.

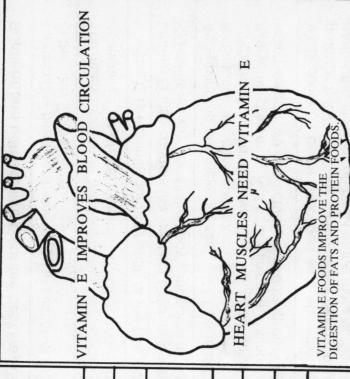

VITAMIN E IMPROVES BLOOD CIRCULATION

HEART MUSCLES NEED VITAMIN E

VITAMIN E FOODS IMPROVE THE DIGESTION OF FATS AND PROTEIN FOODS.

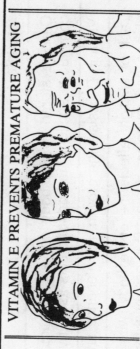

VITAMIN E PREVENTS PREMATURE AGING

Wheat germ oil, Sesame seeds, Tahini, Almonds Hazel nuts, Raw wheat germ, Millet, Rice, Cucumber Brazil nuts, Peanut, Walnuts, Sunflower seeds, Oats Pecan nuts, Asparagus, Peas, Kale, Spinach Brussel sprouts, Apples, Tomato, Banana, Orange Avocado, Pumpkin seeds, Wheat, Rye, Sprouted seeds Carrots, Celery, Lettuce, Lotus root, Grapefruit Chestnuts, Corn, Alfalfa sprouts, Barley, Beans Soya beans, Potato, Triticale

VITAMIN D

— Calciferol — fat soluble

Sunlight and outdoor living are the best ways to obtain Vitamin D.

Vitamin D is produced naturally by the action of Sunlight with the oily substance in the skin (Ergosterol).

The main function of Vit D is to regulate all mineral and, vitamin metabolism, especially that of the minerals Calcium and Phosphorus.

Vitamin D is essential for the health of the Glandular and Nervous system.

Vitamin D also controls the levels of Calcium in the blood and regulates normal glandular activity for all the body's muscles. especially the heart.

As sunlight is our major source of Vit D, it is difficult to state an amount that is suitable for each individual. Such factors as pigment of the skin and strength of sunlight all vary, but a good guide would be to obtain a little everyday, preferably half hour minimum. Excessive amounts lead to sunburn, which means we are actually overdosing on Vit D.

Vit D could be better described as a hormone, rather than a vitamin, as it is produced, by the body, through the action of sunlight with the skin. The darker the pigment of the skin, the more sunlight required to obtain adequate amounts.

Can be stored by the body for a short time. When you are subjected to continuous sunlight the body protects itself, by changing to a darker pigment.

Vitamin D assists the growth, maintenance and repair of all bones and teeth.

Lack of sunlight affects the entire body, with poor conditions of all the vital glands and muscles. Vitamin D is essential for growth of children.

The Vitamin D content of foods is relatively stable to heat and lengthy storage.

Vitamin D is a fat–soluble vitamin, which can be stored by the body.

Vitamin D is stored in the skin, brain, liver and bones.

Vitamin D is required by the Thyroid gland, to manufacture hormones which are essential in control of body metabolism processes, such as digestion.

Vitamin D in combination with vitamin A, offsets colds and flus.

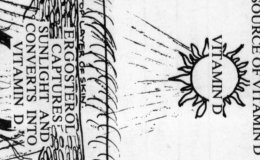

THE SUN PROVIDES THE ULTIMATE SOURCE OF VITAMIN D

VITAMIN D

TOP LAYER OF SKIN

ERGOSTEROL CAPTURES SUNLIGHT AND CONVERTS INTO VITAMIN D.

VITAMIN D AND THE PARATHYROID GLANDS WORK TOGETHER IN REGULATING CALCIUM DISTRIBUTION THROUGHOUT THE BODY.

THE THYROID GLAND NEEDS VITAMIN D TO PRODUCE HORMONES

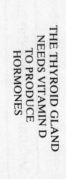

Vit D

VITAMIN D ASSISTS THE GROWTH OF CHILDREN.

MUSCULAR DEVELOPMENT.

NERVOUS SYSTEM.

GLANDULAR SYSTEM.

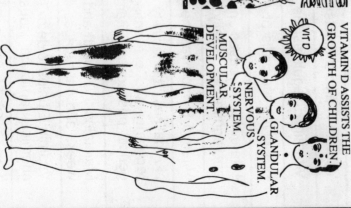

Sunshine, Outdoor living, Sunflower seeds Sunflower meal, Fish oils, Fresh fish, Alfalfa Fresh vegetables, Fresh fruits, Milk, Butter, Celery Spinach, Sprouted seeds, Corn

VITAMIN K

— Antihemorrhagic — fat soluble

Is essential in the process of blood coagulation, that is the clotting time of the blood. When a blood vessel is broken, Vit K has the ability to stop continuous bleeding.

This process of blood coagulation formation takes place in the liver, where the blood is then prepared to go to the site of bleeding and form a mesh like substance, which will prevent further bleeding.

Is essential for the good functioning of the circulatory system, assisting the functions of the heart and liver especially.

Protects the liver against lead pollution which is emmited by car exhausts.

Is destroyed by the taking of aspirin and other salicylates and antiobiotics.

The older we are, the more Vit K required.

The Vit K content of foods is greatly reduced by refrigeration and freezing.

Vitamin K is required for the conversion of Carbohydrates into the form of Glycogen, which is re−converted by the Liver into Glucose: (usuable energy).

Vitamin K is termed the anti−hemmorahagic vitamin.

Vitamin K in combination with Vit.C has been effective in prevention and also improving various types of Hemorrages after surgical operations.

Vitamin K can be synthesized by intestinal bacteria, if the right conditions exist.

Vitamin K is absorbed from the upper section of the Intestines, in combination with Bile and then transported to the Liver, where it is required for the formation of Prothrombin and other related Amino Acids (Protein), which control clotting time of the blood. If the Liver is unable to produce sufficient Bile, the absorption and production of Vitamin K will be greatly limited. Vitamin K has also proved effective in reducing blood loss during times of prolonged menstruation. Vitamin K foods have a vital effect, by improving health and total lifespan.

Vitamin K may also be beneficial to prevent any of the following conditions; Easy bruising, Gallstones, Jaundice and Ulcers.

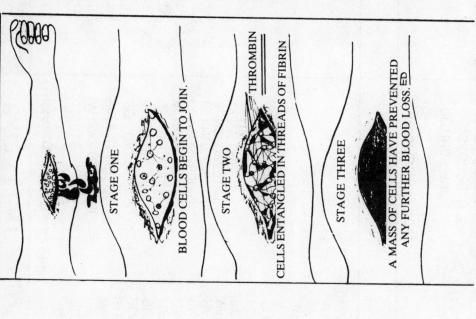

VITAMIN K IS ESSENTIAL IN THE PROCESS OF BLOOD COAGULATION

STAGE ONE

BLOOD CELLS BEGIN TO JOIN.

STAGE TWO

THROMBIN

CELLS ENTANGLED IN THREADS OF FIBRIN

STAGE THREE

A MASS OF CELLS HAVE PREVENTED ANY FURTHER BLOOD LOSS. ED

VITAMIN K IS REQUIRED FOR THE FORMATION OF A SUBSTANCE CALLED THROMBIN, WHICH TRAPS RED BLOOD CELLS INTO A MESH, WHICH PREVENTS FURTHER BLEEDING

Spinach, Lettuce, Parsley, Watercress, Celery Broccoli, Beetroot greens, Green beans, Kelp Cucumber, Leek, Dandelion, Endive, Chives Sprouted seeds, Other sprouts, Fresh fruits

FRESH VEGETABLES

RECENTLY DISCOVERED VITAMINS

VITAMINS	EXCELLENT	GOOD SOURCE	
VITAMIN F FAT SOLUBLE	**(Unsaturated Fatty Acids)** WHEAT GERM OIL SAFFLOWER OIL SOY OIL CORN OIL SESAME OIL ALMOND OIL COTTONSEED OIL PEANUT OIL SUNFLOWER OIL OLIVE OIL TAHINI	GARBANZO BEANS PISTACHIO NUTS AVOCADOS WHOLE GRAINS. MILLET STRAWBERRY BLACKBERRY BLUEBERRY RASPBERRY CASHEWS PECAN NUTS HAZEL NUTS WHEAT GERM BRAZIL NUTS EGG YOLK. FISH SOYA BEANS ALMONDS SUNFLOWER SEEDS SESAME SEEDS MARGARINE WALNUTS	Vitamin F is a fat soluble vitamin which consists of unsaturated fatty acids, which are mainly obtainable from liquid vegetable oils. Vitamin F is essential for effective tissue respiration and the transfer of Oxygen throughout the body, via the bloodstream. Vitamin F combines with Protein & Cholesterol to form Collagen, the cement like substance which joins all living skin tissue together. Vitamin F combines with Vitamin D to provide the minerals Calcium & Phosphorus to al the body's tissues and bones. Vitamin F also stimulates the conversion of Carotene, into the form of Pro Vitamin A. Vitamin F assists in regulating the rate of blood coagulation. Vitamin F is also required for the break down of Cholesterol particles. Vitamin F assists in maintaining resilience and lubrication of all cells. Vitamin F is essential for healthy Glandular functioning. (Adrenal). A deficiency of Vitamin F, may lead to a high Cholesterol level, Colitis, Diabetes, Diarrhea, Mental disorders, Multiple Sclerosis, Constipation Arthritis, Asthma, Acne, Dermatitis, Common cold and Obesity.
VITAMIN P WATER SOLUBLE	**(BIOFLAVIONOIDS)** CITRUS FRUITS BLACKCURRANTS FRESH FRUITS FRESH VEGETABLES	WHOLE GRAINS SPROUTED SEEDS	Vitamin P is a water soluble vitamin, mainly obtainable from fresh fruits and vegetables. Vitamin P is also known as Bioflavonoids. Vitamin P was first discovered from the white pulp of all Citrus fruits. There is 10x the concentration of Vit P in the white pulp of the citrus fruit in comparison to the juice. Vitamin P improves all the functions of Vitamin C. Vitamin P assists Vitamin C for the maintenance of Collagen, the inter cellular substance that joins all health skin tissues together. Vitamin P & C are most beneficial in relieving cases of Rheumatism. Vitamin P may also be beneficial for any of the following ailments: Artheriosclerosis, Easy bruising, High Cholesterol, Hemophilia, Hyper-Tension, Leukemia, Varicose veins, Arthritis, Pheunomia, Ulcers, Common Cold and Scurvy.

RECENTLY DISCOVERED VITAMINS

VITAMINS.	EXCELLENT	GOOD SOURCE	
VITAMIN B 13 OROTIC ACID	ROOT VEGETABLES	FRUITS YOGHURT VEGETABLES	*Vitamin B13, has been used effectively to treat cases of Multiple Sclerosis.* *Vitamin B13, is required for the effective use of Folic acid & Vit B12.* *A deficiency of B13, may lead to liver disorders, cell degeneration and premature aging.* *Vitamin B13 is also required for the health of the nervous system and for efficient brain functioning.*
VITAMIN T	SESAME SEEDS TAHINI	EGG YOLKS	*Vitamin T assists to normalize blood coagulation time.* *Vitamin T is also valuable in restorin health to patients with Anemia.* *Vitamin T assists in the formation of blood platelets, which protect the body against Anemia & Haemophilia (a hereditary disease.)* *Vitamin T may also improve a failing memory and poor concentration.*
VITAMIN U	CABBAGE JUICE	SAUERKRAUT	*Vitamin U, is a recently discovered vitamin, that has shown to promote healing in cases of Peptic & Duodenal Ulcers. Raw Cabbage juice is the best known source of Vitamin U and also abundant in the green magic Chlorophyl. Freshly made Chlorophyl juices are one of the best natural medicines avaible. Chlorophyl is closely related to the structure of Human blood and is one of the easiest absorbed nutrients avaible for the body. Lettuce, Spinach, Cabbage and Parsley are all magic.*

VITAMINS FOOD CHARTS

	EXCELLENT SOURCE	GOOD SOURCE	FAIR SOURCE
VITAMIN A ESSENTIAL ASSOCIATED NUTRIENTS FOR EFFECTIVE ABSORPTION: Calcium, Phosphorus and Zinc. Vitamins: C, D, E, F, B group. NUTRIENT INHIBITING FACTORS: Strenuous exercise, stress and Alcohol.	Dandelion greens, Carrot juice Carrots, Apricots (dr.), Kale Collard, Sweet potato, Parsley Spinach, Turnip greens, Chives Watercress, Mango, Peach (dr.) Cantaloupe, Endive, Apricot Broccoli, Lettuce, Papaya, Prune Pumpkin, Peach, Asparagus Dried banana, Peas (fr.), Loquat	Watermelon, Green beans, Okra Capsicum, Sweet corn, Tangerine Black walnut, Avocado, Lima bean Guava, Cucumber, Black currant Celery, Pistachio nuts, Broad bean Artichoke, Cabbage, Pigeon pea Raspberry, Pecan nut, Currants Blueberry, Grapes, Cashew nuts	Rhubarb, Apple, Strawberry, Fig Grapefruit, Mung bean, Olives Pear (dr.), Pineapple, Lentils Pumpkin + Sunflower seeds, Dates Chick pea, Red Cabbage, Cranberry Jujube, Honeydew melon, Quince Leek, Lemon, Melons, Sesame seed Walnut, Parsnip, Pear, Raisins Eggplant, Radish, Lime, Kelp
VITAMIN C ESSENTIAL ASSOCIATED NUTRIENTS FOR EFFECTIVE ABSORPTION: Calcium and Magnesium. Vitamins: P, A. NUTRIENT INHIBITING FACTORS: Heat, Oxidation, Cigarettes, Pollution, Aspirin and Alcohol.	Acerola cherry, Guava, Capsicum Black currants, Kale leaves Parsley, Collard leaves, Kale Orange peel, Turnip greens, Dock Broccoli, Brussel sprouts Mustard greens, Watercress Cauliflower, Jujube, Strawberry Lemon, Orange, Spinach, Lychee	Currants, Pigeon pea (fr.), Lime Grapefruit, Kumquat, Turnip Cantaloupe, Asparagus, Radish Tangerine, Fennel, Granadilla Okra, Fresh beans, Peas, Melon Loganberry, Tomato, Blackberry Sweet potato, Mung bean sprouts Lettuce, Pineapple, Leek, Parsnip	Quince, Garlic, Sapodilla, Avocado Blueberry, Artichoke, Sweet corn Cucumber, Apricot, Banana, Endive Beetroot, Onion, Celery, Pumpkin Rhubarb, Carrot, Lettuce, Apple Peach, Pear, Watermelon, Eggplant Grapes, Coconut, Mushroom, Figs Raisins
VITAMIN D ESSENTIAL ASSOCIATED NUTRIENTS: Calcium and Phosphorus. Vitamins: A, C, F, B group.	Sunshine, Outdoor living	Sunflower seeds, Sunflower meal Fish oils, Fresh fish, Alfalfa	Fresh vegetables, Fresh fruits Milk, Butter, Celery, Spinach Sprouted seeds, Corn
VITAMIN E ESSENTIAL ASSOCIATED NUTRIENTS FOR EFFECTIVE ABSORPTION: Manganese and Sulphur. Vitamins: C and B group.	Wheat germ oil, Sesame seeds, Tahini, Almonds, Hazel nuts Raw wheat germ, Millet, Rice Cucumber, Brazil nuts, Peanut	Walnuts, Sunflower seeds, Oats Pecan nuts, Asparagus, Peas Kale, Spinach, Brussel sprouts Apples, Tomato, Banana, Orange Avocado, Pumpkin seeds, Wheat	Rye, Sprouted seeds, Carrots Celery, Lettuce, Lotus root Grapefruit, Chestnuts, Corn Alfalfa sprouts, Barley, Beans Soya beans, Potato, Triticale
VITAMIN K ESSENTIAL ASSOCIATED NUTRIENTS Vitamin C. Frozen foods, Aspirin and Pollution.	Spinach, Lettuce, Parsley Watercress, Celery, Broccoli	Beetroot greens, Green beans Kelp, Cucumber, Leek, Dandelion	Endive, Chives, Sprouted seeds Other sprouts, Fresh fruits

VITAMINS   FOOD CHARTS

	EXCELLENT SOURCE	GOOD SOURCE	FAIR SOURCE
VITAMIN B1 ESSENTIAL ASSOCIATED NUTRIENTS FOR EFFECTIVE ABSORPTION: Vitamins: C and B group. NUTRIENT INHIBITING FACTORS: Alcohol and tobacco, stress, refined foods and drinks.	Rice bran, Wheat germ, Soya bean Sunflower seeds, Cowpea, Peanut Sesame seeds, Brazil nut, Pecan Pinto bean, Millet, Wheat bran Pistachio nut, White bean, Wheat Red bean, Broad bean, Lima bean Hazel nuts, Wild rice, Cashew nut Rye, Pigeon pea, Sorghum, Mung Lentils, Peas (fr.), Macadamia nut Rice, Walnuts, Chestnut, Chick pea	Garlic, Almonds, Pumpkin seeds Soya bean sprouts, Turnip greens Barley, Artichoke, Dandelion Asparagus, Okra, Collard, Kale Sweet corn, Mung bean sprouts Parsley, Avocado, Raisins, Figs Cauliflower, Oranges, Broccoli Beetroot greens, Brussel sprouts Mushroom, Potato, Dates Prunes, Kumquat	Artichoke, Snap beans, Chives Parsnip, Capsicum, Watercress, Endive, Carrot, Lettuce, Tomato Banana, Black currants, Grapes Guava, Coconut, Cabbage, Onion Eggplant, Pumpkin, Grapefruit Cantaloupe, Melons, Papaya Turnip, Apple, Apricot, Berries Watermelon, Beetroot, Celery Cucumber, Radish, Rhubarb, Pear Peach, Jujube, Quince, Limes
VITAMIN B2 ESSENTIAL ASSOCIATED NUTRIENTS FOR EFFECTIVE ABSORPTION: Vitamin C and B group. NUTRIENT INHIBITING FACTORS: Alcohol and tobacco, stress, refined foods and drinks.	Almonds, Wheat germ, Wild rice Mushroom, Safflower seed, Millet Turnip greens, Wheat bran, Kelp Collards, Soya bean, Broad bean Dandelion, Kale leaves, Parsley Cashew nut, Rice bran, Broccoli Sesame seeds, Sunflower seeds White bean, Lentils, Mung bean Rye, Pinto bean, Cowpea, Avocado	Asparagus, Spinach, Red bean Peach, Soya bean sprouts, Prune Lima bean, Broad bean, Pigeon pea Apricot (dr.), Brussel sprouts Chick pea, Sorghum, Endive, Pecan Walnuts, Chive, Mung bean sprouts Peanut, Brazil nut, Sweet corn Wheat, Macadamia nut, Pumpkin Snap beans, Dates, Figs, Kumquat	Cauliflower, Raspberry, Parsnip Raisins, Garlic, Lettuce, Rhubarb Capsicum, Turnip, Barley, Banana Blueberry, Cherry, Sweet potato Currants, Leek, Figs, Guava Oranges, Peaches, Artichoke Beetroot, Carrot, Eggplant, Onion Rice, Apricot, Blackberry, Jujube Papaya, Pear, Cucumber, Potato Tomato, Grapes, Cantaloupe, Melon
VITAMIN B3 ESSENTIAL ASSOCIATED NUTRIENTS FOR EFFECTIVE ABSORPTION: Vitamins: C and B group. NUTRIENT INHIBITING FACTORS: Alcohol and tobacco, stress, refined foods and drinks.	Rice bran, Wheat bran, Peanut Wild rice, Sesame seeds, Kelp Sunflower seeds, Rice, Wheat Mushroom, Wheat germ, Sorghum Barley, Almonds, Mung bean Pumpkin seeds, White bean, Dates Millet, Pinto bean, Cowpea	Soya bean, Kale leaves, Lentils Chick pea, Lima bean, Cashew nut Collards, Sweet corn, Avocado Prune, Brazil nut, Broad bean Rye, Asparagus, Potato, Artichoke Pistachio, Macadamia, Guava Parsley, Mango, Peach, Okra Raspberry, Hazel nut, Pecan nut	Walnut, Broccoli, Brussel sprouts Watercress, Mung+Soya sprouts Turnip greens, Banana, Cauliflower Figs, Tomato, Apricot, Cantaloupe Melons, Strawberry, Carrot, Eggplant, Spinach, Turnip, Plum Raisins, Coconut, Chive, Endive Garlic, Cherry, Oranges, Grapes

VITAMINS FOOD CHARTS

	EXCELLENT SOURCE	GOOD SOURCE	FAIR SOURCE
VITAMIN B5	Peanuts, Cashew nuts, Almonds, Brewers yeast, Torula yeast, Soya beans, Wheat germ, Walnuts, Rice bran, Wheat bran, Pecan, Chestnuts, Pumpkin seeds, Peas	Sesame seeds, Brussel sprouts, Lotus root, Collards, Dates, Cauliflower, Celery, Parsley, Yoghurt, Lentils, Millet, Rice	Royal jelly, Capsicum, Parsnip, Kale, Wheat, Carrots, Barley, Oats, Oranges, Banana, Currants, Dates, Leek, Grapefruit, Grapes
VITAMIN B6	Walnuts, Hazel nuts, Yoghurt, Brewers yeast, Torula yeast, Rice bran, Wheat germ, Millet, Soya beans, Sunflower seeds, Sesame seeds, Wheat bran, Rye	Almonds, Brazil nuts, Chestnut, Peanuts, Pumpkin seeds, Barley, Buckwheat, Oats, Bulgar, Rice, Figs, Olives, Potato, Banana, Cabbage, Lettuce, Celery, Kale	Spinach, Avocado, Capsicum, Broccoli, Watercress, Tomato, Pineapple, Apricots, Grapes, Melons, Black currants, Orange
VITAMIN B12	Yoghurt, Cheese, Fresh fish, -plankton, Milk, Eggs	Fermented foods	Organically grown produce Cauliflower-buds Comfrey, Alfalfa
VITAMIN B15	Apricot kernels, Pumpkin seeds, Brewers yeast, Torula yeast, Rice bran, Sesame seeds, Oats	Wheat germ, Wheat bran, Wheat, Rice, Millet, Rye, Barley, Soya beans, Lentils, Raisins	Sprouted seeds-Grains-Legumes, Fresh vegetables, Fresh fruits
BIOTIN	Walnuts, Almonds, Peanuts, Sesame seeds, Sunflower seeds, Brewers yeast, Torula yeast	Mushrooms, Raisins, Soya beans, Rice, Cucumber, Apples, Wheat, Rye, Bulgar, Black currants, Grapefruit, Melons, Tomato	Cauliflower, Watercress, Leek, Lettuce, Avocado, Banana, Strawberries, Oranges, Corn, Dates, Peas, Beetroot
CHOLINE	Lecithin, Spinach, Asparagus, Green beans, Corn, Soya beans, Brewers yeast, Torula yeast, Sesame seeds, Tahini, Pecan	Wheat, Oats, Wheat germ, Peas, Cabbage, Carrots, Turnips, Peanuts, Rice bran, Potato	Millet, Dates, Sprouted seeds, Sunflower seeds, Almonds, Fresh vegetables, Fresh fruits
FOLIC ACID	Green leafy vegetables, Fresh fruits, Potatoes, Almonds, Cauliflower, Sprouted seeds, legumes	Whole grains, Wheat germ, Asparagus, Beetroot, Peas, Parsnips, Kale, Broccoli	Pears, Apples, Avocado, Sweet corn, Brewers yeast, Soya beans, Lima beans

VITAMIN B1

– Thiamine – water soluble

Essential for the health of the entire nervous system.

The body can only store limited amounts of Thiamine, and it must be obtained regularly from the diet, so as to remain in good health. During times of depression, worry, and any negative emotional stress, the body rapidly uses its reserves of this vitamin. These negative emotions cause a substance to leave the body's glands which destroys B1 on contact.

Essential for the proper functioning of the digestive system, especially when carbohydrates and fats are eaten. The more starches and sugars that are eaten, the more Thiamine required.

Assists the body to utilize energy from carbohydrate foods.

Soluble in water, insoluble in fats. and easily lost by heat and cooking.

Aids growth of young children and teenagers. Vit B1 helps the young.

As a result of strenuous exercise, the amounts of thiamine should be increased. White rice and refined foods are Thiamine deficient.

During fevers or periods of pregnancy and lactation, the amounts of Vit B1 should be increased. Thiamine prevents accumulations of fat in the arteries.

Alcohol, depletes the reserves of this vitamin from the body. Try a B1 drink.

The heart may also suffer, due to a deficiency, resulting in shortness of breath and irregular heartbeat.

Usual symptoms are, lack of initiative, poor appetite, depression, irritability, poor memory, tendency to tire easily, lack of concentration, swelling of the ankles. A Vitamin B1 deficiency can affect your entire health.

A Thiamine deficiency may also result in a lack of Oxygen absorption by the blood, which leads to poor mental alertness and inability to learn and concentrate. Thiamine is required by the Stomach to produce Hcl, essential for the digestion of protein foods. Wheat germ is a protein food also rich in Thiamine. Most fresh vegetables provide adequate supplies of Thiamine.

VITAMIN B1 FOR HEALTHY NERVES.

SOMATIC NERVES	AUTOMATIC NERVES.	
CONTROLS THE SENSE ORGANS AND MUSCULAR ACTION.	CONTROLS THE GLANDS, HEART, INTESTINES AND SEX ORGANS.	

SENSORY	MOTOR	SYMPA-THETIC	PARA-SYMPA-THETIC
EYES	MUSCULAR ACTION	DIGESTION	RELAXATION
SKIN		HEART	
EARS		LIVER	
NOSE		LUNGS	SLEEP
MOUTH		PROTECTION	

THIAMINE IS THE MORALE VITAMIN

Rice bran, Wheat germ, Soya bean, Sunflower seeds Cowpea, Peanut, Sesame seeds, Brazil nut, Pecan Pinto bean, Millet, Wheat bran, Pistachio nut White bean, Wheat, Red bean, Broad bean, Lima bean Hazel nuts, Wild rice, Cashew nut, Rye, Pigeon pea Sorghum, Mung bean, Lentils, Peas (fr.) Macadamia nut, Rice, Walnuts, Chestnut, Chick peas Garlic, Almonds, Pumpkin seeds, Soya bean sprouts Turnip greens, Barley, Artichoke, Dandelion Asparagus, Okra, Collard, Kale, Sweet corn Mung bean sprouts, Parsley, Avocado, Raisins, Figs

VITAMIN B2

— Riboflavin — water soluble

Vitamin B2 is essential for good eyesight, healthy skin and cellular growth, which promotes a youthful complexion and makes it easy to stay and look young.

Soluble in water, stable to heat and oxidation and fairly sensitive to light.

Only a limited amount can be stored by the body and therefore it should be obtained regularly from the diet.

Vitamin B2 is required by the stomach to assist the secretion of essential Gastric juices, absorption of all nutrients — Proteins, Carbohydrates, Fats.

Vitamin B2 is essential for cell respiration and nerve tissue repair.(Spinal Cord).

Vitamin B 2 increases life expectancy, promotes general health, promotes rate of growth for children and provides extra stamina and vitality for adults.

Riboflavin is absorbed through the walls of the small intestine and then carried by the blood to all tissues of the body. Any excess is excreted in the urine. Of all the B Group Vitamins, Riboflavin is most likely to be deficient.

A deficiency of Vit. B2, exists amongst people who regularly consume alcohol.

A lack of can result in retarded growth, premature ageing, skin disorders, dimness of vision, cataract symptoms and intolerance to bright light.

A lack of can also result in baldness and falling hair. 'B2 for you Sir.'

A deficiency can also lead to dermatitis, cracked lips and sore mouth, acne, oily skin and ulcers.

Riboflavin is essential, especially during periods of lactation, otherwise a hair and weight loss will result, also affecting the early development of the child.

The daily requirements of Riboflavin are closely related to body size, metabolism rate, growth rate and intake of Protein & Carbohydrate foods and body stress. Brewers yeast is the richest natural source of Riboflavin or Vitamin B2.

A Riboflavin deficiency, promotes the formation of Arthritic conditions, Parkinsons disease, Influenza, Stomach ulcers, Cancer, Retarded growth, Acne, Dermatitis, various nervous disorders, Diabetes, eye fatigue, Sensitivity to light, Diarrhea and physical exaustion. Vitamin B2 is most important.

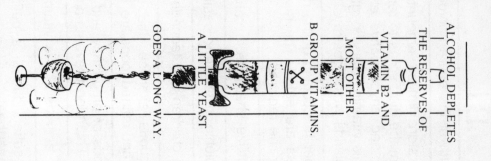

ALCOHOL DEPLETES THE RESERVES OF

VITAMIN B2 AND MOST OTHER

B GROUP VITAMINS.

A LITTLE YEAST

GOES A LONG WAY.

VITAMIN B2 IMPROVES GROWTH OF CHILDREN PROMOTES GOOD EYESIGHT HEALTHY SKIN & HAIR.

VITAMIN B2 HELPS TO SUSTAIN YOUTHFULNESS.

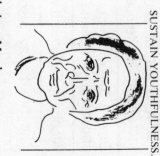

Almonds, Wheat germ, Wild rice, Mushroom Safflower seed, Millet, Turnip greens, Wheat bran Kelp, Collards, Soya bean, Broad bean (dr.) Dandelion, Kale leaves, Parsley, Cashew nut Rice bran, Broccoli, Sesame seeds, Sunflower seeds White bean, Lentils, Mung bean, Rye, Pinto bean Cowpea, Avocado, Asparagus, Spinach, Red bean Peach, Soya bean sprouts, Prune, Lima bean Broad bean, Pigeon pea, Apricot (dr.) Brussel sprouts, Chick pea, Sorghum, Endive, Pecan Walnuts, Chive, Mung bean sprouts, Peanut

VITAMIN B3

— Niacinamide — water soluble

Vitamin B3 assists the body to perform energy producing reactions in all cells.

Vit.B3 activates enzymes in the body, nourishes the nerves, brain, skin and hair.

Essential for normal functioning of the stomach and intestines. A lack of can result in varied digestive disturbances such as vomiting, diarrhea, constipation and indigestion. Niacin assists the functions of digestive enzymes.

Vitamin B3 helps to control the release of fats from the body and regulates the fat levels of the blood, which can prevent high Cholesterol and heart attacks.

Is essential for the efficient use of protein. (Meat, Fish, Nuts, Seeds, Grains.)

Vit.B3 helps promote a peaceful nights sleep. No need for sleeping tablets.

Strenuous exercise depletes the reserves of B3. (Mental & Physical)

A deficiency of Vit.B3 can result in mental depression, personality changes and an extreme deficiency can result in promoting various mental disorders.

Niacin is slightly soluble in water, stable to heat, oxidation, light, acidity and alkalinity. Niacin is not as easily destroyed by cooking as other B group vitamins.

Niacin is essential for good blood circulation and reducing blood cholesterol levels. An excess consumption of refined sugar and Carbohydrate refined products, will lead to a Niacin deficiency. Green vegetables will restore health.

Niacin is an essential ingredient for the production of both male and female sex hormones. Wheat germ is also an excellent source of Niacin.

A mild Niacin deficiency, may show as, Muscular weakness, general fatigue, indigestion, poor appetite and numerous types of skin allergies.

The Amino Acid Tryptophan can be converted by the body into Niacin.

Niacin is an essential ingredient for nearly every reaction, in the process of : Digestion and normal Metabolism of Carbohydrates, Fats and Proteins.

A severe Niacin deficiency, may lead to Ulcers, irritability, recurring headaches, dermatitis, diarrhea, Cancer sores, Artheriosclerosis, Diabetes, loss of hair, Arthritis and Parkinsons disease. A whole grain breakfast cereal will supply B3.

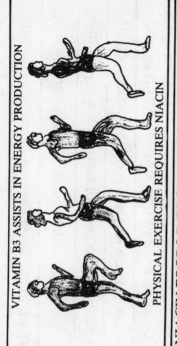

VITAMIN B3 ASSISTS IN ENERGY PRODUCTION

PHYSICAL EXERCISE REQUIRES NIACIN

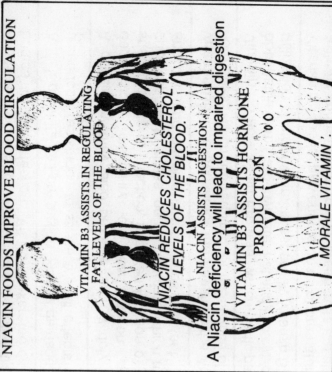

NIACIN FOODS IMPROVE BLOOD CIRCULATION

VITAMIN B3 ASSISTS IN REGULATING FAT LEVELS OF THE BLOOD

NIACIN REDUCES CHOLESTEROL LEVELS OF THE BLOOD.

NIACIN ASSISTS DIGESTION. A Niacin deficiency will lead to impaired digestion

VITAMIN B3 ASSISTS HORMONE PRODUCTION

'MORALE VITAMIN'.

Rice bran, Wheat bran, Peanut, Wild rice Sesame seeds, Kelp, Sunflower seeds, Rice, Wheat Mushroom, Wheat germ, Sorghum, Barley, Almonds Mung bean, Pumpkin seeds, White bean, Dates Millet, Pinto bean, Cowpea, Soya bean, Kale leaves Lentils, Chick pea, Lima bean, Cashew nut, Collards Sweet corn, Avocado, Prune, Brazil nut, Broad bean Rye, Asparagus, Potato, Artichoke, Pistachio Macadamia, Guava, Parsley, Mango, Peach, Okra

VITAMIN B5

— Panthothenic acid — water soluble

Vitamin B5 is found in every living cell of the body. Panto means 'everywhere'.

Vitamin B5 is essential for proper digestion, especially the breakdown of fats.

Vitamin B5 is important for the body's control and use of Cholesterol from fats.

Vit.B5 improves a poor memory and protects the body in times of stress.

Vitamin B5, taken daily, can improve the condition of skin, eyes, hair and nerves.

A deficiency leads to, ulcers in the digestive tract and failure to produce anti-bodies to fight infection. Vit.B5 is excreted daily via the urine.

A lack of white cell production, kidney damage, heart trouble, headaches and a reduced resistance to stress are all effects of a deficiency of Vitamin B5.

A deficiency may also produce such widely varied symptoms as, apathy, depression, instability of heart action, abdominal pains, increased susceptability to infection, impaired function of the adrenal glands which help one respond to stress, nerve disorders which may produce muscle weakness and pins and needles in the hands and feet. Vit.B5 is required daily.

Vitamin B5 is essential for the health of the Adrenal glands and the Adrenal hormones, which are required for maintenance of healthy skin and nerves.

Vitamin B5 acts as an Enzyme, which participates in the utilization of energy, obtainable from Carbohydrate, Fat and Protein foods. B5 is also essential for the utilization of other vitamins especially Vitamin B2. Sesame seeds are excellent.

Vitamin B5 foods prevent the onset of premature aging, wrinkly skin, baldness, Arthritis and retarded growth. Fresh fruits are also a good source of Vitamin B5.

Vitamin B5 has been used effectively in reducing the toxic side effects of many antibiotics and also protects the body against cellular damage, from radiation.

Be sure to obtain some Vit B5 natural foods daily. If you have never tried the taste of Sunflower seeds, Sesame seeds, Tahini , you'll be in for a real treat . Their not just health foods, but foods which have and give a whole lot of Life.

Vitamin B5 has beneficial effects for the following ailments: Anemia, Hypoglycemia, Epilepsy, Insomnia, Arthritis, Asthma, Cancer and Tuberculosis.

Frozen foods are deficient in Vit.B5.

A DEFICIENCY OF VITAMIN B5 MAY LEAD TO LOSS OF HAIR AND MUSCULAR WEAKNESS.

VITAMIN B5 IMPROVES DIGESTION.

VITAMIN B5 STIMULATES THE ADRENAL GLANDS TO PRODUCE *NATURAL CORTISONE* 'AND OTHER ADRENAL HORMONES, WHICH ARE ESSENTIAL FOR HEALTHY NERVES AND SKIN.

ADRENALIN PROTECTS THE BODY IN TIMES OF STRESS AND SHOCK.

ADRENAL GLANDS.

VITAMIN B5 IS ESSENTIAL FOR THE HEALTH OF THE ADRENAL GLANDS

Sesame seeds, Brussel sprouts, Lotus root, Collards Dates, Cauliflower, Celery, Parsley, Yoghurt, Lentils Millet, Rice, Royal jelly, Capsicum, Parsnip, Kale Wheat, Carrots, Barley, Oats, Oranges, Banana Currants, Dates, Leek, Grapefruit, Grapes

VITAMIN B6 — *Pyridoxine Hydrochloride — water soluble*

Vitamin B6 assists in the formation of red blood cells and the healthy activity of the nervous system. Vit B6 is also essential for the production of Anti—bodies.

Vitamin B6 is water soluble and required regularly from the diet.

Vitamin B6 is often termed the VITALITY VITAMIN.

Vitamin B6 is essential for the conversion of Protein foods into Amino—Acids.

Especially important in the first few months of infancy and protects the mother and child against the effects of anaesthetics and nausea of pregnancy.

Protects against the formation of kidney stones, as B6 is involved in converting Oxalic acid into a harmless form. Also helps to produce the hormone Adrenalin, which is used up under stress.

Vitamin B6 foods control pre—mensturation problems of acne.

Vit B6 is required for the conversion of the Amino Acid Tryptophan, into Niacin.

Vit B6 protects against the harmful effects of Gamma radiation and X rays.

Alcohol, oral contraceptives and the Pill all cause a severe loss of Vitamin B6.

A lack of B6 may lead to irritability, oversensitivity, adrenal exaustion and Ulcers.

A lack of results in headaches, weak concentration, poor memory, general decline of intelligence and unhealthy nerves. The master gland of the body, the Pituitary gland, is also affected when B6 is not properly supplied through the diet, by abnormal metabolism, which affects the entire body's health.

A lack of may result in anaemia, convulsions, nervousness of the hands, numbness, tender gums and has been used effectively in cases of Parkinsons disease, arthritis, visual fatigue and cataracts.

Vitamin B6 is required for the absorption of Vitamin B12 and for the production of vital Gastric juices (Stomach). Wheat germ is an excellent source of Vit B6.

Vitamin B6 helps to maintain a balance of minerals, Potassium & Sodium, which is essential for the health of the entire nervous system. Fresh fruits contain B6.

75% OF THE B6 CONTENT OF WHOLE WHEAT IS LOST DURING PROCSSING.

VITAMIN B6 IS ESSENTIAL FOR THE HEALTH OF THE NERVOUS SYSTEM

VITAMIN B6 IS VITAL FOR EFFICIENT FUNCTIONING OF THE BRAIN

PITUITARY GLAND

VITAMIN B6 Is ESSENTIAL ESPECIALLY DURING PREGNANCY

FASTING AND WEIGHT REDUCING DIETS WILL QUICKLY DEPLETE YOUR BODY RESERVES OF VITAMIN B6 AND MOST OTHER WATER SOLUBLE VITAMINS.

VITAMIN B6 PROTECTS MOTHER AND CHILD

Vit B6 is essential for the synthesis and proper functioning of D.N.A. & R.N.A. which are genes that are capable of passing on hereditary characteristics.

Walnuts, Hazel nuts, Yoghurt, Brewers yeast Torula yeast, Rice bran, Wheat germ, Millet Soya beans, Sunflower seeds, Sesame seeds Wheat bran, Rye, Almonds, Brazil nuts, Chestnut Peanuts, Pumpkin seeds, Barley, Buckwheat, Oats Bulgar, Rice, Figs, Olives, Potato, Banana, Cabbage Lettuce, Celery, Kale, Spinach, Avocado, Capsicum Broccoli, Watercress, Tomato, Pineapple, Apricots Grapes, Melons, Black currants, Orange

VITAMIN B12

— Cyanocobalamin — slightly water soluble

Vitamin B12 is required for normal functioning of the nerves and also for the metabolism of Fats, Proteins and Carbohydrates. Vitamin B12 also assists the action of Vitamin C, B5 and the mineral Iron.

Required amounts per day are only, 141 thousand-millionth of an ounce.

A dietary deficiency of Vit.B12 may not show up for 5–10 years as the body is capable of re–absorbing sufficient amounts of B12, from the intestinal tract, which therby reduces the need for a regular supply. An abundance of Folic Acid foods, such as green leafy vegetables, Brewers yeast and nuts, can prevent the possibility of blood cell retardation, when a diet is low in Vit.B12

Vitamin B12 is the only Vitamin that plants cannot synthesize and their source of B12 is not essential but often available from bacteria & fungi in the soil. All animals except Humans, can synthesize their own supply of Vit.B12.

Vitamin B12 is the only vitamin which contains a mineral element – Cobalt.

Essential for the normal functioning of all the body's cells. A severe deficiency will lead to a case of pernicious anaemia, a condition in which the body produces insufficient or defective red cells. Vitamin B12 is water soluble

Vitamin B12 is a heat sensitive vitamin. Up to 85% of the B12 content of meat is lost in the process of cooking. It has recently been discovered that the ultimate source of B12, was with certain bacteria which are formed in the lower Intestines, by the eating of natural foods, which encourage the development and absorption of Vitamin B12.

Laxatives can seriously deplete the reserves of B12 and many other nutrients.

Vitamin B12 has been used effectively in providing relief from the following symptons: Fatigue, Nervous irritability, poor memory and concentration.

Vitamin B12 may also be effective in treating conditions of Anemia, Asthma, Ulcers, Angina Pectoris, Diabetes and Neuritis.

Vitamin B12 is essential for the functioning of most body cells and for control of the Genetic Nucleic acids, such as D.N.A. & R.N.A. A deficiency of Vit.B12 may prevent genetic cells from dividing properly. Immature red blood cells are a often the result and also fewer red blood cell production occurs, resulting in muscular weakness. Folic Acid especially is closely related to efficient functioning of B12.

VITAMIN B12 IS ABSORBED FROM THE SMALL INTESTINE AND THEN STORED IN THE LIVER

VITAMIN B12 ASSISTS IN THE FORMATION OF RED BLOOD CELLS, WHICH MAINLY OCCURS IN THE BONE MARROW.

Vitamin B12 has been a most controversial topic, with many ideas related to the eating of meat. A Strict Vegetarian: one who never eats meat or any Animal Origin produce will surely have an imbalance of Vit B12 in relation to all other vitamins. On the other hand a person who regularly eats meat has even more problems to worry about. Vit B12 canbe stored by the body for up to three years, which relates closely to evolutionary progress of man. from the times of being a pure vegetarian animal and the slow transition into the slaughter of animals for food and survival. Nowadays meat eating is on the increase and often excessive, with hospitals full of proof. If your family has been eating meat for many generations, your body and mind might also be adjusted to continue without any hesitation. Changes in human nutrition are slow but steady. The occasional eating of meat with a well balanced meal is a good way to get Vit B12 and Protein. Excess eating of meat is a dangerous way to live.

Yoghurt, Cheese, Fresh fish -plankton, Eggs, Milk, Comfrey, Alfalfa, Green leafy vegetables Fermented foods, Organically grown produce Cauliflower-buds

VITAMIN B15

— Pangamic acid — water soluble

Vitamin B15 improves the body's capacity to utilize energy from food thereby providing extra strength, physical & mental energy and self repair abilities.

Vitamin B15 is a good preventative of premature aging, as it improves the body's ability to use oxygen and also improves the circulation of the blood.

Protects against possible hardening of the arteries, as it prevents fat particles from accumulating in the bloodstream. Vit B15 assists the heart muscles.

Vitamin B15 Assists the healing of abrasions and cuts.

Vitamin B15 is more effective when all other B group Vitamins are also

Works as a detoxyfying agent against possible cancer causing chemicals and other forms of environmental poisons and pollutants. (Plastic Containers).

Helps to stabilize emotional and mental problems with its beneficial qualities and effects on the nervous system. (Brewers yeast is excellent).

Beneficial qualities are closely related to all of the B group vitamins.

Vitamin B15 is a water soluble vitamin required regularly from the diet.

Vitamin B15 prevents against the harmful effects of carbon monoxide pollution.

The effectiveness of Vitamin B15 is improved and reliant on Vitamin A & E.

Vitamin B15 stimulates the glandular system, which improves the entire body's performance. Sunflower seeds are also a valuable source of B15.

Vitamin B15 has proved effective in treatment of high blood pressure and for lowering cholesterol levels of the blood. Fresh vegetables contain Vitamin B15.

Excessive perspiration causes a great loss of Vitamin B15.

Vitamin B15 has provided good results in the treatment of Rheumatism, Angina heart troubles, asthma, hypertension, Emphesema, alcoholism and Cancer.

Vitamin B15 may also be beneficial for the treatment of Cirrhosis of the Liver, Hepatitis, High Cholesterol, Arteriosclerosis, Headaches, Emotional & Mental Stress and Hypertension. Freshly made vegetable juices are most beneficial.

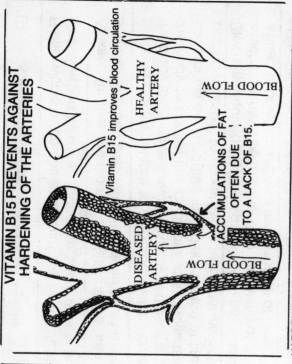

VITAMIN B15 PREVENTS AGAINST HARDENING OF THE ARTERIES

Vitamin B15 improves blood circulation

HEALTHY ARTERY

BLOOD FLOW

ACCUMULATIONS OF FAT OFTEN DUE TO A LACK OF B15.

DISEASED ARTERY

BLOOD FLOW

HARDENING OF THE ARTERIES LEADS TO HIGH BLOOD PRESSURE.

Vitamin B15, was originally found and extracted from apricot kernels.

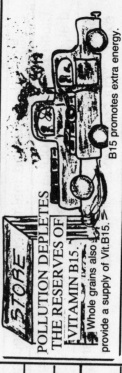

B15 promotes extra energy.

POLLUTION DEPLETES THE RESERVES OF VITAMIN B15.

Whole grains also provide a supply of Vit.B15.

VITAMIN B15 HAS SHOWN TO BE A PREVENTATIVE SUBSTANCE IN THE TREATMENT OF CANCER. NORMAL BODY CELLS NEED OXYGEN. CANCER CELLS CAN LIVE WITHOUT OXYGEN. VIT B15 INCREASES THE BODY'S ABILITY TO USE OXYGEN.

Apricot kernels, Pumpkin seeds, Brewers yeast Torula yeast, Rice bran, Sesame seeds, Oats Wheat germ, Wheat bran, Wheat, Rice, Millet, Rye Barley, Soya beans, Sprouted seeds-Grains-Legumes Lentils, Raisins, Fresh vegetables, Fresh fruits

BIOTIN

— Vitamin H — water soluble

Biotin is essential for normal cellular growth of all body tissues.

Biotin works in combination with the Amino Acid Lysine, for the distribution of CO_2, Carbon Dioxide around the body, mainly from the lungs.

Assists in the breakdown of fatty foods into glucose, a usable energy source. A Biotin deficiency may lead to an overweight condition.

Biotin is closely related to all Bgroup Vitamins, especially Choline. They assist the body to produce a natural supply of the substance.Lec i thin,which is used by the body to control the levels of Fat & Cholesterol in the bloodstream. Lec i thin is an important ingredient for the entire nervous system & brain. Lec i thin assists the body to produce Energy. Soy Milk & Beans contain Lec i thin

Biotin is required for those people who have continual problems with digestion, which may have been caused by the taking of Antibiotics, Mineral oil or Raw egg white, all of which deplete the reserves of Biotin.

Most modern cereals and refined food products have their Biotin content removed entirely by the processes of refinement. (Whole foods give Life).

Biotin is essentiaI for normal cellular growth of all body tissues and cells.

Biotin foods assist the maintenance, repair and growth of bones.

Biotin is a water soluble vitamin which should be obtained regularly from the diet, to ensure maximum health. Green leafy vegetables are excellent.

Biotin can be synthesized from intestinal bacteria, when favourable conditions exist. Your body needs fruit to keep clean inside.

Biotin is required for the utilization of nutrients from protein, Folic acid, Vit B5 and Vitamin B12. There's no use eating meat for protein when the body is incapable of using it. Biotin and all the B vitamins work in harmony.

Additional amounts of Biotin are required for mothers, during pregnancy and times of lactation. Do your baby a favour and eat the right foods.

A deficiency may lead to lack of appetite, inability to sleep, muscular pains, and nervousness. A Biotin deficiency may also lead to cot—death.

A Biotin deficiency can also lead to dermatitis, mental depression and baldness.

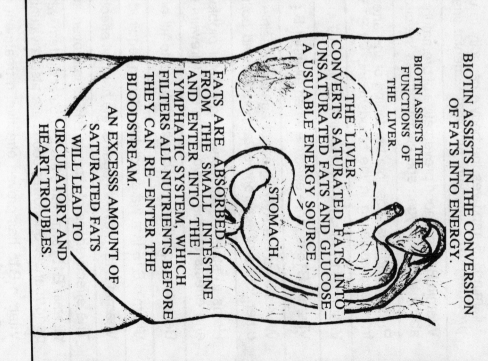

BIOTIN ASSISTS IN THE CONVERSION OF FATS INTO ENERGY.

BIOTIN ASSISTS THE FUNCTIONS OF THE LIVER.

A USABLE ENERGY SOURCE.

CONVERTS SATURATED FATS INTO UNSATURATED FATS AND GLUCOSE—

THE LIVER

STOMACH.

FATS ARE ABSORBED FROM THE SMALL INTESTINE AND ENTER INTO THE LYMPHATIC SYSTEM, WHICH FILTERS ALL NUTRIENTS BEFORE THEY CAN RE-ENTER THE BLOODSTREAM.

AN EXCESSS AMOUNT OF SATURATED FATS WILL LEAD TO CIRCULATORY AND HEART TROUBLES.

Walnuts, Almonds, Peanuts, Sesame seeds Sunflower seeds, Brewers yeast, Torula yeast Mushrooms, Raisins, Soya beans, Rice, Cucumber Apples, Wheat, Rye, Bulgar, Black currants Grapefruit, Melons, Tomato, Cauliflower, Watercress Leek, Lettuce, Avocado, Banana, Strawberries Oranges, Corn, Dates, Peas, Beetroot

CHOLINE

— very soluble in water

Choline assists in the digestion of all types of fatty foods.

Assists the rebuilding of damaged kidneys, liver and the muscles of the brain and heart. Choline foods also strengthen weak blood capilaries.

Is required for the storage of many vitamins and minerals, especially Calcium and Vit A. Protein is also essential for effective Choline intake.

A lack of Choline has a direct relationship to the cholesterol levels of the blood. Lecithin is a substance that the body produces only when there is sufficient amounts of Choline and the other B complex vitamins.

A deficiency is a factor responsible for high blood pressure, hardening of the arteries and also a tendency for accumulation of excessive weight.

Alcohol consumption increases the need for extra Choline intake.

Is usually found in good amounts and combination with all Vit B enriched foods. Choline is only effective when combined with other B complex vitamins.

Choline foods prevent the accumulation of fats in the Liver and promote even distribution of fats around the body, to all the various cells.

Choline is essential for the health of the entire nervous system. Choline plays an important role in the transmitting of nerve impulses, throughout the entire body.

Choline foods assist the functions of the Liver and Gallbladder and prevent the formation of gall stones. Lecethin is an excellent source of Choline.

Choline can be synthesized by intestinal bacteria with the essential ingredients Folic acid, B12 and the amino acid Methinone.

Choline foods are a natural fat and cholesterol dissolver.

Choline foods may also be beneficial for any of the following ailments: High High Cholesterol, Hepatitis, Hypoglycemia, Dizziness, Multiple Sclerosis, loss of hair, Glaucoma, Asthma, Excema, Alcoholism and Muscular dystrophy.

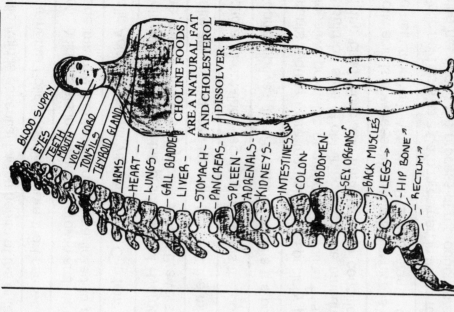

CHOLINE FOODS ARE A NATURAL FAT AND CHOLESTEROL DISSOLVER.

BLOOD SUPPLY
EYES
TEETH
MOUTH
VOCAL CORD
TONSILS
THYROID GLAND
ARMS
HEART
LUNGS
GALL BLADDER
LIVER
STOMACH
PANCREAS
SPLEEN
ADRENALS
KIDNEYS
INTESTINES
COLON
ABDOMEN
SEX ORGANS
BACK MUSCLES
LEGS
HIP BONE
RECTUM

CHOLINE IS REQUIRED FOR THE TRANSMITTING OF NERVE IMPULSES, FROM THE SPINAL CORD TO ALL AREAS OF THE BODY.

Lecithin, Spinach, Asparagus, Green beans, Corn Soya beans, Brewers yeast, Torula yeast Sesame seeds, Tahini, Pecan, Wheat, Oats Wheat germ, Peas, Cabbage, Carrots, Turnips Peanuts, Rice bran, Potato, Millet, Dates Sprouted seeds, Sunflower seeds, Almonds Fresh vegetables, Fresh fruits

FOLIC ACID

— Vitamin Bc — M — water soluble

Folic Acid is essential for the health of the entire nervous system. (Spinal cord).

The name Folic is derived from the Latin word for Foliage or leaf, (Folium).

Folic acid assists in the proper growth and reproduction of red blood cells, in the bone marrow. Leukemia has been linked to a severe deficiency of Folic acid.

Folic Acid works with Vitamin B12 & C to form body Protein and red blood cells.

Folic acid stimulates the production of Hydrochloric acid, which is essential for the conversion of any protein foods. Brewers yeast is an excellent source.

Folic acid is required for absorption of the minerals Iron and Calcium.

Folic acid obtained regularly, prevents the possibility of fatal anemia.

Contraceptives, the Pill rapidly deplete the body's reserves of Folic acid.

Infants require more than adults, especially premature babies and those with digestive problems or when an infection has developed. All pregnant women should be sure of obtaining adequate amounts to assist healthy development of the child. Folic acid improves the condition of the hair and skin.

Folic acid is a water soluble vitamin, which is required regularly from the diet in combination with Vitamins B12 and vitamin C, to breakdown protein foods.

Folic acid acts as a Carbon carrier, in the formation of new red blood cells and is also needed in the process of reproduction and all cellular growth.

Folic acid is essential in the formation of genetic cells, D.N.A. & R.N.A. These cells cannot divide properly if Folic acid is lacking from the diet.

Folic acid is destroyed by high temperatures, cooking and lengthy storage.

Folic acid is required for the prevention of blood disorders. A prolonged Folic acid deficiency may lead to Leukemia, Arthritis, Arteriosclerosis, Mental and physical fatigue, Glandular exaustion and Ulcers.

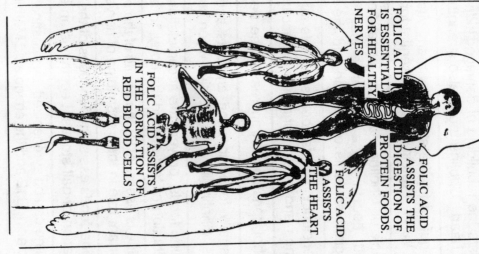

FOLIC ACID FOR HEALTHY NERVES

FOLIC ACID IS ESSENTIAL FOR HEALTHY NERVES

FOLIC ACID ASSISTS THE DIGESTION OF PROTEIN FOODS.

FOLIC ACID ASSISTS THE HEART

FOLIC ACID ASSISTS IN THE FORMATION OF RED BLOOD CELLS

Green leafy vegetables, Fresh fruits, Potatoes Almonds, Cauliflower, Sprouted seeds, legumes Whole grains, Wheat germ, Asparagus, Beetroot Peas, Parsnips, Kale, Broccoli, Pears, Apples Avocado, Sweet corn, Brewers yeast, Soya beans Lima beans

INOSITOL
— soluble in water

Assists the action of the heart by cleansing the blood of excessive fats.

A lack of Inositol has a deteriorating effect on the health of the nerves.

Is destroyed by a continual use of caffeine drinks.

Insufficient amounts of Inositol, may lead to loss of hair and baldness.

A common ingredient of modern pesticides is called Lidane, which kills insects by paralyzing the vital amounts of Inositol in their bodies. Similar affects are caused to the human body's supply of Inositol, which is severly depleted by the effects of insect sprays.

Inositol promotes the body's ability, to produce Lecethin, which assists in disolving fats and reducing blood cholesterol levels.

An Inositol deficiency, may also lead to: constipation, eczema and heart disease. Inositol foods have a stimulating effect for digestive action.

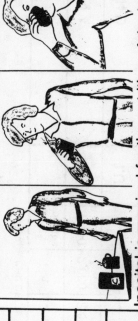

INOSITOL IS DESTROYED WITH CONTINUAL COFFEE DRINKING

Inositol is required for the nutrition of the brain cells

Oranges, Grapefruit, Lemons, Brewers yeast Tomato, Sprouted seeds, Watermelon, Beetroot Banana, Apples, Wheat, Wheat germ, Lecithin Green leafy vegetables, Fresh fruits, Molasses Whole grains, Legumes

P.A.B.A.
— Para-aminobenzoic acid — water soluble

When this B group vitamin is lacking from the diet its main effect is on the colour of the hair, which usually tends to turn a shade of grey or even completely white.

P.A.B.A. is essential for the synthesis of Folic acid, which combines in preventing such problems as fading hair colour and skin pigment disorders.

P.A.B.A. assists the breakdown and use of Protein foods.

Is effective in treating the skin condition known as Vitiligo, where the skin pigment is completely lost leaving large patches of white skin.

P.A.B.A. is a water soluble vitamin, required regularly from the diet.

P.A.B.A. is also required in the formation of red blood cells.

P.A.B.A. can be synthesized, when favourable conditions exist.

P.A.B.A. is often used in some modern suncreams.

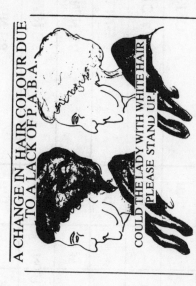

A CHANGE IN HAIR COLOUR DUE TO A LACK OF P.A.B.A.

COULD THE LADY WITH WHITE HAIR PLEASE STAND UP.

UNEVEN SKIN PIGMENT DUE TO A LACK OF P.A.B.A.

EXCELLENT SOURCE	GOOD SOURCE
CITRUS FRUITS BLACK CURRANTS FRESH VEGETABLES SPROUTED SEEDS	FRESH FRUITS WHOLE GRAINS

VITAMINS – R.D.A. CHART

		CHILDREN			GIRLS							BOYS			MEN	
		0–6 months	1–3	4–6	11–14	15–18	19–22	23–50	Pregnant	Lactating	51+ over.	11–14	15–18	19–22	23–50	51+
VITAMIN A	I.U.	1,400	2,000	2,500	3,300	—	4,000	—	5,000	6,000	4,000	—	—	—	5,000	—
VITAMIN D	I.U.	400	—	—	—	400	—	—	—	400	—	400	—	—	400	—
VITAMIN E	I.U.	4	7	9.0	10	12	12	—	15	15	12	15	15	—	15	15
VITAMIN C	mg.	35	40	40	40	45	45	45	60	80	45	45	45	45	45	45
VITAMIN B1	mg.	0.3	0.7	0.9	1.2	1.2	1.1	1.0	+.3	0.5	1.1	1.4	1.5	1.5	1.2	1.2
VITAMIN B2	mg.	0.4	0.8	1.1	1.2	1.3	1.4	1.4	1.2	+.3	0.5	1.1	1.5	1.5	1.6	1.5
VITAMIN B3	mg.	9.0	12	16	16	14	14	13	+2	+4	12	18	20	18	16	16
VITAMIN B5	mg.	No R.D.A. available.					5–10								5–10	
VITAMIN B6	mg.	0.3	0.6	0.9	1.2	1.6	2.0	2.0	2.5	na.	2.0	2.0	2.0	2.0	2.0	2.0
CHOLINE	mg.				500–900				500–900						500–900	
FOLIC ACID	mg.	0.5	0.1	0.2	0.3	0.4	0.4	0.4	0.8	0.5	0.4	0.4	0.4	0.4	0.4	0.4
INOSITOL	mg.						1,000mg.			1,000mg.					1,000mg.	
P.A.B.A.	mg.	NO R.D.A. available.							NO R.D.A. available.						NO R.D.A. available.	
BIOTIN	mcg.				150–300				150–300						150–300	
VITAMIN B12	mcg.	0.3	1.0	1.5	2.0	3.0	3.0	3.0	4.0	4.0	3.0	3.0	4.0	4.0	3.0	3.0
VITAMIN K	mcg.	300–500			300–500				300–500						300–500	

CHAPTER SEVEN

SUMMARY

DIETARY GUIDE INTRODUCTION

GUATEMALA

CARROTS
GUICOY
PAPAYA
PINEAPPLE

BLACK BEANS
TORTILLAS

CHEESE

CHARD
BLACK BEANS
TORTILLAS

CHEESE
CHICKEN

AFRICA

MILK

MEAT

MILK

BLOOD

MEAT

MILK

WILD FRUITS

POLYNESIA

TARO
TARO LEAVES COCONUTS
BREAD-FRUIT LIMES

BANANAS

COCONUTS

FISH

UNITED STATES

SOFT DRINKS
PROCESSED FOOD

BUTTER
MILK

CORN

WHEAT
BREAD CARROTS ORANGES
CORN CUCUMBERS
POTATOES TOMATOES
STRING-BEAN

APPLES

BREAD CORN

BEEF
CHEESE
CHICKEN MILK

Central circle

FATS & OILS. 15 – 20%

CARBOHYDRATES. 50% DAILY INTAKE.

PROTEIN. 30 – 40% DAILY INTAKE.

FATS. OILS.
OLIVES. WHEAT GERM OIL. MAYONNAISE.
AVOCADOS. SUNFLOWER OIL. PEANUT OIL.
MACADAMIA NUTS OLIVE OIL.
POLY UNSATURATED OILS.
COCONUT. COTTON SEED OIL.
SEED OILS. SESAME OIL.
VEGETABLE OILS. SOY OIL.
FISH OILS. ALMOND OIL.
COD LIVER OIL.
BACON FAT.
SAFFLOWER OIL.
MARGARINE.
LIVER OIL.

STARCHES.
WHEAT.
CORN.
RICE RYE.
MILLET.
OATS BARLEY.
LENTILS BEANS.
MUNG BEANS.
KIDNEY BEANS.
BROAD BEANS.
POTATOES.
PUMPKIN.
BUCKWHEAT.
CAROB. LIMA BEANS.
WHOLE GRAINS.

VEGETABLES.
ASPARAGUS.
ARTICHOKES.
BEETROOT.
BRUSSEL SPROUTS.
BROCOLI.
CABBAGE.
CAULIFLOWER.
CARROTS.
CELERY.
CORN.
CUCUMBER.
LETTUCE.
MUSHROOMS.
ONIONS.
PARSLEY.
PEAS.
CAPSICUM.
RADISH.
SPROUTS.
TURNIPS.
WATERCRESS.
ZUCCHINI.

Sweet FRUITS.
BANANAS.
DATES RAISINS.
FIGS SULTANAS.
PERSIMMONS.
DRIED FRUITS.

Sub Acid FRUITS.
APPLES.
APRICOTS.
BLACKBERRIES.
BLUEBERRIES.
CHERRIES.
GRAPES.
LYCHEES.
LOGANBERRIES.
RASPBERRIES.
STRAWBERRIES.
NECTARINES.
PAW PAWS.
PEACHES.
PEARS.

Acid FRUITS.
GRAPEFRUIT.
KIWI FRUITS.
LEMONS.
LIMES.
MANDARINS.
ORANGES.
PASSION FRUIT.
PINEAPPLES.
TOMATOES.

MELONS.
CANTELOPES.
WATERMELONS.
HONEYDEW.
MELONS.

PROTEINS. Primary.
ALMONDS. SUNFLOWER SEEDS.
BRAZIL NUTS. BREWERS YEAST TORULA YEAST.
CASHEW NUTS. SESAME SEEDS LIMA BEANS. WHOLE GRAINS.
HAZEL NUTS. SOY BEANS. SOY MILK. TAHINI.
WALNUTS. LECITHIN PUMPKIN SEEDS.
PISTACHIO. CHESTNUTS MACADAMIA NUTS. PECANS.
SPROUTED SEEDS. PEANUTS. WHEAT GERM OIL.

PROTEINS. Secondary.
ANCHOVY. BASS. COD. FLOUNDER. HADDOCK. HERRING. MACKEREL. PERCH PIKE.
SALMON. SHRIMP. SWORDFISH. TROUT. TUNA. HALIBUT. SCALLOPS. WHITEFISH.
CATFISH. CAVIAR. CLAMS. CRAB. DULSE. EEL. FLOUNDER. PRODLESS. KELP.
LOBSTER. OYSTERS.
BEEF. PORK. CHICKEN. LAMB. RABBIT. TURKEY. VEAL. DUCK. QUAIL. GOOSE.
CALF. BACON.
PARMESAN. SWISS. RICOTTA. BLUE VEIN. GOUDA. FETA. COLBY.
CREAM. MOZZARELLA. CHEDDAR. LEYDEN. MEUNSTER. SAMSOE.
ROQUEFORT. PORT. NEUFCHATEL. TILSIT. SKIM MILK.
YOGHURT. EGGS. BUTTER. MILK. GOAT MILK.

AUSTRALIA

SOFT DRINKS
PROCESSED FOOD

BUTTER
CHEESE
MILK

WHEAT
CORN APPLES
BREAD CABBAGE
BEER CARROTS ORANGES
LETTUCE PINEAPPLE
POTATOES TOMATOES

MILK

BEEF
CHEESE
CHICKEN
EGGS
LAMB

INDIA

CHAPATI
DAHL

BUTTER
CHEESE
MILK

CABBAGE ORANGES
CARROTS PEARS
POTATOES MANGOES

GHEE
LAMB

RICE

LAMB

DAHL CURDS
CHAPATI

FRANCE

WINE

CHEESE

BREAD
BLETTE

ARTICHOKES
CARROTS
LETTUCE
POTATOES TOMATOES
TURNIPS

BREAD
CHEESE

CHICKEN
SNAILS

JAPAN

SOYA BEAN
-KELP

RAW-COOKED FISH

RICE

SOYA
BEAN SOUP

ONIONS

MANDARIN
ORANGES

STRAWBERRIES

RAW-COOKED FISH
SHRIMP
SEAWEED-KELP

SOYA BEAN

YOUR DIET CHART

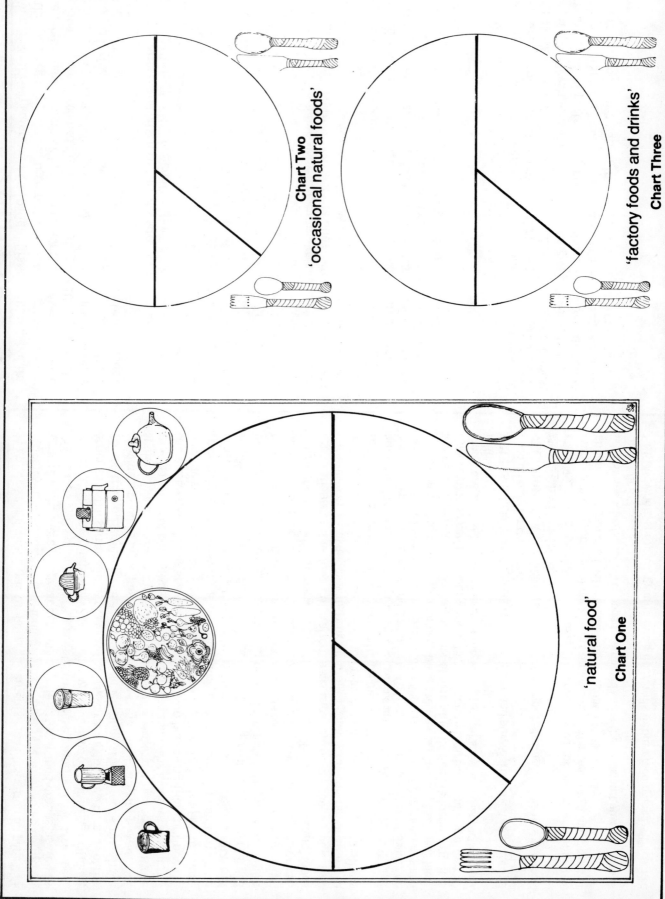

'natural food'

Chart One

Chart Two
'occasional natural foods'

'factory foods and drinks'
Chart Three

DIETARY GUIDE INTRODUCTION

In order to obtain your own summary of nutrition, firstly make a list of the basic foods that you regularly obtain, then place those foods into either the carbohydrate food group, protein or lipid group, some foods are associated with more than one group, refer to the illustration on page 16 for full details on food groups. After placing those 'basic foods' into chart one, also place those natural foods that you may occasionally eat, into chart two. For those people who are obtaining 'other food': processed, refined and snack foods, place those foods into chart three. Most processed and refined foods are grouped as carbohydrates and fats, if you are not sure of the food group, think about the origin of the food, possibly a combination of a few foods and related to one main natural-food-ingredient. After listing those foods in their groups; you will obtain a valuable visual understanding of the diet you have and by refering to the pages describing the natural foods you obtain (the main nutritional benefits are mentioned) there may be numerous other benefits associated with those natural foods and by referring to the nutrient evaluation charts and the chapters on minerals and vitamins, you can obtain a better understanding about the benefits of those natural foods in relation to their nutritional qualities. Apart from the nutrients in food, the taste-appeal of food has an important role in guiding your dietary intake and as many 'factory foods' are specially prepared to excite the taste buds, often due to an excess sugar and fat content. You may be tempted to over-indulge in those foods and unfortunately obtain a poor supply of natural whole foods and their essential life nutrients: minerals, vitamins and enzymes. Once the taste buds have become addicted to such 'factory food products', there may be little chance for natural foods to provide their unique, often subtle taste qualities, as well as their valuable supply of nutrients and living benefits, unless, a better understanding of health is recognized and the variety of natural foods used as the alternative.

Introduction to food combination charts: this last chapter of the book is designed to assist you with the preparation of natural meals, drinks and snacks. There are five main food combination charts – pages 203, 205, 207, 209 and 211; these charts display those food combinations that are most suitable for human digestion and also for their taste-appeal. On pp. 18, 19, 85, 125 and various other parts of this book, the processes of food digestion and metabolism are explained and that will provide vital knowledge about the reasons for proper food combination in order to obtain maximum benefits from a meal.

'We all have individual nutritional requirements', the illustration on page 209 provides a basic idea of the 'food groups' that peop;e from some countries survive with, there is a great difference in those 'basic food groups' as well as the various types of lifestyle that people from those countries have developed, to suit their environment. With such a wide variety of cultures, including other countries throughout the world, it is fascinating to take a glimpse of the 'foods that other people eat' and for generations, these foods may have provided good health, possibly long before the word 'nutrition' was first spoken. We are now in the 'nutrition conscious era' and it has become more than a matter of curiosity to know a little more about the foods we are eating, the western world has sparked off the nutrition boom and that continues to provide not only answers and questions about the 'right foods to eat' but also considerable controversy about the value of some foods in comparison to others and more precisely, the question of the 'balanced diet' and the intake of minerals and vitamins. Also on page 200, the centre illustration (enlarged view on page 13) over 150 natural foods are mentioned, the most common foods are illustrated and evaluated in this book for their nutritional qualities, all based on precise nutrient evaluation charts and combinations of various nutrients. Throughout many parts of the world, a wide variety of natural foods are available and as food cultivation areas expand, the availability of a wide variety of natural foods will provide more people with the opportunity to experience 'new foods', some of which may become 'staple foods' and others may provide the occasional variety to the diet.

Summary: the four main charts: (Fruits, Grains and Legumes), (Fruits, Nuts and Seeds), (Vegetables, Grains and Legumes), (Grains, Legumes, Nuts and Seeds) on pp. 203, 205, 207 and 209 provide a total, over 500 basic meal combination ideas and when compatible foods are combined, there are over 2,000 complete meal ideas available, if you can obtain the majority of natural foods that are mentioned. It is important to remember that the individual natural foods that are mentioned, over 60 foods, are all designed to be used in the 'whole natural state' and that includes the following:

FRUITS: whole, grated, sliced, chopped, juiced and pureed from the fresh state and used directly for that time.

VEGETABLES: whole, grated, sliced, diced, chopped, steamed, baked, freshly juiced, from freshly picked produce.

GRAINS: whole-sprouted, pre-soaked, steamed, boiled for less than 5 minutes, (simmer the legumes or allow 2 hours on low heat), prepared into a flour, milk or chopped form, all obtained from the whole Legume.

NUTS: unshelled, shelled, chopped, combined with other nuts, nut butter, nut milk or nut flour.

SEEDS: whole-sprouted, ground into a flour, milk or butter, combined with cooked meals or fresh produce.

FRUITS, NUTS & SEEDS FOOD RECIPES CHART

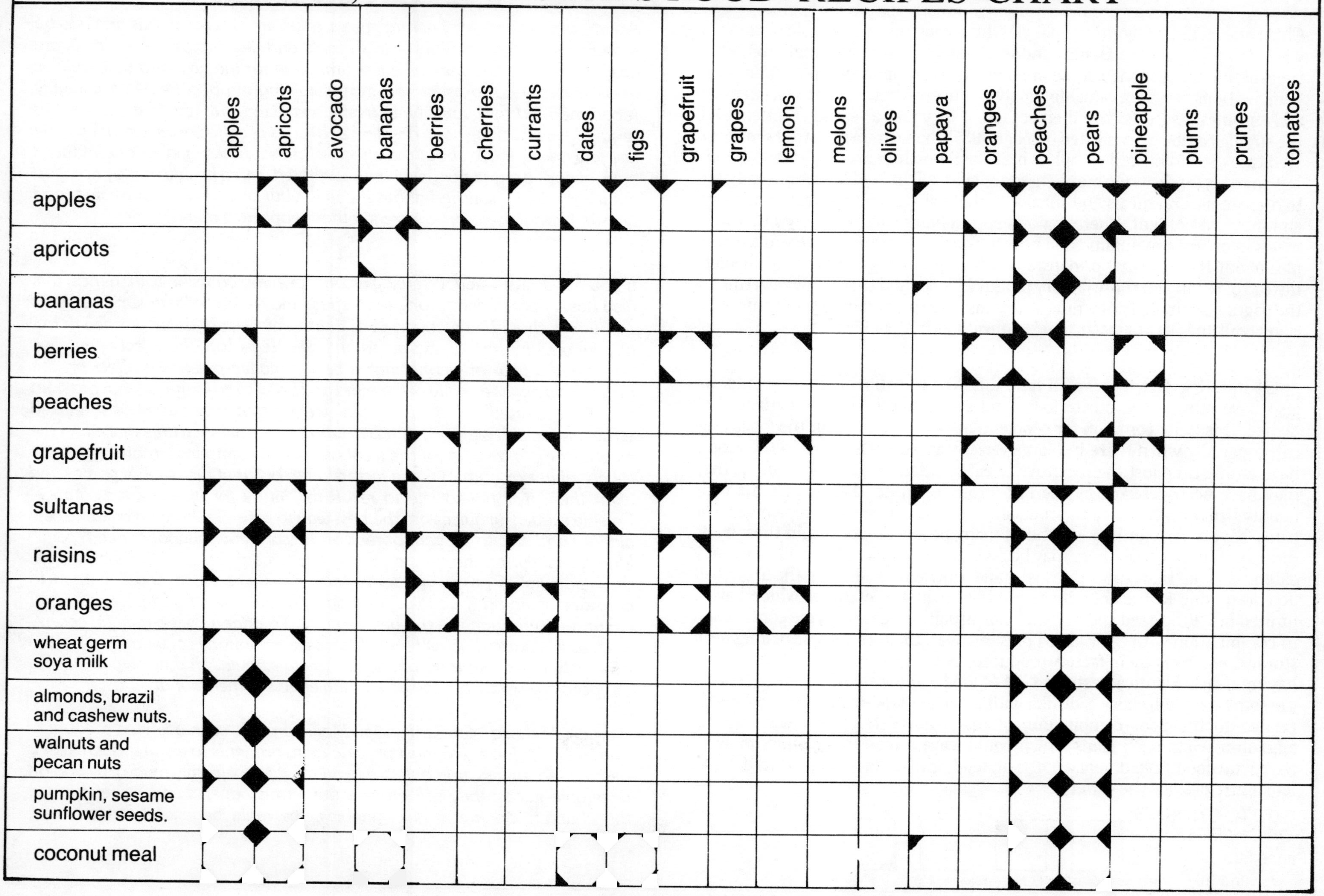
apples
apricots
avocado
bananas
berries
cherries
currants
dates
figs
grapefruit
grapes
lemons
melons
olives
papaya
oranges
peaches
pears
pineapple
plums
prunes
tomatoes
apples
apricots
bananas
berries
peaches
grapefruit
sultanas
raisins
oranges
wheat germ soya milk
almonds, brazil and cashew nuts.
walnuts and pecan nuts
pumpkin, sesame sunflower seeds.
coconut meal

DIETARY GUIDE INTRODUCTION

Chart one: page 203. For those people who are fortunate to be able to obtain a wide variety of fresh fruits, nuts and seeds, there are over 80 simple combinations of those foods to try, some providing a good supply of protein and most combinations provide a valuable supply of glucose-energy, minerals, vitamins and enzymes. As fruits have their season, it may take a year to experience all the simple combinations listed on page 203. When compatible fruits, nuts or seeds are used to make a complete breakfast, lunch or evening meal, there are over 200 individual simple and easy to prepare natural meals and snacks, each having a different taste sensation and nutrient content. There is no need to obtain such a variety of natural meals in order to maintain good health; these charts are to give you a better idea about the potential of natural foods in providing variety to your diet, instead of relying on those factory produced foods and snacks. By referring to the pages describing fruits, nuts and seeds, you can obtain valuable information about the benefits that these natural foods provide.

Apart from the fact that we all have different nutritional requirements, we also have our own favourite foods and some that we have experienced to dislike. It is quite common for people to be very choosy about the foods they eat, especially when there is a large variety, and unfortunately, some people have at one time lost the incentive to eat some fruits, nuts or seeds, as they may have been deterred by the taste from 'one bite' that was from a poor quality fruit or other natural produce. It is most important to remember that fruits have a very limited life and as many people do not obtain their fruits directly from the tree, there may be several weeks before the fruit is actually eaten, during that time the taste and nutrient quality of the fruit will deteorate, due to the abundance of life-elements — enzymes which have a limited life. Processed and refined foods usually have no enzyme content and in combination with their added preservatives, they are capable of long term storage, retaining their 'factory produced taste' for many months, each packet having nearly identical taste and list of food additives. Another main reason for some people to have a dislike with a certain food-fruit could be directly related to the poor combination of that fruit with other foods, causing after-dinner stomach pains which could leave a life-long memory to avoid that fruit-food, avoid replacing that food with a 'factory produced food', let Nature provide the variety!

CODE TO SYMBOLS:
FOR CHARTS.
Pages 203, 205
and 207

Breakfast   Lunch   Evening Meal   Snacks

Apart from the variety of natural meals, there are also numerous drinks to be made from a combination of fresh fruits and vegetables, these drinks are easy to prepare and they take less time than for the 'water to boil'. As this book is designed to assist you in maintaining the best health, it is highly recommended that you obtain freshly extracted fruit and vegetable juices regularly. If you have been drinking 2-10 cups of coffee or tea per day for the last few years, think about the effects of those drinks, if even one of those cups of coffee or tea per day were substituted with a freshly made juice, you could be slightly satisfied about the way your body has been treated, and possibly about the way you 'treat' other people to a friendly drink.

If you are accustomed to serving alcohol at every occasion with friends, you also has a very negative long term effect and the sincerity of such alcoholic gatherings should be recognized as detrimental to not only your health but also for your friends. As explained on pages 166-168, the effect of regular-prolonged intake of alcohol has a very negative-poisoning effect on the body, reducing the ability of the mind and body to co-ordinate, that provides the 'light-hearted' — 'light-headed' feeling that may promote a relaxed atmosphere with plenty of things to talk about, until such time that either the alcohol supply runs dry or the alcohol-poisoning imparts a more aggressive touch, either or both of those factors often occur at the alcohol parties and even then, it is not to late to resort to Nature for effective reassurance. Freshly made fruit juices are the best way to assist the body to utilize excess alcohol and also to prevent or reduce the common 'hangover head' pains. Unfortunately, by the time a person has become effected by the alcohol, their powers of proper reasoning are greatly reduced and for them to consider having a 'fruit juice' instead of another alcohol drink may never occur, even though it is the best remedy. To offer a coffee may be accept-able; as it is backed up with possible positive memories of what a coffee can do in situations like that; providing a new stimulation that may assist in a temporary revival from the deadening effects of the alcohol.

As most of those 'standard social drinks' provide such a limited amount of nutrients, the food-diet must provide extra nutrients to ensure that health is maintained, unless, you obtain a regular supply of freshly made fruit and or, vegetable juices; they will provide numerous benefits and by referring to the chapters on fruit and vegetables, the main benefits are mentioned.

The chart lists grains/legumes as columns (left to right): barley, corn-maize, millet, oats, rice, rye, wheat, buckwheat, bulgar, sorghum, triticale, soya milk, wheat germ, lecethin meal and powdered yeast. Fruits are listed as rows. A filled mark (◆) indicates a combination.

Fruit	barley	corn-maize	millet	oats	rice	rye	wheat	buckwheat	bulgar	sorghum	triticale	soya milk	wheat germ	lecethin meal and powdered yeast
apples	◆	◆	◆	◆	◆	◆			◆	◆	◆	◆	◆	◆
apricots	◆	◆		◆	◆	◆	◆	◆	◆	◆	◆	◆	◆	◆
avocadoes				◆	◆		◆			◆		◆		◆
bananas					◆	◆			◆		◆	◆	◆	◆
berries														
cherries														
currants				◆	◆			◆	◆	◆	◆	◆		◆
dates									◆	◆	◆	◆	◆	◆
figs			◆						◆	◆	◆	◆	◆	◆
grapefruit														
grapes														
raisins			◆	◆	◆	◆	◆		◆	◆	◆	◆	◆	◆
sultanas			◆	◆	◆	◆	◆		◆	◆	◆	◆	◆	◆
olives		◆			◆		◆		◆	◆	◆		◆	◆
oranges														◆
peaches			◆	◆	◆		◆		◆	◆	◆	◆	◆	◆
pears			◆	◆	◆	◆		◆	◆	◆	◆	◆	◆	◆
powdered yeast			◆	◆	◆	◆	◆	◆	◆	◆	◆	◆	◆	◆
soya grits			◆	◆	◆	◆		◆	◆	◆	◆	◆	◆	◆
soya milk			◆	◆	◆	◆	◆	◆	◆	◆	◆		◆	◆
coconut meal			◆	◆	◆		◆	◆	◆	◆	◆	◆	◆	◆
wheat germ			◆	◆	◆	◆		◆	◆	◆	◆	◆	◆	◆

FOOD COMBINATION CHART — RECIPE GUIDE INFORMATION

Chart Two: page 205. The variety of simple meal combinations that are provided by the group of fruits, whole grains and legumes is abundant. Over 270 basic single combinations are available — see chart, and by combining a few compatible fruits with either whole grains or legumes, over 500 individual complete breakfast, lunch or evening meals are possible, all depending on your accessibility to such natural produce. If there is a natural food store in your local area, you can obtain the majority of those whole food products are supplied by supermarkets and for the best value, and best products, your local natural food store is well worth a visit for your weekly shopping requirements.

Most whole grain and legume produce is very economical when compared to the price of processed and refined breakfast foods and various other canned products, and even though the packaged food may seem to be larger, the contents are greatly reduced when considering nutritional value. It may take some time for you to get used to buying natural whole grains and legumes instead of those over-advertised packaged foods, firstly you may want to finish the packet of breakfast cereal that is on the kitchen shelf, then you may have to make a special note to include a visit to the natural food store, and once you get there it may be difficult to decide about what foods to buy, as there are so many natural foods displayed. To be sure that you have the basic whole grain and legume foods, refer to the chapter on whole grains and legumes for a list of these foods and also for information about their benefits and method of preparation. As the most common 'staple food' is bread, you should always obtain the best quality whole grain bread and be careful about the imitations, some so-called whole grain bread may also include numerous additives — see page 156 for a list of common food additives. Over a dozen food additives — chemicals may be included with some mass produced bread, bread improver and mould inhibitors are very common additives and the effects of all those additives may not seem to do any harm today but when used regularly over a prolonged period, the effects are made obvious. The price of a good quality whole grain bread may be a few cents more than a mass produced chemical bread but instead of eating five or six slices of flour-chemicals, a good whole grain bread will satisfy the appetite with a couple of slices as well as providing those nutrients to assist digestion and maintain positive health. The bread you eat effects the life you live!

Breakfast   Lunch   Evening Meal   Snacks

If you are interested in promoting your health, both freshly made fruit and vegetable juices provide a simple and most effective health restoring power as well as their delicious taste, when properly prepared and served.

Comparing the ways in which people have their own favourite drinks: coffee, tea or alcohol, it is quite obvious that they are fairly particular in the way those drinks are prepared and served, to suit their taste. As people are so particular about the way to serve such drinks as coffee, tea or alcohol, it becomes a routine to expect a certain taste in order to obtain contentment and even though those drinks have no positive health benefits, they have become part of the 'standard diet', especially in America and Australia, where the society is especially geared to cater for those 'demanding-drinks'.

As the society is providing those drinks as the 'standard social drinks', people who may not particularly enjoy those customs, take part in some way to maintain their friendship and social presence. A bottle of soft drink for the children, a glass of beer for dad, a glass of wine for mum and a cup of coffee for granny. Everybody having a different drink and all of them obtaining no effective nutrition, just a stimulation that become addictive and with which, the body must continually compete with in order to provide the stimulation.

As mentioned throughout the chapters on minerals and vitamins, the glandular system provides the main areas of stimulation and for the stimulation to occur, the glands have to be given certain nutrients, none of which are provided by coffee, tea, alcohol or soft drinks. The only reason those drinks can provide their various forms of stimulation is due to their individual ingredients: caffeine, tannin, alcohol and sugar, all of which have different effects upon the body's glandular system.

Everybody can obtain numerous benefits from freshly made juices and even though they may not completely take the place of coffee, tea, alcohol or soft drinks, freshly made juices will be the best assistant to provide the vital balance of nutritional needs and they will protect against numerous 'social diseases'. If you have no juice extractor, do not rely on packaged fruit or vegetable juices as an alternative, they are more expensive and do not supply the valuable life elements — enzymes. Without enzymes, there would be no life! The main benefit of freshly made juices is that they provide an abundance of life elements, very few life elements are obtained from cooked food and those 'social drinks'. Only fresh natural produce can give you life and the juices will help you to obtain more life so as you may overcome the effects of those 'social drinks and foods', most of which are lacking in the real thing — life! A fresh juice now will help you live better today and more tomorrow, have at least one fresh juice a day to 'help your body live again'!

VEGETABLES, GRAINS & LEGUMES RECIPES CHART

	asparagus	beetroot	green beans	broccoli	brussel sprouts	cabbage	carrots	capsicum	cauliflower	celery	cucumber	garlic	leek	onions	lettuce	parsley	peas	parsnips	potatoes	pumpkin	radish	watercress	spinach
barley	▶			▶		▶	▶	▶	▶		▶	▶	▶	▶	▶	▶	▶		▶	▶	▶		
corn-maize	▶	▶		▶		▶	▶	▶		▶	▶	▶		▶	▶	▶	▶		▶	▶	▶		▶
millet	▶	▶					▶		▶		▶	▶		▶									
oats	▶	▶					▶		▶		▶	▶		▶							▶		
rice	▶	▶	▶	▶		▶	▶	▶	▶	▶	▶	▶	▶	▶	▶	▶	▶				▶	▶	▶
rye	▶	▶					▶		▶		▶	▶		▶							▶	▶	
wheat	▶	▶					▶		▶		▶	▶		▶							▶		
Bulgur, sorghum and triticale	▶	▶		▶		▶	▶	▶	▶	▶	▶	▶	▶	▶	▶	▶	▶				▶	▶	▶
chick peas	▶		▶	▶	▶	▶	▶	▶	▶	▶	▶	▶	▶	▶	▶	▶	▶			▶	▶	▶	▶
kidney bean	▶		▶	▶	▶	▶	▶	▶	▶	▶	▶	▶	▶	▶	▶	▶	▶				▶	▶	▶
lentils	▶		▶	▶	▶	▶	▶	▶	▶	▶	▶	▶	▶	▶	▶	▶	▶				▶	▶	▶
lima bean	▶		▶	▶	▶	▶	▶	▶	▶	▶	▶	▶	▶	▶	▶	▶	▶		▶	▶	▶	▶	▶
mung bean	▶		▶	▶	▶	▶	▶	▶	▶	▶	▶	▶	▶	▶	▶	▶	▶			▶	▶	▶	▶
soya beans	▶		▶	▶	▶	▶	▶	▶	▶	▶	▶	▶	▶	▶	▶	▶	▶				▶	▶	▶

FOOD COMBINATION CHART — RECIPE GUIDE INFORMATION

Chart Three: page 207, Vegetables, Grains and Legumes combination chart. Of all the combination charts, this chart provides the most abundant variety of combinations, over 500 simple combinations are available and by combining a few compatible foods, you could prepare over 2,000 individual complete meals, mainly for lunch and the evening meals. One of the most common lunch ideas is the sandwich and if you are fortunate enough to obtain a good quality whole grain bread, made from wheat, rye, oats, corn or triticale, there are over 200 different sandwich ideas available, by combining a variety of freshly prepared vegetables with a few slices of 'whole grain bread'.

By referring to pp. 128–129, there is valuable information about the benefits of butter and margarine and you will find that it is recommended that you make the effort to prepare 'better-butter', a combination of natural butter with a good quality cold pressed oil and by adding small amounts of lecithin granules, brewers yeast and some vegetable salt, you can be sure that the butter you use is well worth spreading on the whole grain bread. Make the effort to prepare some better-butter, it has very good keeping qualities and it will 'spread even better than margarine'. Once you have obtained a good quality whole grain bread and some better-butter, your sandwich idea is on an excellent start to providing positive nutritional value and by combining a few fresh vegetables: grated carrot, beetroot, cucumber and some outer green lettuce leaves, that sandwich will be an excellent take-away lunch, prepare some at home today. Apart from adding freshly prepared vegetables, you could add some soya mayonnaise or other good quality mayonnaise, seasoning, tahini, alfalfa sprouts and finely chopped onion and parsley, that sandwich will not only satisfy the appetite but also provide a major portion of your daily nutrient requirements and a valuable supply of enzymes — life. If you have never tried a sandwich like that before, you will be surprised to find that it may give you an excellent alternative to any tasty take-away meals and that the price is far less, when you prepare the sandwich at home. Every meal you have at home can save considerable expense and as the 'standard diet' obtainable from most shops would not include all the natural benefits that a sandwich can provide, regularly prepare your sandwich/lunch at home, it should take no more than 5 minutes once you have become accustomed to the preparation and when considering take-away foods, you may have to wait longer than that, just to be served, a lunch that is not worth waiting for as the nutritional potential may be greatly reduced with any added food-chemicals, excess fat content, poor produce and lack of essential life elements. Be sure to try the complete natural sandwich this week.

Numerous other lunch ideas are possible with the variety of natural foods mentioned on chart three, you can prepare over 50 different types of soup, ideal for a winter lunch at home or take some along to work in a thermos, a most suitable take-away alternative. Home made soups are also ideal for the start to an evening meal, especially in winter. There are 14 main natural foods listed in the right hand columns on page 207; all of these are suitable as a base for soup, when obtained in the natural – whole state, they can be pre-soaked to reduce cooking time and also to promote a valuable increase in nutritional value, see section on sprouting (pp. 103–106) for details. If you intend to prepare a soup, always pre-soak the whole grain for a few hours before cooking, a few days is highly recommended for the best nutritional value. You can prepare a large quantity of pre-soaked grains or legumes and apart from soups, there are numerous recipes that require pre-soaked grains and legumes, they keep very well in the fridge after they have been pre-soaked or sprouted. By combining a whole grain with a legume, for example rice with lima beans, the protein availability – N.P.U. (see pages 41, 82, 87 and 88 for details), is greatly improved and so can obtain a fair portion of your daily protein requirements, even from a soup, especially if you use soya beans (see pages 89–91 for methods of preparation and some delicious recipes).

Whole grains and legumes are also the main ingredients for over 200 individual evening meals, they require about half an hour preparation time and combine very well with all types of fresh vegetables, steamed and grated. Such main meals as casseroles, vegetable pies, vegetable-bean loaf, vegetable-burgers, vegetable rolls and a large variety of other recipes, check through the recipes on pp. 32, 41 and 91 and discover some basic and delicious combinations of vegetables with whole grains and legumes. For more ideas, look at the chart, page 207, and you will discover a world of natural recipe ideas, prepare for a complete evening meal today.

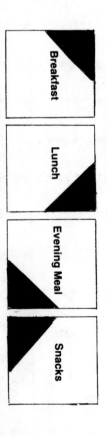

Breakfast | Lunch | Evening Meal | Snacks

These four groups of symbols refer to the following pages: 203, 205 and 207; each represents a suitable recipe combination, for breakfast, lunch, evening meal or snacks, some combinations may be suitable for all four groups, refer to the charts for details. Natural foods provide the best variety of recipes.

GRAINS, LEGUMES, NUTS & SEEDS PROTEIN CHART

Amounts based on 100 gram portions 50-50, for a person weighing 70-80 Kg. Approximate protein value.

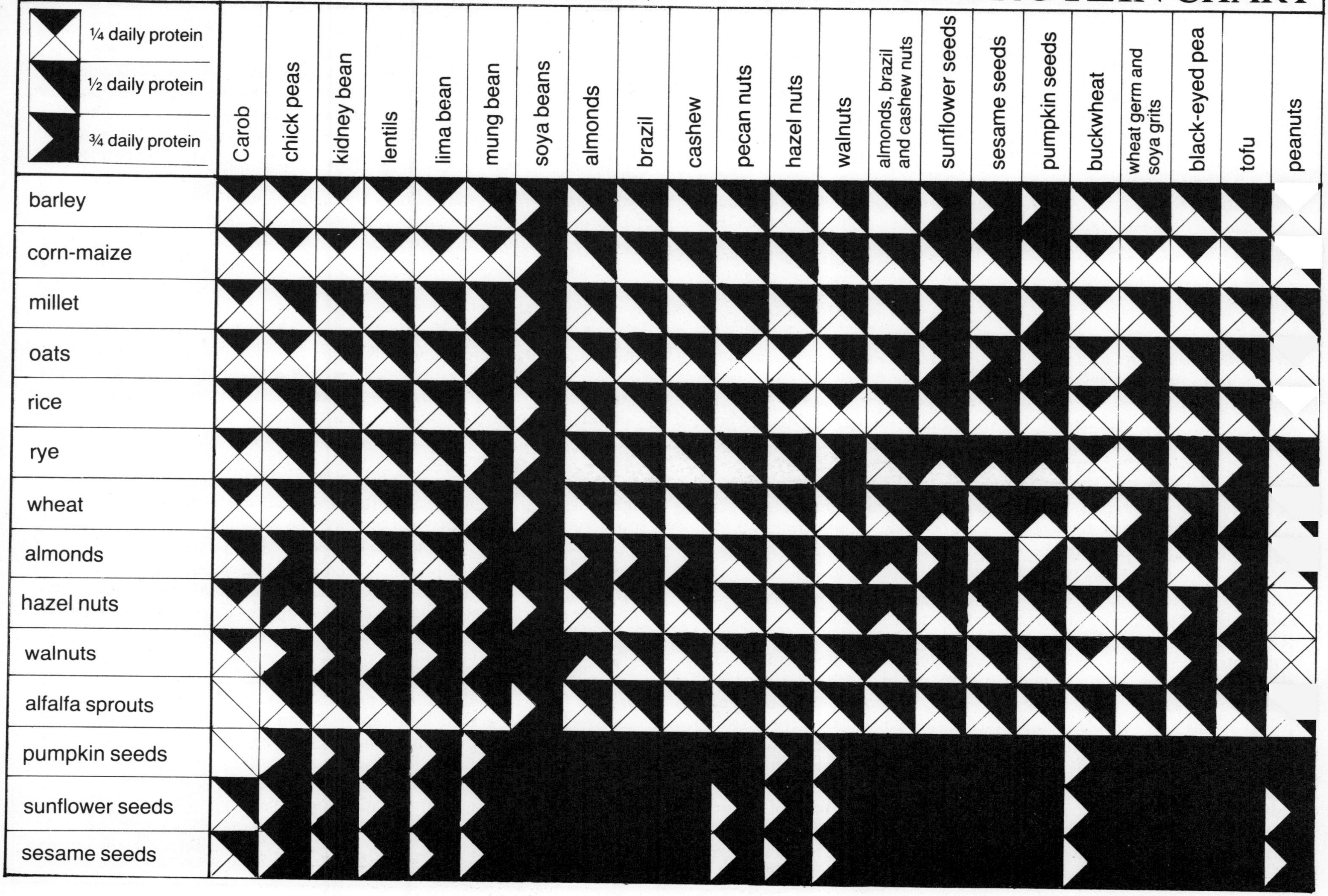
¼ daily protein
½ daily protein
¾ daily protein
Carob
chick peas
kidney bean
lentils
lima bean
mung bean
soya beans
almonds
brazil
cashew
pecan nuts
hazel nuts
walnuts
almonds, brazil and cashew nuts
sunflower seeds
sesame seeds
pumpkin seeds
buckwheat
wheat germ and soya grits
black-eyed pea
tofu
peanuts
barley
corn-maize
millet
oats
rice
rye
wheat
almonds
hazel nuts
walnuts
alfalfa sprouts
pumpkin seeds
sunflower seeds
sesame seeds

Chart Four: page 209. Grains, Legumes, Nuts and Seeds Protein chart. This chart is designed to give you an approximate visual display of natural primary protein food combinations and their ability to supply varying amounts of the essential daily protein requirements. As explained throughout the protein chapter and various pages of the grains and legume sections, all the essential amino acids — protein are obtainable from a wide variety of foods, apart from animal products (refer to pages 41, 82, 83, 84, 87, 88, 98 and 99). Throughout many parts of the world, people rely on the protein contained in whole grains, legumes, nuts and seeds for their daily require-ments and without any doubt, there are more benefits obtainable from those natural primary protein foods in comparison to animal protein foods.

Throughout other parts of the world, especially Australia and America, the animal protein foods have become the dominant protein providers, even though the variety of natural primary protein foods are also obtainable. Everybody needs protein value, the group of whole grains, legumes and especially nuts and seeds should provide a majority of the daily protein requirements. As the 'standard diet' throughout Australia and America is based on animal protein foods, the variety of delicious, healthful primary protein recipes are often stored in the kitchen cupboard, and rarely given the chance to take an active part in supplying daily protein requirements. The chart on page 209 provides over 300 individual natural protein combinations, and as with the other charts on combination, when the compatible foods are used to prepare a complete meal, there are over 600 natural primary protein breakfast, lunch and evening meals as well as over 50 simple protein snacks, ideal for any occasion that requires a convenient easy-to-pack snack.

One of the main obstacles in 'starting to use natural foods' for complete meals is often due to a lack of 'thinking about natural foods' first, instead of the often automatic decision to combine an animal protein food and/or factory food, to make a meal. Once you become accustomed to thinking about natural foods first, you will surely require a few good recipes to start with, numerous basic protein recipes are provided throughout this book and if you retrieve some of those 'cupboard recipe books', and ensure that your weekly shopping includes 'only natural foods', you then appreciate the potential of natural foods in the best way possible — regularly. Before the days of the 'factory foods', people lived entirely on natural foods and even though in some parts of the world animal protein foods were the basic protein providers, in the majority of countries natural protein foods: whole grains, legumes, nuts and seeds were the protein foods and they continue to provide millions of people with protein.

If you intend to start using more natural protein foods and less animal protein foods, you should check through the charts on combination and make a list of the foods that you require to have the 'basic protein foods', to start with, you require no more than a dozen main primary protein foods and you may have over half of them hidden in the cupboard. In combination with the primary protein foods, you should obtain at least three different seasonal fruits and fresh garden vegetables, without the fruits and vegetables it is difficult to prepare complete, delicious and well presented meals, even though you will obtain good protein value. Check through the other charts to find out what discover numerous fruits and vegetables that will enhance the total appeal and nutritional value of the breakfast, lunch or dinner recipe idea, as well as fruits or vegetables combine with your 'protein meal idea', then you will such recipes as protein bread, protein snacks, protein party dips, protein drink ideas and delicious protein sweets.

As each combination is presented in a way to provide an approximate guide to the amount of protein obtained (based on 100 gram edible portions — 50% of one food and 50% of the other food, for a person weighing between 70-80 kg), you can look though the list of compatible foods and discover their protein potential, and even though you may not use a 50-50 combination of two foods, you can obtain a good idea about compatible protein foods and within a few minutes, you may find that a start to a simple recipe idea is already in your mind, from then onwards, if you need a little more assistance, check through the other food combination charts on the previous pages and there will be numerous other foods that will combine very well and make it easy to prepare a complete breakfast, lunch, evening, snack or party recipe.

It is unfortunate that throughout such developed countries as Australia and America, where the availability of natural foods is abundant, many children are given animal protein foods exclusively, and for those children to start life so adapted to animal protein foods, it becomes very difficult for them to later on, change their eating habits.

Another main obstacle to overcome when deciding to use natural primary protein foods instead of animal protein foods and factory foods is that, the group of whole grains, legumes, nuts and seeds may appear to be very unattractive when stored in their bare-form and that may not at all excite your appetite or give you the incentive to continue with the idea of natural primary protein preparation. If you have prepared such a meal before, you can then appreciate the delightful and most appetising appeal of a completed recipe idea, and with the assistance of these charts, you may discover even more, suitable appetising recipe ingredients and continue to obtain full contentment from the world of natural foods, daily.

FOOD EXPENSE & DAILY DIET COMPARISON CHART

natural food diet

Breakfast — $

$	
.10	
.20	
.60	
.90	

- drink of water, add a squeeze of lemon or orange juice. Cup of herbal tea or coffee, or, make a freshly extracted orange and pineapple juice.
- 1 bowl of freshly grated fruits, (depending on seasonal availability): apple, pear, sultanas and raisins and combine with a half a cup of chopped almonds or walnuts. Add a tsp. of tahini for extra protein value.

(pie chart: Carbohydrate, Total Fat, Protein)

Lunch — $

$
.40
.90
1.30

- freshly made apple and apricot juice, or, carrot, celery and parsley juice.
- equal portions of almonds, brazil and cashew nuts — 100 gram total, combine with a crisp apple or ripe peach. An ideal take-away substitute and an excellent source of complete protein.

Evening meal — $

$
.60
.10
.70

- vegetable-barley soup (see page 36), including, broccoli, carrot, capsicum, celery and leek, with a slice of whole grain rye bread. As the lunch-time meal supplied 75% of your protein, breakfast supplied 15%, this meal will provide the extra protein required as well as a valuable supply of nutrients.

Snacks-Drinks — $

$
.30
.40
.20
.90
$3.80

- glass of freshly extracted grape juice.
- 1 apple, 3 apricots.
- 2 cups of herbal tea or coffee.
- optional: to obtain a simple and extra complete source of protein-snack, try a handful of sunflower seeds or pumpkin seeds, they will greatly re-vitalize your health, or, try a protein milk shake: soya milk, banana, carob and wheat germ.

'standard diet'

Breakfast — $

$
.10
.30
.10
.50
1.00

- glass of milk, cup of coffee or tea with milk and sugar.
- 1 bowl of refined — packaged breakfast cereal with milk and sugar, plus, tinned fruits.
- 2 slices of toast and jam — or other spread.
- 2 eggs plus 1 piece of bacon (this breakfast is very acid forming and supplies no vitamin C or essential enzymes — life).

(pie chart: Carbohydrate, Total Fat, Protein)

Lunch — $

$
.50
.40
.50
.10
.40
1.90

- bottled or canned soft drink, glass of beer, wine or pasteurized milk.
- sandwich: 1 slice of ham, 1 slice of processed cheese, onions, tinned beetroot and pale lettuce leaves (served on white-refined bread-starch).
- 2 small cakes or sausage rolls.
- cup of coffee or tea with milk and sugar.
- chocolate, candy bar or potato chips.

Evening meal — $

$
.50
1.20
.60
.10
2.40

- soft drink, beer, wine, milk, cup of tea or coffee.
- 3oz. steak (100 gram), frozen peas and potato chips — cooked, canned asparagus and mushrooms, one pale lettuce leaf.
- pre-frozen apple pie and cream with added gelatin and preservatives.
- cup of coffee or tea.

Snacks-Drinks — $

$
1.20
.30
.30
.30
2.10
$7.40

- 3 cans of soft drink or beer.
- 1 packet of potato chips or 2 cheese biscuits or sweet biscuits.
- 3 cups of coffee or tea with sugar and milk.
- 3 pieces of chocolate or candy.

RECIPE GUIDE INFORMATION — WEIGHT CONTROL — DIET

These charts are designed to show the basic difference between the standard diet and the natural food diet. Both diets are placed into four groups: breakfast, lunch, evening meal and snacks and drinks.

At the start of the day, the circle would be empty, and once the breakfast meal is obtained, the approx. food value is shown as the dark areas (top circles). The circles are based on the three main food groups: Carbohydrates 50% daily diet. Protein 30-40% daily diet and the Lipids 15-20% daily diet (see page 13 for details). By adding the food value of the breakfast with the lunch food value, the dark area increases and when the evening meal is added, the circle may be full, thereby showing a complete intake of the three main food groups for one day. An additional circle (below) is provided for any snacks or drinks obtained as an extra intake. An excess intake may occur because of the snacks and drinks, unless extra exercise is obtained. These charts are a guide to the way every meal or snack will contribute food value, they are based on the average man and women (see page 14 for details).

Also provided with these charts are the approx. cost of the meals obtained and without doubt, the natural food daily diet is the best value. Processed, refined and canned foods are more expensive than the fresh, natural produce. Only natural foods can provide natural meal satisfaction and natural weight control.

The natural diet day is the best way to obtain all the essential daily nutrients, to help you live and Laugh with Health.

As mentioned throughout this book, natural whole foods provide all the essential nutrients to assist digestion and metabolism of the food eaten. When processed and refined foods are added to the diet, various nutrient deficiencies will occur (see minerals and vitamins chapter), causing an imbalance of nutrients to assist digestion and metabolism. Over a time of a few years, the body metabolism will degenerate at a rate equal to the intake of processed-factory foods, slowly leading the way to a slow metabolism and the adding on of extra weight. At this stage, it is advisable to eliminate all forms of factory foods, if you intend to lose weight in the best way possible — naturally. To replace all forms of factory foods with natural whole foods may seem a difficult and unnattractive method of losing weight, for someone who may greatly rely on those factory foods for their daily meals, however, the variety of complete, sustaining natural meals (see combination — recipe charts, pp. 203, 205, 207 and 209), provide a delicious alternative that with practice and determination, you will discover the natural way to enjoy every meal and promote a renewed vitality and the 'state of natural weight'.

The 'standard diet' has developed over the past twenty years, and today, factory foods, have become very popular especially in Australia and America. Special techniques and ingredients are added to factory foods, to make them popular, however, as the essential nutrient requirements are often lacking, a person may attempt to obtain their daily nutrient requirements and at the same time, eat too much food. Only natural foods can supply all your daily nutrient requirements, the standard diet will promote excess eating without supplying the essential active nutrients: enzymes, minerals and vitamins to assist digestion of the food, the result is dissatisfaction and an attempt to satisfy with another dose of factory-foods, drinks and alcohol, never obtaining a correct daily balance of life supporting happiness — health elements.

As can be seen from the 'natural food diet' lists, pages 211 and 213, regular use of fresh fruits and vegetables is obvious, for breakfast, have some fresh fruits with the whole grain — cooked, for lunch have a variety of freshly prepared vegetables in combination with cooked grains — bread, or combine fresh fruits with a variety of nuts, for the evening meal, combine fresh and cooked vegetables with legumes — cooked or whole grains — cooked. The balance between the intake of cooked — fresh foods is vital for maintenance of good health and natural weight.

An overweight person may have developed such a condition due to a number of reasons and may also at some times, consider ways and means to reduce weight. The basic reason that is often given is narrowed down to the point that, 'most overweight people eat too much food in relation to physical expended energy'! However, what makes a person eat too much food or obtain insufficient physical energy is more the cause than the actual amount of food eaten. Food is one of the basic needs and it is often the most easily obtained, a basic need is a natural desire and because most people can obtain a good supply of food, they may overdose in comparison to their 'basic need'. When the other basic needs are hard to obtain, food may take the place of those 'missing needs'. The most content people do not rely just on food for their daily satisfaction! Numerous other psychological reasons may also provide reasons for the development of an overweight condition, 'does your body control your mind, or, your mind control your body this interrelationship between mind and body harmony is a vital factor in maintaining a healthy lifestyle. Food is part of the life cycle of this planet-earth when food is eaten, an overweight person may have developed a genuine desire to take part in as much earth-life as possible, especially when their lifestyle is not at all related to 'working with the earth'.

FOOD EXPENSE & DAILY DIET COMPARISON CHART

natural food diet

Breakfast

$	$
	.40
	.60
1.00	

- drink of water.
- carob and banana milkshake or an apple and peach juice – freshly extracted.
- 1 bowl of whole oats – (pre-soaked overnight), 1 tbl.sp. wheat germ, ¼ cup of chopped hazel or walnuts, soya milk or fresh milk, sultanas, raisins and freshly grated apple.

Lunch

| .60 |
| .20 |
| .30 |
| .20 |
| **1.30** |

- apricot and peach juice, or, apple and strawberry juice, or, carrot juice with celery, or, have a fresh fruit – (all fruits contain at least 60% mineral water).
- sandwich: whole grain rye bread or home made wheat bread – (see page 31), 2 slices. **Add:** freshly grated carrot and beetroot. chopped capsicum, green lettuce leaves, chives, alfalfa sprouts and one slice of natural cheese, use tahini butter.

Evening meal

| .50 |
| .60 |
| .30 |
| **1.40** |

- glass of freshly extracted apple and pineapple juice, or, strawberry and pineapple juice, or, carrot, cucumber and celery juice, or, cup of herbal tea or coffee, or carob-chocolate drink.
- lima bean loaf – (see page 38), plus, a fresh garden salad with sweet corn, grated carrot and cucumber and green lettuce leaves with soya mayonnaise or tahini salad dressing.

Snacks-Drinks

| .60 |
| .10 |
| .60 |
| **1.30** |
| **$ 5.00** |

- 2 crisp apples, 1 orange, 1 banana.
- 2 glasses of water, or, 2 cups of herbal tea.
- handful of almonds, cashew and brazil nuts, or, handful of sunflower seeds or pumpkin seeds, or, 2 home made millet or oatmeal cookies.

(Pie charts labelled Carbohydrate, Total Fat, Protein for Breakfast, Lunch, Evening meal, and Snacks-Drinks.)

'standard diet'

Breakfast

$	
10	
.50	
.30	
.90	

- glass of milk, cup of coffee or tea (none of these supply the essential life vitamin – C, the glass of processed orange juice is lacking in those nutrients that assist vitamin C activity).
- scrambled, fried or poached eggs. (supplies protein, however it is completely lacking in enzymes — the spark of life). (2 eggs.)
- 3 pieces of refined bread – toast. (lacks essential B group vitamins and is loaded with chemical additives).

Lunch

| .50 |
| .80 |
| .10 |
| .30 |
| **1.70** |

- glass of water, beer, wine, milk or sugar soft drink (very few nutrients are supplied by these drinks).
- 1 meat pie or hot-dog – hamburger, serve of fat-coated potato chips.
- 1 fruit (should be eaten first).
- 1 packet of candy or biscuits.

Evening meal

| .80 |
| .30 |
| .30 |
| .50 |
| **1.90** |

- 100 gram serve of chicken, plus, one serve of packaged-frozen potato chips – cooked. Small serve of tinned beetroot and asparagus with a leaf of lettuce. Salt added. (This type of meal supplies a limited amount of essential nutrients, apart from the protein content of the factory-fed chicken.)
- glass of beer, wine or soft drink, all are refined Carbohydrates, they easily promote weight problems.

Snacks-Drinks

| 1.00 |
| .20 |
| .40 |
| **1.60** |
| **$7·10** |

- milk shake, 2 glasses of beer or 2 cans of soft drink.
- 2 cups of coffee or tea.
- handful of chocolate coated glazed fruits (all of these snack foods and refined drinks do not supply the nutrients that are lacking from this days – sample meal, the body's nutrient needs are not obtained and that leads to dissatisfaction — sickness.

(Pie charts labelled Carbohydrate, Total Fat, Protein for Breakfast, Lunch, Evening meal, and Snacks-Drinks.)

DAILY DIET COMPARISON — WEIGHT CONTROL — DIET

Apart from psychological reasons for food, there are a few basic physical reasons. They can be summarized into the following: Food is essential for life, a simple statement that is based on more intricate grounds. The three main food groups are Carbohydrates, Proteins, and Lipids. When those individual food groups are obtained from the diet, and after the process of digestion, the end-products that can be used for the maintenance of life are basically: Glucose, Amino Acids, and Fatty Acids. These nutrient require-ments will provide the initial, or more precisely, the essential desire to ensure that those basic nutrients are obtained.

As all parts of the body require those three basic food groups, an overweight person will have to provide extra food-nutrients to feed all those extra body-cells, unless they have adjusted their 'state of security', and recognize that for those extra pounds or kg. to be lost, they must live with less! The inspiration for such a change to develop has to be powerful or attractive enough to sustain those early stage 'hunger hang-ups'. Once your body-metabolism has become accustomed to obtaining less food, or a more suitable diet, those extra heavy cells will begin to disappear; only the essential living cells should remain. Depending on the types of food a person is eating, various benefits could be obtained by ensuring that any food that is eaten must be used directly from the natural-whole state.

It also must be mentioned that regular use of cooked meals, especially those with added fats and oils, are a main cause of obesity. Depending on the type of cooked meat, your body metabolism may also degenerate, especially if no 'live-food' is eaten at the same meal. There are over 200 complete meals to be prepared from fresh fruits, vegetables, sprouted foods and numerous other combinations that include a small portion of cooked food with a larger portion of fresh food. The balance between intake of cooked food in comparison to fresh foods is vital for maintenance of positive health and for regulation of weight. For maximum benefits, at least 75% of the daily diet should be fresh foods, the other 25% cooked food. By maintaining such a balance, natural weight control will quickly develop, making it easy to lose weight and also obtain satisfying complete meals. The easiest fresh foods to prepare and serve are fruits and vegetables.

It may be difficult to change your diet traditions today, but within a few months, and using suitable alternative complete meals (pages 202–210), the natural freshly prepared meals will delight the taste buds, provide a correct balance of essential human nutrients, and promote natural weight control. No other weight-losing program could be as complete as the 'natural weight—natural foods' method.

A cooked meal is a compact meal, lacking in some nutrients, providing a large portion of food, often double the actual food requirement. It is easy to eat more cooked food and less fresh food. Cooking prepares food sub-stance into an easy-to-digest form. If the cooked food was able to be eaten raw, it could take more energy to prepare, chewing the food several more times, also taking more time to have the meal and far less food could actually be eaten at the one meal. Don't let the cooked meals take over your diet. Always combine some fresh foods or drinks with the cooked meals. As mentioned throughout the fruits and vegetable chapters and on pp. 206 and 208, the use of freshly made juices can greatly assist in controlling weight.

All the essential active nutrients are supplied by freshly made fruit or vegetable juices and they are easy to digest, when properly combined, and they will provide an abundance of enzymes to assist in replacing the daily loss of enzymes from cooked meals. To lose weight may take several months, depending on the time the overweight condition has developed and the type of diet that is maintained, as well as the type of exercise obtained. If a person has been overweight for several years, it may also take several years to obtain normal weight. If a complete natural food diet is maintained, loss of weight will occur more often and more effectively, with no health risks attached.

Complete fasting diets are not recommended. Every day the body requires some nutrients. If they are not obtained, numerous health risk factors will develop. Both the B group vitamins and vitamin C are required daily. Without them, you may feel miserable, tired, and most upset about having to lose weight. If you ensure that you obtain a small portion of any food that is an excellent source daily (see food charts), your attempts at losing weight will be made more pleasant. There is no doubt that 'starving the body' or complete fasting does cause rapid loss of weight. However, the nutrient deficiencies that occur are not worth the effort. Always ensure that you obtain freshly made juices when fasting, and any food that is eaten should be an excellent source of those essential daily nutrients. Fasting promotes an effective cleansing of the body; it regenerates body metabolism and allows the digestive organs to have a rest. Always be moderate in the type of fasting you attempt, slowly obtaining less food, not just an abrupt shortage. Your body is used to a regular pattern. If that is disrupted, your mind will also be affected. Have a fast from food for six hours, twice a week, preferably after the intake of freshly made juices, in the morning. Also remember that you can have a small fast with every meal. Never overload the stomach with food and poor combinations. Be content to know that you have more food available if you need it. A meal should give you energy, not make you tired. Always prepare natural meals.

COMBINATION GUIDE

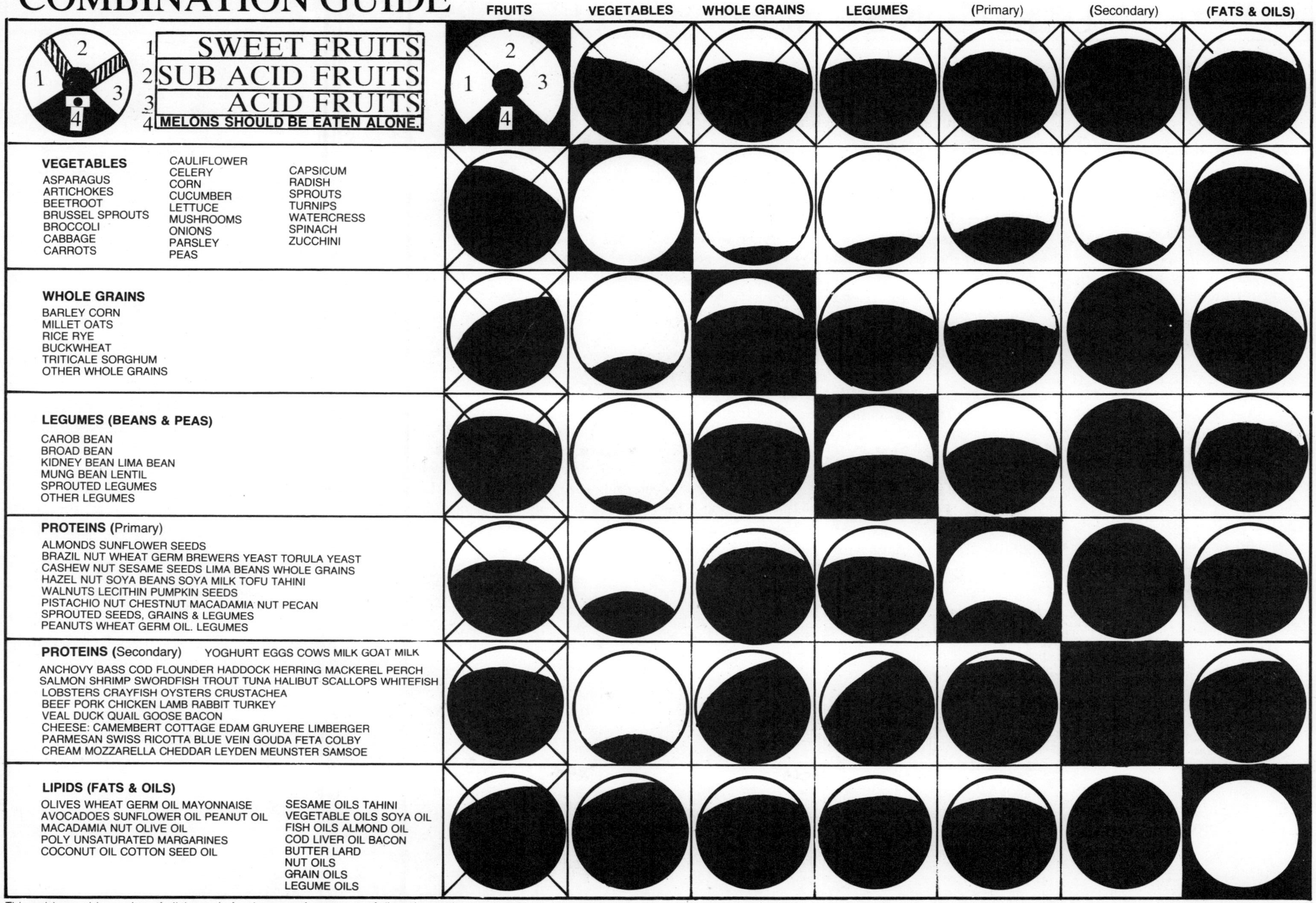

	FRUITS	VEGETABLES	WHOLE GRAINS	LEGUMES	(Primary)	(Secondary)	(FATS & OILS)

Legend:
1 SWEET FRUITS
2 SUB ACID FRUITS
3 ACID FRUITS
4 MELONS SHOULD BE EATEN ALONE

VEGETABLES
ASPARAGUS
ARTICHOKES
BEETROOT
BRUSSEL SPROUTS
BROCCOLI
CABBAGE
CARROTS
CAULIFLOWER
CELERY
CORN
CUCUMBER
LETTUCE
MUSHROOMS
ONIONS
PARSLEY
PEAS
CAPSICUM
RADISH
SPROUTS
TURNIPS
WATERCRESS
SPINACH
ZUCCHINI

WHOLE GRAINS
BARLEY CORN
MILLET OATS
RICE RYE
BUCKWHEAT
TRITICALE SORGHUM
OTHER WHOLE GRAINS

LEGUMES (BEANS & PEAS)
CAROB BEAN
BROAD BEAN
KIDNEY BEAN LIMA BEAN
MUNG BEAN LENTIL
SPROUTED LEGUMES
OTHER LEGUMES

PROTEINS (Primary)
ALMONDS SUNFLOWER SEEDS
BRAZIL NUT WHEAT GERM BREWERS YEAST TORULA YEAST
CASHEW NUT SESAME SEEDS LIMA BEANS WHOLE GRAINS
HAZEL NUT SOYA BEANS SOYA MILK TOFU TAHINI
WALNUTS LECITHIN PUMPKIN SEEDS
PISTACHIO NUT CHESTNUT MACADAMIA NUT PECAN
SPROUTED SEEDS, GRAINS & LEGUMES
PEANUTS WHEAT GERM OIL. LEGUMES

PROTEINS (Secondary) YOGHURT EGGS COWS MILK GOAT MILK
ANCHOVY BASS COD FLOUNDER HADDOCK HERRING MACKEREL PERCH
SALMON SHRIMP SWORDFISH TROUT TUNA HALIBUT SCALLOPS WHITEFISH
LOBSTERS CRAYFISH OYSTERS CRUSTACHEA
BEEF PORK CHICKEN LAMB RABBIT TURKEY
VEAL DUCK QUAIL GOOSE BACON
CHEESE: CAMEMBERT COTTAGE EDAM GRUYERE LIMBERGER
PARMESAN SWISS RICOTTA BLUE VEIN GOUDA FETA COLBY
CREAM MOZZARELLA CHEDDAR LEYDEN MEUNSTER SAMSOE

LIPIDS (FATS & OILS)
OLIVES WHEAT GERM OIL MAYONNAISE
AVOCADOES SUNFLOWER OIL PEANUT OIL
MACADAMIA NUT OLIVE OIL
POLY UNSATURATED MARGARINES
COCONUT OIL COTTON SEED OIL
SESAME OILS TAHINI
VEGETABLE OILS SOYA OIL
FISH OILS ALMOND OIL
COD LIVER OIL BACON
BUTTER LARD
NUT OILS
GRAIN OILS
LEGUME OILS

This guide provides a view of all the main food groups; for reasons of digestion and proper nutrition, some groups may not be suitable when combined—for example, Legumes and Secondary Protein foods (dark circle). Such combinations as whole grains and vegetables are usually very suitable. With fruits there are four separate areas, as each fruit group has different combining abilities. The white area of the circles denotes a suitable combination. This chart is a summary of the food combining information provided earlier. A proper combination will give the best food value.

NUTRITION SUMMARY — EFFECTS OF TIME

Time gives us the opportunity to live, and with continuous energy, life keeps on going. Every living creature has one main common characteristic: Life, the duration of which is only relevant when one can comprehend the 'sense of time'. Nowadays, people are taught from childhood to relate their 'existence with time', often without appreciating that as time goes on, so does the 'gift of life'. When so much emphasis is placed on Time, it should be 'only natural' that every effort be made, by everybody, to promote their life and to provide those 'life-promoting ingredients' for all who are alive. Life is a gift and as any gift, it should be respected and appreciated. For thousands of years, people have gathered valuable survival knowledge and today, we have sufficient knowledge to provide everyone with a comfortable supply of the 'basic survival needs': food, clothing, shelter, water and knowledge. The peak of natural living is possible today, in comfort, however many people are losing touch with the 'natural world' and in thousands of different ways, an increasing number of 'anti-natural elements': chemicals, factory foods, pollution, city stress etcetera (see pp. 217–218) all have the ability to destroy the benefits of natural living and for many people, sickness and impaired health are more prevalent than their 'times of good health'. When considering the increased amount of knowledge from the past 50 years, there must be a far greater opportunity these days to live in good health and not to be attacked by regular sickness throughout life and to spend the last decade or so in a state of total sickness. We don't like to be sick, our life has taken so long to develop, just the expense of a lifetime food supply should provide incentive to consider life as a great investment and because of an increasing life-value, the effort you make to obtain better nutrition: complete natural food diet and lifestyle (see pp. 217–218) will promote a longer life and with every moment of life, your body is always happy to know that every meal will provide complete natural energy, life promoting abilities and a total variety of taste sensations that are greatly appreciated when you become 'naturally hungry'. "If you think they have a good life, think about the foods they eat". Every page of this book is a summary, the total view and appreciation of natural foods and their benefits can only be expressed in terms of positive life-participating experiences and the happiness that good health provides, Laugh with Health.

9,000 B.C.
Bow and arrow first used.
Dog domesticated.

8,000 B.C.
NEOLITHIC STONE AGE
(New Stone Age)

7,000 B.C.
Sheep domesticated.

5,000 B.C.
Wheat cultivated –
Middle East.

4,500 B.C.
Boomerang used by
Australian Aboriginals
for hunting.

3,500 B.C.
Bees domesticated in
Euroasia and Africa.
Grapes Grown.

3,000 B.C.
Egyptian farming flourishes.
Potatoes cultivated in
South America.

2,500 B.C. – BRONZE AGE
Plow and Beast used
for farming.

2,200 B.C.
Peruvians grow Beans.
Papyrus-Paper used
by Egyptians.

2,000 B.C.
Farming developed
in Malaya.

2,000 B.C.
Cooking pots first used
– China.

1,700 B.C.
Chinese writing developed.

Chickens domesticated.
Horses domesticated in Asia.
Tobacco growing in Mexico
and South America.

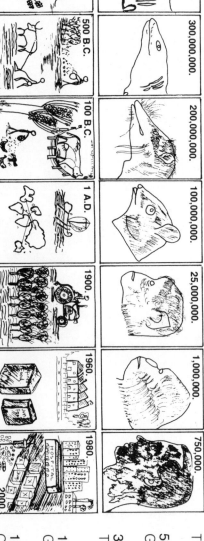

1,000 B.C.
Chinese use coal as fuel.

800 B.C.
Agriculture reaches U.S.A.

776 B.C.
First Olympic Games.

400 B.C. – IRON AGE
Starts in Europe.

323 B.C.
Alexander the Great – dies
of fever.

310 B.C.
Greek scientist.
(Theophrastus), writes a
study on Minerals.

300 B.C.
Alexandrian Physician,
(Herophilus), investigates
the brain and pioneers in
post-mortem studies.

272 B.C.
Artistarchius – Greek
Philosopher, declares that
the Earth revolves around
the Sun.

20 B.C.
Chinese Revolution.

6 B.C.
Thought to be the exact
birth date of Jesus Christ.

50 A.D.
Greek Philosopher describes
– medicinal plants.

350 A.D.
Tea drinking begins (China).

1000 A.D.
Golden Age.

1980 A.D.
Chemical Age.

Natural steps to health chart

1: Complete natural food diet, including seasonal fruits and a wide variety of fresh vegetables throughout the year, including freshly made fruit juices and vegetable juices, in regular small amounts: 7ozs, per day of each fruit and vegetable juice. Sprouted Legumes, Grains and Seeds. Nuts and Seeds, ground and eaten raw. Regular short fasting, at least six hours between large meals, 1 hour between different fruits and six hours between nut and seed meals with either whole grains or legumes. Daily sunshine, at least 3 hours moderate sunlight. Dairly work in the fields, gardening and long walking, deep breathing outdoor exercise. Yoga, relaxation and various types of meditation. Swimming and regular natural river or sea baths, hobbies related to natural creativity: painting, music, sculpture, carving, weaving, carpet-making, plant cultivation, food preparation, making clothes and home building. Climate ranging between 10-30 Celcius, over the four seasons, natural scenery and regular adventures to other beautiful areas, by long walking and a few days away from the main home, surviving on fresh water, fresh fruits, nuts, seeds, whole grains, legumes, fresh vegetables and sprouted foods, prepared for the journey. Seasonal love making and sharing regularly all types of human desires and emotions with a positive approach and direction. Survival based on a wide variety of foods all grown organically and obtained as mentioned above. Proper chewing of food and food combination. No types of environmental pollutants, car exhaust fumes or other toxic elements, just clean fresh mountain or country air, forest air for a real treat. Comfortable living and sleeping areas, no television or other mind-distracting appliances, no alcohol, cigarettes, processed foods and drinks. No animal-origin food, except, a weekly serve of natural bacteria yoghurt. Regular use of blended fruits, nuts and seed drinks, one per day. Lifestyle based on self-sufficiency with barter-trading for other local produce.

2: Mainly natural food diet, including a variety of seasonal fruits and fresh garden vegetables, occasional market produce. At least one freshly extracted fruit or vegetable juice daily, 7ozs. Occasional use of sprouted foods, once a week. Occasional nut protein meals, blended nut, seed or fruit drinks. Daily sunshine, at least one hour moderate light. Occasional gardening, long walking, deep breathing, yoga, relaxation and meditation. Occasional swimming, use of warm showers and baths. Climate ranging between 10-30 Celcius, throughout the seasons. Mixture of country and city lifestyle and activities. Occasional television viewing, radio and hi-fi equipment. Basic application of food preparation and combination, mainly fresh produce, some whole grain bread obtained from the natural food store, regular use of whole grains and legumes with vegetables, a limited intake of animal protein foods: yoghurt and natural cheese. No processed or refined foods: tinned food, packaged breakfast foods or sugar drinks, no added sugar with meals, no alcohol except on rare occasions, no cigarettes, the occasional coffee or tea, mainly herbal teas and freshly extracted juices. Limited amount of toxic inhalation: car exhaust, air pollution, factory smoke or other sprays. Regular exercise, good sleeping and living conditions, regular natural-seasonal love making and a desire to share positive experiences. Lifestyle based on both self-sufficiency and other essential goods obtained from other stores. Use of car occasionally, for long distance travelling. Occasional fasting — once per week, for 8 daylight hours, including juices only. Occupation based on self-sufficiency with occasional city work for reasons of improved country living.

1	'complete natural food diet and natural environment' Life expectancy: 90-100 and over
2	'mainly natural food diet and natural environment' Life expectancy: 80-90
3	'occasional processed foods and drinks and mainly city environment' Life expectancy: 70-80
4	'mainly processed foods and drinks and city environment' Life expectancy: 60-70
5	'limited natural food diet and complete city environment' Life expectancy: 50-60
6	'depleted natural food diet, city environment' Life expectancy: 40-50

"Take six big steps and then discover the seventh"

NATURAL STEPS TO HEALTH INFORMATION

3: Natural food diet with occasional processed foods and drinks. Occasional use of freshly extracted juices, once per week. Occasional use of nut and seed protein meals and blended drinks, once per week, basic food combination and natural food preparation practised regularly, occasional sprouted food, once per month. Occasional gardening, relaxation and meditation, once a week. Regular use of warm showers and the occasion swimming, once a month. Daily television viewing, an hour per day, regular hi-fi and radio music. Occasional natural whole grain bread, mainly refined bread, occasional use of whole grains, once a week, legumes once every two weeks, occasional meat eating, regular use of natural yoghurt and cheese and occasional poultry, once a month, eggs once a week. Occasional tinned foods, once a week, small amounts of added sugar, no more than 100grams per week. Occasional alcohol, once a week, four glasses, occasional cigarette, two a day, one coffee or tea per day, mainly herbal teas. Occasional exercise, good sleeping conditions and regular love making, using contraceptives and natural methods. Mainly city lifestyle with regular visits to the countryside, seaside or mountains. Occasional fasting, once per week, 6 daylight hours, including fresh juices only. Occupation based on city work, housing in city environment, pollution and car exhaust fumes prevalent. Regular use of fresh vegetables, cooked and raw, daily. Climate between 10-30 Celcius, throughout the seasons. Occasional fresh fish meal.

4: Mainly processed, refined and supermarket foods and drinks, regular purchase of a limited amount of fresh fruits and vegetables, occasional freshly extracted juice, once a month, no sprouted foods. Occasional whole grain and legume meals, every two weeks, mainly packaged and tinned foods used as the basic foods with some fresh vegetables obtained twice per week. Irregular sunshine, 3 days per week, limited amount of gardening and deep breathing exercises. Regular warm-hot showers, swimming only at holiday time. Limited food combination and preparation, mainly with cooked meals. Meat eating, once per week, regular use of cheese, poultry, eggs and fresh fish, occasional use of natural yoghurt, occasional fasting for weight control. Regular alcohol, 2 glasses per day, coffee, 2 glasses per day, regular cigarette smoking, 10 cigarettes per day, over 100 grams of sugar per week. Limited amount of proper exercise. Regular loving making, using contraceptives. Regular use of car for travel to countryside or beach. Mainly city air environment, car exhaust and factory fumes prevalent. Occasional use of fresh fruit meals or vegetables with whole grains or legumes. Daily television, 3 hours per day, hi-fi and radio music and the news, advertisements, 4 hours per day. Occasional herbal teas. Comfortable sleeping and living conditions, occasional adventures to the country for the weekend.

5: Limited natural food diet, mainly processed and refined supermarket foods and drinks, less than six pieces of fresh whole fruits per week, occasional fresh garden salad, once per week, no freshly extracted juices, mainly hot drinks, coffee, 4 cups per day, or tea. Irregular sunshine, 2 days per week, 1 hour per day. Regular alcohol, 4 glasses per day, more on the weekend. Over 200 grams of sugar added to foods, per week. No effort with regular exercise, occasional quick run around the city block. Daily use of car for travel, city pace. Regular excess intake of polluted city air, car exhaust and factory smoke. Regular cigarettes, over 10 cigarettes per day. Daily television, over 3 hours per day, radio and hi-fi, over 3 hours per day, including news and advertisements. Occasional exciting movie viewing, mainly serial television programs. Regular use of soft sugar drinks and sugar foods, chocolate, candy or lollies. Comfortable sleeping conditions and living area. Daily eating of meat, cheese and eggs, regular eating of poultry and take-away hot foods, batter-fish, pies, pasties, hamburgers and other fat-coated foods. No proper food combination or preparation methods. Regular annual holidays and lifestyle reliant on city living.

6: Depleted natural food diet, over 90% of foods obtained from packets, tins or bottles, processed and refined diet. No understanding of basic foods for health. Irregular outdoor living and sunshine, 1 day per week, 2 hours sunlight. No fasting, daily use of meat, twice per day, regular use of processed cheese, factory eggs and poultry, no fresh fish, only the occasional batter pre-frozen fish and canned fish meals. Over 6 eggs per week, fried in poor quality oil. Regular use of salt, over 200 grams of sugar added to coffee or tea drinks, per week, over 100grams of sugar added to meals. Regular eating of white bread, refined breakfast cereals, eggs and meat for breakfast, canned meat products, sausages and frozen meat products. Regular meals obtained from take-away shops, over 4 glasses of soft drink per day, over 6 glasses of alcohol and excessive amounts on the weekend. Over 20 cigarettes per day, every day. Reasonable sleeping and living conditions. Lack of regular exercise, excess intake of polluted air, car exhaust fumes and factory smoke, the occasional drink of polluted water. Occasional restaurant meals, mainly meat. No intake of natural yoghurt. Over 6 eggs per day, occasionally. Use of poor quality cooking oils and fats. Daily television watching, over 5 hours per day and night. Regular radio listening, advertisements and news. Less than six fresh fruits per week, mainly cooked vegetables and the occasional whole grain meal, once in two weeks, rarely preparing food for good health. Hectic city living, rushing to work with a stomach full of meat. Regular doses of city stress, occasional love making, regular annual holiday revival attempts. Lifestyle completely related to city living, the occasional walk in the city parks and gardens, listening to the birds. A limited education on the purpose and effects of food and the diet.

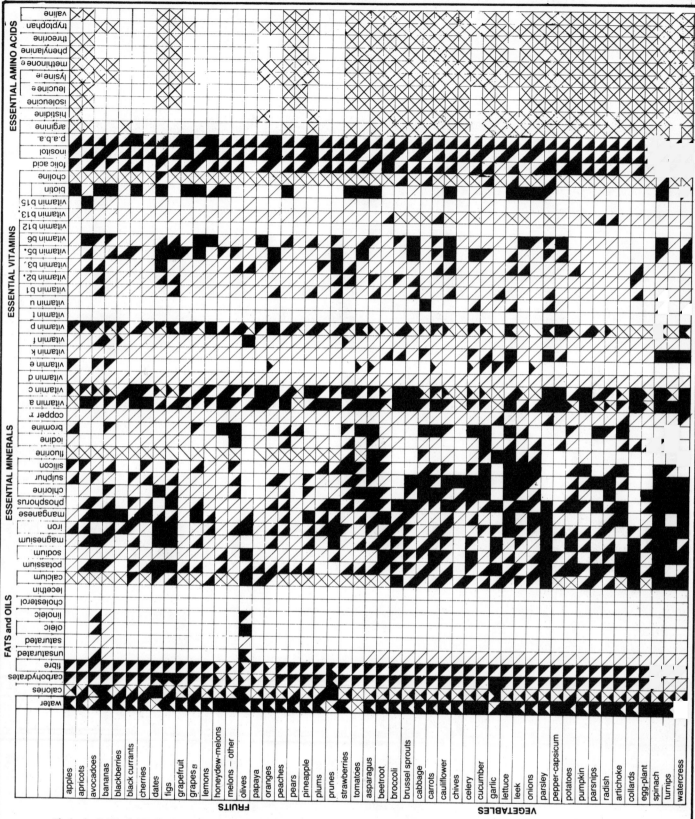

TOTAL NUTRIENT — FOOD CHART

This chart is to provide a visual display of the availability of the essential nutrients from a wide range of natural foods. For full numerical details, refer to pages 43, 61, 79, 97 and 117. There are seven main food-groups: Fruits, Vegetables, Grains, Legumes, Nuts, Seeds and Animal produce. By referring to this total nutrient — food chart, the supply of nutrients from the main food groups can be compared and the main nutrient benefits or deficiencies are made obvious. For full details on the supply of minerals and vitamins, refer to pp. 158–161 and 184–186; these pages will provide food charts for all essential minerals and vitamins. Also refer to the protein chapter, pp. 81–117.

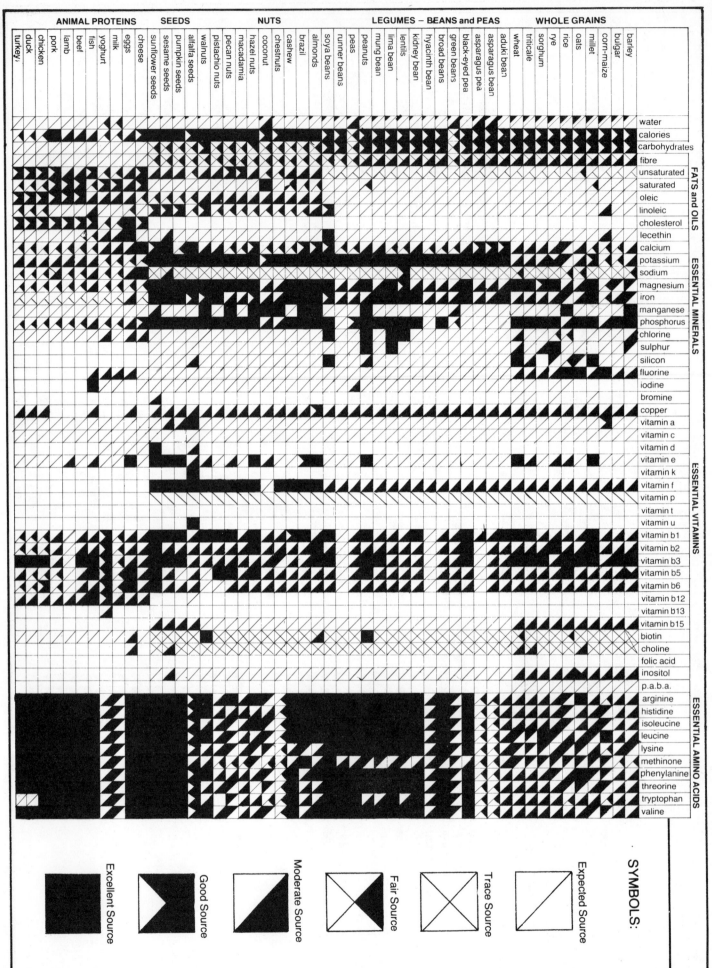

CREDITS

Writing a book, especially for the first time, is a challenge that involves many contributing factors. Love, patience, and understanding, which my mother reflected, gave me energy that is now part and parcel of this entire book. Every day, in every way, with love, many thanks, Liselotte.

I would also like to acknowledge the assistance from the following people, who contributed in a spectrum of ways that now deserve a special mention: Joanne Moore, Ingrid Koch, Glenys Gray, Mark and Jan Heaysman, Tony Murphy, Yvonne Koene, Damian Koch, Andrea Aitken, Bert and Heather Raisbeck, Roy and Beryl Pearce, Fred and Radhika Koch, John and Kim and friends from Metung.

I would like to give special thanks to my father, Mr. Josef L. Koch, for the valuable contribution to my early days of study and education. Every moment together with the sharing of life from those first few steps and all the memories and times still ahead.

As the ingredients of this book, *Laugh with Health*, are based on the knowledge from years of nutritional research, by thousands of people throughout the world, I would like to express my appreciation of their work in the nutrition field; thanking you for your individual contribution, your help has made this book possible and your research has provided the answers to make this book complete.

Additional credits are given to the following people who assisted in the preparation of this book, *Laugh with Health*. Over two years ago, the original typeset manuscript was completed, with assistance from E. Gee printers Bairnsdale, many thanks to both Neil Crawford and Dennis McNamara for their assistance during the early stages of this project and special thanks for printing the first edition book covers.

The printing of this book was greatly assisted with the help of Mr. and Mrs. D. Yeates, Mr. Alan Truscott, Mr. David Hamilton, Mr. Eric Yeates and all the friendly people at James Yeates, Bairnsdale.

The typesetting for this book was mainly completed by Allegro Graphics, Burwood, special thanks Corrie for providing such an excellent service and also to Janette, for your combined efforts in typesetting, preparation and advice. Other typesetting was also completed by Sunstrip printers, Nambour, thanks to you, Mr. Allen Halling and staff.

Other people who provided valuable assistance during the publishing stage of this book, *Laugh with Health*, are as follows: many, many thanks to Marc and Lyz Hall, your assistance gave inspiration and also the typewriter to complete this revised edition copy, thanks also to Mr. Nigel Egan, Mr. John Miles, John Saxon, Les and Jan Kershaw, Mary and Judd Zychinski, Roland and Barbara Koch, Rick van Beek and friends from Ontos village and Sunrise farm.

Special thanks to Rick for his assistance during the early stage of book publishing. Thanks to everyone who helped in any way.

Many thanks also to the following people who have contributed the essential financial resources, to make this book, *Laugh with Health*. Dr. and Mrs. F. Lustenberger-Koch, Mr. and Mrs. H. Hug-von Werdt, Fred and Radhika Koch, Mr. J. L. Koch, Mr. Don Kugelman, Mr. Vivian Lees, Jim Donovan, Mrs. Liselotte Seelig, Mr. Ward, Mr. Langenbacher. Thanks also to Professor Dr. H. Aebi, for a rewarding recommendation.

BIBLIOGRAPHY

1 — Anatomy and Physiology for Nurses — W. Gordon Sears
— Arnold Book Publishers.

2 — Nutrition in Action — Ethel Martin — Holt, Reinhart and Winston.

3 — Introduction to Nutrition — Henrietta Fleck — McMillan Publishing.

4 — Understanding Food — Lendal H. Kotschevar
— John Wiley & Sons Publishing.

5 — Composition and Facts about Food — Ford Heritage
— Health Research Centre.

6 — Feast and Famine — Lord Boyd Orr. — Rathbone Books.

7 — Raw Juice Therapy — Susan Charmine — Baronet Books.

8 — Healthful Eating Without Confusion — Paul G. Bragg, N.D. P.H.D.
— Health Science Books.

9 — Protein for Vegetarians — Gary Null — Jove Books.

10 — Scientific Vegetarianism, Book of Survival, Essene Science of Life,
The Book of Minerals, Treasury of Raw Foods — Academy Books.

11 — Natures Healing Grasses — H. E. Kirshner — H. C. White Publications.

12 — Become Younger — N. W. Walker, M.D. D.S.C. — Norwalk Press.

13 — Food Combining Made Easy — H. M. Shelton — Shelton Publications.

14 — Seeds and Sprouts for Life — Dr. Bernard Jensen, D.C.
— Jensen Nutritional Health Products.

15 — Nuts and Bolts of Nutrition — Ontario Dietic Association
— Ontario Dietic + Hospital Association.

16 — Natures Incredible Foods — Vitaplex — Vitaplex Publication.

17 — Food Remedies — M. Blackmore, N.D. D.C. — Blackmore Publication.

18 — Laurels Kitchen — L. Robertson, C. Flinders, B. Godfrey — Nilgri Press.

19 — Family Health Care — Readers Digest — Readers Digest Publication.

20 — Basic Knowledge of Esthetics — H. Pieranti.

21 — Concise Oxford Dictionary — Clarendon Press.

22 — Relax and Survive — Anne Wigmore, D.D. N.D. Naturama — Anne Wigmore.

23 — Energy, Evolution, Universe, The Mind, The Body, Health & Disease,
Water, Time, The Cell, Growth — Time Life Books — Publication.

24 — Vitamin C and the Common Cold — Linus Pauling

25 — Natures Healing Agents — R. S. Swinburne — Philadelphia
— Dorrance Publishing.

26 — Family Guide to Better Food and Health — R. M. Decith
— Meredith Corporation.

27 — Your Body is Your Best Doctor — M. E. Page, H. L. Abrams
— Keats Publishing.

28 — Lets Get Well, Lets Have Healthy Children, Lets Eat Right to Keep Fit
— Adelle Davis — Harcourt, Brace and World Publication.

29 — Basic Nutrition and Diet Therapy — C. H. Robinson
— MacMillan Publishing.

30 — Basic Nutrition in Health and Disease — P. S. Howe
— W. B. Saunders Publishing.

31 — Modern Nutrition in Health and Disease — R. S. Goodhart and M. E. Shils
— Lea & Febiger Publishing.

32 — Beware of the Food You Eat — Ruth Winter — Signet Books.

33 — Fit for Anything — Kekir Sidhwa — Health for all Publishing.

34 — Proteins — Their Chemistry and Politics — A. M. Altschul
— Basic Books Publishing.

35 — Nutrition Almanac — Nutrition Research, Inc.
— McGraw-Hill Book Company.

36 — The Wholefood Catalogue — Vicki Peterson — Grass roots books.

37 — Recipes for a Small Planet — Ellen Buchman Ewald
— Ballantine books, New York.

38 — The Natural Health Book — Dorothy Hall
— Thomas Nelson Australia Pty. Ltd.

39 — The Healing Power of Natural Foods — May Bethel
— Wilshire Book Company.

40 — Diet and Nutrition — Rudolph Ballentine, M.D.
— The Himalayan International Institute, Honesdale, Pennsylvania.

41 — The Natural Foods and Nutrition Handbook — Rafael Marcia
— Harper & Row Publishing.

42 — Are You Confused, How to Get Well — Paavo Airola
— Health Plus Publishing.

43 — Nutrition and Physical Fitness — L. J. Bogert, G. M. Brigs & D. H. Callaway
— Saunders Publishing.

44 — Get Well Naturally — Linda Clark — Devin-Adair Publishing.

45 — Complete Handbook of Nutrition — Gary & Steve Null
— R. Speller Publishing.

46 — Health and Disease — Dubos, Rene & Maya Pines
— The Time Life Books Publishing.

47 — The Save Your Life Diet — David M. Locke — Crown Press.

48 — Cancer — Facts and Fallacies — Emmaus, Pa. — Rodale Books.

BIBLIOGRAPHY

49 – Nutrition: An Integrated Approach – R.L. & M. Pike
   – John Wiley & Sons Publishing.

50 – Diet for a Small Planet – Francis L. Lappe – Ballantine Books.

51 – Vitamin E: The Key to a Healthy Heart – Herbert Bailey – Arc Books.

52 – About Mothers, Children, and Their Nutrition – T.G. Basu
   – Thorsons Publication.

53 – Diet and Disease – E. Cheraskin, W. M. Ringsdorf and J.W. Clark
   – Prevention – Dec. 72.

54 – Sweet and Dangerous – John Yudkin – Peter H. Whyden Publication.

55 – Vitamins and Minerals – Arthur W. Synder – Hansens Publication.

56 – The Get Well Body Book – Mike Samuels & Hal Bennet – Random House.

57 – Food for Better Living – Irene McDermott, M. Trilling & F. Nicholas
   – J. B. Lippincott Co.